Third Edition

BECOMING A HELPER

Third Edition

BECOMING A HELPER

MARIANNE SCHNEIDER COREY
Private Practice

GERALD COREY
California State University, Fullerton

Diplomate in Counseling Psychology,
American Board of Professional Psychology

Brooks/Cole Publishing Company

I**T**P® *An International Thomson Publishing Company*

Pacific Grove • Albany • Belmont • Bonn • Boston • Cincinnati • Detroit • Johannesburg • London
Madrid • Melbourne • Mexico City • New York • Paris • Singapore • Tokyo • Toronto • Washington

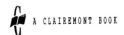

A CLAIREMONT BOOK

Sponsoring Editor: *Eileen Murphy*
Editorial Assistants: *Lisa Blanton and Susan Carlson*
Marketing Team: *Jean Thompson and Margaret Parks*
Production Coordinators: *Fiorella Ljunggren and Tessa McGlasson*
Production: *Cecile Joyner, The Cooper Company*
Manuscript Editor: *Kay Mikel*

Permissions Editor: *Carline Haga*
Interior and Cover Design: *Vernon T. Boes*
Cover Photo: *Michael Ventura, Photo Network*
Indexer: *Glennda Gilmour*
Typesetting: *Bookends Typesetting*
Cover Printing: *Phoenix Color Corp.*
Printing and Binding: *Maple-Vail Book Manufacturing Group*

For more information, contact:

BROOKS/COLE PUBLISHING COMPANY
511 Forest Lodge Road
Pacific Grove, CA 93950
USA

International Thomson Publishing Europe
Berkshire House 168-173
High Holborn
London WC1V 7AA
England

Thomas Nelson Australia
102 Dodds Street
South Melbourne, 3205
Victoria, Australia

Nelson Canada
1120 Birchmount Road
Scarborough, Ontario
Canada M1K 5G4

International Thomson Editores
Seneca 53
Col. Polanco
11560 México, D.F., México

International Thomson Publishing GmbH
Königswinterer Strasse 418
53227 Bonn
Germany

International Thomson Publishing Asia
221 Henderson Road
#05-10 Henderson Building
Singapore 0315

International Thomson Publishing Japan
Hirakawacho Kyowa Building, 3F
2-2-1 Hirakawacho
Chiyoda-ku, Tokyo 102
Japan

Printed in the United States of America

10 9 8 7 6 5 4

Library of Congress Cataloging-in-Publication Data

Corey, Marianne Schneider, [date]–
    Becoming a helper / Marianne Schneider Corey, Gerald Corey.—3rd ed.
        p. cm.
    Includes bibliographical references (pp.   ) and index.
    ISBN 0-534-34794-0
    1. Human services—Vocational guidance—United States. 2. Social service—Vocational guidance—United States. I. Corey, Gerald. II. Title.
HV10.5.C67   1998
361.3'2'023739—dc20
                                                          96-41520
                                                          CIP

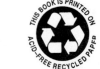

*To our daughters, who are touching the lives
of others in their own special ways—
Cindy through counseling, Heidi through drama*

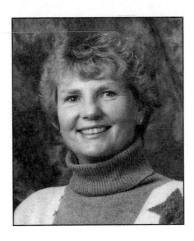

MARIANNE SCHNEIDER COREY is a licensed marriage and family therapist in California and is a National Certified Counselor. She received her master's degree in marriage, family, and child counseling from Chapman College. She is a Fellow of the Association for Specialists in Group Work and a clinical member of the American Association for Marriage and Family Therapy. She holds memberships in the California Association of Marriage and Family Therapists, the American Counseling Association, the National Organization for Human Service Education, the Association for Spiritual, Ethical, and Religious Values in Counseling, and the Association for Specialists in Group Work.

Marianne has been actively involved in providing training and supervision workshops in group process for human-services students and professionals; she regularly facilitates a self-exploration group for graduate students in counseling and co-facilitates weeklong residential workshops in personal growth. She is an adjunct faculty member of the Counseling Department at California State University at Fullerton. With her husband, Jerry, Marianne has conducted workshops, continuing-education seminars, and personal-growth groups in Germany, Belgium, Mexico, and China, as well as regularly doing these workshops in the United States. In her free time Marianne enjoys traveling, reading, visiting with friends, and hiking.

Marianne has co-authored the following books (published by Brooks/Cole Publishing Company):

- *Issues and Ethics in the Helping Professions*, Fifth Edition (1998, with Gerald Corey and Patrick Callanan)
- *Groups: Process and Practice*, Fifth Edition (1997, with Gerald Corey)
- *I Never Knew I Had a Choice*, Sixth Edition (1997, with Gerald Corey)
- *Group Techniques*, Second Edition (1992, with Gerald Corey, Patrick Callanan, and J. Michael Russell)

Marianne and Jerry have been married since 1964. They have two adult daughters, Heidi and Cindy. Marianne grew up in Germany and has kept in close contact with her family there.

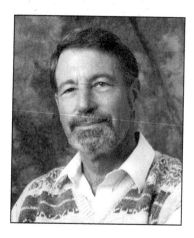

GERALD COREY is professor of human services and counseling at California State University at Fullerton and a licensed psychologist. He was the Coordinator of the Human Services Department at the above university for nine years. A licensed psychologist, he received his doctorate in counseling from the University of Southern California. He is a Diplomate in Counseling Psychology, American Board of Professional Psychology and a National Certified Counselor. He is a Fellow of the American Psychological Association (Counseling Psychology) and a Fellow of the Association for Specialists in Group Work.

Jerry received the Outstanding Professor of the Year Award from California State University at Fullerton in 1991 and was the recipient of an honorary doctorate in humane letters from National Louis University in 1992. He teaches both undergraduate and graduate courses in ethics and professional issues. In addition, he teaches undergraduate human-services courses in the theory and practice of counseling, group counseling, and experiential groups. With his colleagues he has conducted workshops in the United States, Germany, Belgium, Scotland, Mexico, and China, with a special focus on training in group counseling. He often presents workshops for professional organizations and at various universities. Along with his wife, Marianne, and other colleagues, Jerry offers week-long residential personal-growth groups and residential training and supervision workshops each summer. In his leisure time, Jerry likes to travel, hike and bicycle in the mountains, and drive his 1931 Model A Ford.

Recent publications by Jerry Corey, (all with Brooks/Cole Publishing Company) include:

- *Issues and Ethics in the Helping Professions,* Fifth Edition (1998, with Marianne Schneider Corey and Patrick Callanan)
- *Groups: Process and Practice,* Fifth Edition (1997, with Marianne Schneider Corey)
- *I Never Knew I Had a Choice,* Sixth Edition (1997, with Marianne Schneider Corey)
- *Theory and Practice of Counseling and Psychotherapy,* Fifth Edition (and *Manual*) (1996)
- *Case Approach to Counseling and Psychotherapy,* Fourth Edition (1996)
- *Theory and Practice of Group Counseling,* Fourth Edition (and *Manual*) (1995)

- *Group Techniques*, Second Edition (1992, with Marianne Schneider Corey, Patrick Callanan, and J. Michael Russell)

He is co-author, with his daughters Cindy Corey and Heidi Jo Corey, of an orientation-to-college book entitled *Living and Learning* (1997), published by Wadsworth. He is also co-author (with Barbara Herlihy) of *Boundary Issues in Counseling: Multiple Roles and Responsibilities* (1997) and *ACA Ethical Standards Casebook*, Fifth Edition (1996), both published by the American Counseling Association.

CONTENTS

Chapter 1
ARE THE HELPING
PROFESSIONS FOR YOU? 1

Chapter 2
GETTING THE MOST FROM YOUR
EDUCATION AND TRAINING 28

Chapter 6

VALUES AND THE HELPING RELATIONSHIP   153

Chapter 7

CULTURAL DIVERSITY IN THE HELPING PROFESSIONS   174

Chapter 11

UNDERSTANDING LIFE TRANSITIONS   285

Chapter 12

STRESS AND BURNOUT   305

Chapter 13

THE CHALLENGE
OF RETAINING YOUR VITALITY   323

PREFACE

Many books deal with the skills, theories, and techniques of helping. Yet few books address mainly the problems involved in becoming an effective helper or focus on the personal difficulties in working with others. In writing this book, we had in mind both students who are planning a career in human services, counseling, psychology, social work, or related professions and helpers who have just begun their careers. We intend this book to be used as a supplement to textbooks dealing with helping skills and with counseling theory and practice. Earlier editions of *Becoming a Helper* have proved useful for introductory classes in human services, social work, and counseling as well as classes in practicum, fieldwork, and internship.

We focus on the struggles, anxieties, and uncertainties of helpers. In addition, we explore in depth the demands and strains of the helping professions and their effects on the provider. We begin with a discussion of the motivations for seeking a career in the helping professions. We encourage our readers to examine their personal motives and needs for helping, and we challenge them to be honest in assessing what they will get from their work. Because students are often conditioned to be passive learners, we challenge them to take an active stance in their educational program. Being active applies to selecting field placements and internships as well as getting the most from supervision. Therefore, we offer some practical strategies for ensuring quality experiences in fieldwork and profiting from supervision.

We provide an overview of the stages of the helping process, with a brief discussion of the skills and knowledge required to be a successful agent at each of these stages. The focus of this discussion is not on skill development but on the personal characteristics that enable helpers to be effective. Because helpers ask clients to examine their behavior to understand themselves more fully, we ask helpers to be equally committed to an awareness of their own lives. Without a high level of self-awareness, a helper may obstruct clients' progress, especially when these clients are struggling with issues the helper has avoided facing.

Beginning and seasoned helpers encounter common problems in their work, related to dealing with resistance, transference and countertransference, and difficult clients. Forming a sense of ethical awareness and learning to resolve professional dilemmas is a task facing all helpers. We raise a number of challenges surrounding current ethical issues as a way to sensitize readers to the intricacies of ethical decision making.

We explore the belief systems of helpers and discuss the positive and negative effects that a variety of beliefs and assumptions can have on one's practice. Values are an integral part of the client-helper relationship, and we devote considerable attention to an analysis of how values influence helping. We develop the thesis that the job of helpers is not to impose values but to help clients define their own value system. Special consideration is given to understanding and working with culturally diverse client populations.

We also deal with understanding one's role as a helper in the community; we discuss the group process and the value of group work in human-services work; and we examine the importance of reviewing family-of-origin experiences, focusing on how earlier relationships continue to influence the quality of later ones. We look at how helpers deal with their own life transitions and discuss the implications of this process when working with the clients' life crises. Other topics covered in the book are stress and burnout and ways to stay alive and vital, both as a person and as a professional.

Although this book should be useful to any student planning to enter the helping professions, our backgrounds are in the field of counseling, and this orientation comes through in our approach. Therefore, those who want to work in the counseling aspects of the human services are likely to find this book especially meaningful. We have tried to write a personal book that will stimulate both thought and action. At the end of each chapter we encourage readers to commit to some specific action that will move them closer to their goals.

New to This Edition

Below is a brief overview of some of the topics that are new to this edition or that have been revised and expanded.

- Factors to be considered in choosing a career
- The value of journal writing and suggestions for keeping a journal
- Selecting a fieldwork placement
- Viewing education as an investment, becoming an active learner, and dealing with inadequate supervision
- Short-term approaches to treatment; the impact of managed care on the delivery of services by both agencies and private providers and on the training and role of helpers
- Our theoretical orientation, the role of theory in the helper's practice, and an integrated approach to helping
- The importance of termination issues for both helper and client
- Common forms of resistance; transference and countertransference issues
- Ethical decision making
- Multiple relationships and boundary issues
- Bartering, with case example
- Sexual attraction between helper and client
- Dual relationships with former clients and with supervisors or teachers
- Ethical and legal standards

- Ways of preventing malpractice suits
- The role of religious and spiritual values in the helping relationship
- The need for a multicultural emphasis and some of its trends; the development of multicultural competencies and standards; additional self-assessment inventories on cultural diversity and gender equity
- The outreach approach
- Stress and burnout

New to this edition is an *Instructor's Resource Manual.* It contains suggestions for teaching the course, class activities to stimulate interest, transparency masters, and a bank of test items. Included are many multiple-choice, true-false, matching, and short essay questions from which the instructor can choose.

Acknowledgments

A number of reviewers provided insightful comments and reacted to our proposed ideas for the third edition. They include Juli Compton, San Juan College; Marcia Freer, Doane College; Dovie Jane Gamble, University of Florida; Steve Jaggers, Mt. Hood Community College; Sheldon Kleine, clinical psychologist in private practice in Washington; Mary Kay Kreider, St. Louis Community College; Rob Lawson, Western Washington University; Rich Reiner, Rogue Community College; and Guy Wylie, Western Nebraska Community College.

Three individuals gave us helpful feedback on the chapter on the community: Sid Gardner, California State University, Fullerton; Mark Homan, Pima Community College; and Jerome Wright, Savannah State University. Three student reviewers offered insightful comments and suggestions: Sheila Bell, a graduate student in social work at the University of Southern California; Julie Boyer, a graduate assistant in human services at Metropolitan State College of Denver; and Michelle Muratori, a graduate student in counseling at Northwestern University.

We are especially indebted to Lupe Alle-Corliss and Randy Alle-Corliss, who gave generously of their time to make this a better book. As licensed clinical social workers in agency settings and as college instructors, they greatly contributed to our discussion of the basic issues involved in working in a community agency and provided useful case examples and illustrations. We also appreciate Glennda Gilmour's work in compiling the index.

The dedicated members of the Brooks/Cole team continue to offer support for all our projects. It is a delight to work with a dedicated staff of professionals who go out of their way to give their best. They include Eileen Murphy, the editor of counseling and psychology; Fiorella Ljunggren, production services manager; Cecile Joyner, of the Cooper Company, who coordinated the production of this book; and Kay Mikel, the manuscript editor of this edition, whose fine editorial assistance kept this book reader-friendly. We also want to recognize the work of the late Bill Waller, who edited the two previous editions of *Becoming a Helper,* and whose influence has carried over into this edition.

Marianne Schneider Corey
Gerald Corey

Chapter 1

ARE THE HELPING PROFESSIONS FOR YOU?

FOCUS QUESTIONS

1. What has attracted you to the helping professions? Who in your life has been instrumental in your decision to consider this role for yourself?

2. What is your main motivation for wanting to be a helper?

3. What needs of yours are likely to be met through your work as a helper? To what degree do you think that these needs might either enhance your ability to help others or diminish it?

4. Think of a time when you very much needed help from a significant person in your life or from a counselor. What did you most want from this person? What did he or she do that was either a help or a hindrance to you?

5. Think about the attributes of an effective helper. What are a few traits or characteristics that you would identify as being the most important?

6. What do you consider to be some counterproductive attitudes, beliefs, and behaviors of helpers? Can you identify three major personal characteristics that are likely to strain the ability of helpers to form effective relationships with those who are seeking their assistance?

7. At this time in your life, how prepared (from a personal standpoint) do you feel you are to enter one of the helping professions? If you were applying to a graduate program or for a job in the field, you might be asked these questions: "What qualities, traits, attitudes, values, and convictions are central to the person who you are?" "How might these personal characteristics be either assets or liabilities for you as you pursue a career in the helping professions?"

8. What kind of education and training program do you think best fits your interests and talents? How do you see this program as a means to attaining your career objectives?

9. If you could pursue a career in one of the helping professions at this time, what would your ideal vision be? What work particularly appeals to you? With what clients would you most like to work? What kind of human-service work would bring you the greatest meaning and satisfaction?

AIM OF THE CHAPTER

As you consider a career in one of the helping professions, you are probably wondering: "Are the helping professions for me? Do I know enough to help others? Will I be able to apply what I'm learning in my education to my job? Will this career be satisfying in the long run?" This book is intended to help you answer these and other questions about your career. The focus of the book is on *you* and on what you need personally and professionally to be the best helper possible. We also emphasize the realities you are certain to face when you enter the professional world. You will be best able to cope with the demands of the helping professions if you get an idea now of what lies ahead.

We begin in this chapter by inviting you to examine your diverse motives for becoming a helper. We challenge you to clarify what you get from helping others as well as what you are able to give them. Ideally, you will be able to meet your own needs and the needs of your clients through the helping process. We share our own experiences as beginning helpers to demonstrate that learning to become a helper is a process, with its ups and downs. This chapter also introduces you to the attributes of an effective helper. Although we do not think that there is one perfect pattern of characteristics that identifies "ideal" helpers, we do present some attributes as a catalyst to encourage you to think about the characteristics you possess that could either help or hinder you in your work with others. Because most students express concerns about what professional program will best help them attain their career objectives, we explore the differences among various educational routes. We also examine some of the major factors to consider in selecting a career in the helping professions. Although you may think you know the career path you want to pursue, we encourage you to keep your options open while you are reading this book and taking this course. You will probably work in several different positions within a career area, and many human-services professionals change careers at different points in their lives. For instance, they may begin by providing direct services to clients in a community agency and then shift to administering programs.

Finally, keep in mind as you read this book that we use the terms *helper* and *human-services professional* interchangeably to refer to a wide range of practitioners, including social workers, clinical and counseling psychologists, marriage and family therapists, pastoral counselors, community mental-health workers, and rehabilitation counselors.

EXAMINING YOUR MOTIVES FOR BECOMING A HELPER

In choosing a career in the helping professions, you would do well to begin by examining your motivations for pursuing this path. It is critical that you be honest with yourself about the needs you will satisfy by entering this field. Your motives and needs can work either for or against both you and your future clients. In fact, the same need or motive has the potential to become either a productive or a counterproductive force in your helping style. As you reflect on the needs described in this section, ask yourself: "Do I deny having certain needs? How might I be able to satisfy both my own needs and those of the people who seek my help? What needs of mine, if any, might I be inclined to meet at the expense of my clients? Are some of my needs so intense that they cannot be met?"

Typical Needs of Helpers

Below are some motivations that we have observed in our own students and trainees in the helping professions. We encourage our students to recognize their needs, to accept them, and to become aware of how these needs influence the quality of their interactions with others.

The need to make an impact.   Perhaps you are hoping that you will exert a significant influence on the lives of those whom you touch. Many helpers profess altruistic desires to make the world a better place. Yet it is all too rare that we hear students and trainees admit that they are entering a helping profession because they want to satisfy a diverse range of their own needs. They may want to know that they are important and that they have the power to help people help themselves. Although they recognize that they won't be able to change the world in dramatic ways, they still want to make a dent in some corner of that world. When clients are not interested in changing or don't want their help, however, they sometimes become frustrated. Your entire worth as a person should not be tethered to the need to make an impact on the lives of others.

The need to return a favor.   The desire to emulate a role model often plays a part in the decision to be a helper. Someone special may have entered your life in a very influential way. This role model may be a teacher or a therapist. Many one-time clients in counseling, for example, decide to become counselors themselves. Or the influential person may be a grandmother, uncle, or parent. Many therapists whom we know have acknowledged that they were greatly influenced by their experience in personal therapy to seek the education needed to become therapists themselves.

The need to care for others.   You may have been a helper from a very early age. You were the one in your family who attended to the problems and concerns of other family members. Your peers and friends found it easy to come to you to unload their burdens. You heard that you were a "natural helper." Based on these life experiences and some of your early decisions, you sought out training to capitalize on your talent. One of the pitfalls of being a caregiver to significant people in your life has been that no one attended to your needs, and thus you never learned to ask for what you needed. While you were so busy making sure that others were taken care of, you forgot that you, too, needed someone to listen to you and understand your situation. You can easily become personally and professionally burned out, or emotionally exhausted, if you don't learn to ask for help when you need it.

One of the professionals who reviewed the manuscript of this book reported that out of 33 psychologists in the training program at his institute half identified themselves as "rescuers" in alcoholic families. In his view, they were recruited at birth and trained daily to stabilize the family. Many of our own students are adult children of alcoholics who adopted the role of peacemaker in their families. Although this pattern is not necessarily problematic, it is important that such helpers become aware of their dynamics and learn how they operate in both their personal and their professional lives.

If the pattern described here fits you, you may profit from reevaluating your early decision to focus on taking care of others to the exclusion of taking care of yourself. If you burden yourself with the full responsibility of always being available for everyone who might need your help, you are likely to find that you will soon have little left to give.

The need for self-help. You may want to go into the helping professions, at least in part, to work on personal issues. For example, you may have experienced the difficulties of growing up in an alcoholic family, and you may still be vulnerable due to your early wounding. In your professional work you are likely to encounter a number of individuals who have struggled with similar concerns. Helpers who specialize in abused children may have been victims of child abuse. Some women who were involved in abusive marriages eventually become counselors who specialize in working with battered women. Your interest in helping others often stems from an interest in dealing with the impact of your own struggles.

The main point is that the motivation for selecting a specialty can be the wellspring of creativity for you. It is not necessarily important that you be "adjusted"; rather, what is useful is to be aware of your own personal issues. As Rollo May has said, healers are most often able to heal others out of their own experience with psychological struggle. It is the wounded healer, not the adjusted helper, who can be authentically present for others searching to find themselves. If you have struggled successfully with a problem, you are able to identify and empathize with clients who come to you with similar concerns.

This motivation could also work against you and your clients. Consider the case of a female counselor who works with women who are the victims of spousal abuse. The counselor may try to work out her own unfinished business and conflicts by giving plenty of advice and pushing these women in certain directions. Because of her unresolved personal problems, she may show hostility to the abusing husband, especially if she becomes overinvolved with family dynamics.

The need to be needed. Very few helpers are immune to the need to be needed. The problem arises when you deny that you want to feel needed. It may be psychologically rewarding to you to have clients say that they are getting better because of your influence. These clients are likely to express their appreciation for the hope that you have given them. You may value being able to take care of other people's wants, and you may get a great deal of satisfaction from doing so. To us, satisfying this need is perhaps one of the greatest rewards of being helpers. We hope that you will not be apologetic about having this need and will not deny that you like being needed and appreciated. If this need is consistently in the forefront, however, it can overshadow the needs of your clients. Some helpers foster dependency by encouraging their clients to call them often. Perhaps they need their clients more than their clients need them.

Wanting to feel appreciated for what you are doing for others can be perfectly all right. The danger exists when you *must* receive appreciation and recognition to feel worthwhile. If you depend exclusively on your clients to feel like a useful human being, your self-worth is on shaky ground. The reality is that many clients will not express appreciation for your efforts. Furthermore, agencies often do not give recognition or positive feedback. Instead, you may get feedback when your performance does not meet with the expected standards. No matter what you accomplish, the institution may expect more of you. Eventually, you may feel that whatever you do will not be enough.

Some helpers love their work because they have so many opportunities to feel needed. In many ways their work becomes their life. The possible danger with relying completely on your work to satisfy your need to feel needed is that your purpose and meaning in life might vanish if you could no longer work.

The need for money.   Some helpers have come to enjoy the financial rewards of their work. We usually suggest that if students need to make a great deal of money they look elsewhere than the helping professions. In most cases, beginning helpers are not likely to get rich. Many professionals feel that they are not adequately compensated financially for their contributions.

You certainly do not need to feel guilty for wanting to earn a good living. If you were to donate most of your services and had to struggle to make ends meet, you might soon find yourself resenting all that you were giving to your clients. However, financial motives can work against establishment of therapeutic relationships. If you make how much you are earning from each client your primary concern, you are likely to keep clients coming to you when it is no longer in their best interest.

The need for prestige and status.   You may have hopes of acquiring a certain level of prestige, if not a certain income level. Yet if you work in an agency, many of the consumers of the services you offer will be disadvantaged. You will be working with people on probation, those with various addictions, poor people, and people who are sent to you. Because of this clientele, you will frequently not be given the prestige and the status you deserve. In fact, society may not even respect you. For this reason, it is important that you evaluate status within yourself rather than measuring it by what others give you.

Conversely, you may work in a setting where you can enjoy the status that goes along with being respected by clients and colleagues. If you have worked hard and become good at what you do, allow yourself to accept the prestige you have earned. You can be proud yet still be humble. If you become arrogant as a result of your status, however, you may be perceived as unapproachable, and clients may be put off by your attitude. You become prone to accepting far more credit for your clients' changes than you deserve. Some clients will put you on a pedestal, and you may come to like this position too much. Remember, those on a pedestal have only one place to go—down. If you want your self-esteem to rest on a solid foundation, it is essential that you look within yourself to meet your status needs rather than looking to others to provide you with affirmations that you are indeed a worthwhile person.

The need to provide answers.   Many of our students seem to have a strong need to give others advice and to provide the "right answers." For example, some of our students say they feel inadequate if their friends come to them with a problem and they are not able to give them concrete advice. Yet their friends may really need to be listened to and cared for rather than to be told "what they should do." Although you may find satisfaction in influencing others, it is important to realize that your answers may not be best for them. Your purpose is to provide direction and to assist clients in discovering their own course of action. If you find that your need for providing advice and answers sometimes gets in the way of effectively relating to others, we encourage you to tell people that your tendency is to offer answers but that you hope they can look within themselves for a possible answer that will help them.

The need for control.   Related to the need to provide others with advice and answers is the need to control others. Most of us have some need for self-control and also the need to control others at times. Although some degree of control of our lives is essential for our security and sanity, when we overcontrol, we allow very little spontaneity into our lives. If we are overly attracted to schedules and planning, there is not much room for surprises. Some have a great need to control what others are thinking, feeling, and doing. You might ask yourself these questions: Are you convinced that some people should think more liberally (or more conservatively)? When people are angry, depressed, or anxious, do you sometimes tell them that they should not feel that way and do your best to change their state of mind? Do you at times have a strong need to change the way people who are close to you behave, even if what they are doing does not directly affect you? If you honestly search inside yourself for these answers, you may find that you have a need to control the attitudes, beliefs, emotions, and behaviors of friends, family members, and those with whom you work. The more you attempt to control them, the greater the chances are that they will find a variety of ways to resist your control. Although some helpers have a need to control under the guise of being helpful, it can be a productive exercise to reflect on what the outcomes might be if you gave more and more control to those you encountered. After all, is your purpose in helping to control the lives of others, or is it to teach others how to regain effective control of their own lives?

How Your Needs and Motivations Operate

We often say that in the ideal situation, your own needs are met at the same time that you are meeting your clients' needs. Most of the needs and motives we have discussed can work either for or against a client's welfare. There is nothing wrong with most of these needs, nor do they have to get in the way of effective helping. When you are unaware of them, however, there is a much greater likelihood that they will determine the nature of your interventions. If you are attempting to work through unconscious personal conflicts by focusing on the problems of others, for example, there is more chance that you will use your clients to meet your needs. In addition, you may be in trouble if some of these needs assume such a high priority that you become obsessed with satisfying them. For instance, if your need for control is so high that you consistently attempt to determine the path that others take, this influence could easily interfere with their development of independence and freedom. Helpers who meet their own needs at the expense of their clients are depriving their clients of the quality of care to which they are entitled. If you feel a strong need to provide answers to every problem a client presents, for example, this giving of advice is not so much in the best interest of the client but, rather, is meeting your need for giving answers and advice to others. As you reflect on the needs we have discussed, think about how they might either enhance or interfere with your helping of others. If you have not worked with clients yet, think of situations when you talked with friends or family members who were struggling with some problem. Recall how you related to them as they were searching for the best course of action. Do your best to identify how any of these needs can become problematic if you deny them, become obsessed with them, or meet them at the expense of others.

Examine Your Own Motives for Helping

At this point we encourage you to reflect on your own motivations for considering a career as a helper. Ask yourself these questions, and strive to answer them as honestly as you can: "Have I given much thought to why I'm considering a helping career? How aware am I of my own needs and motivations? Am I able to meet my needs and at the same time meet the needs of those I help? Do I feel guilty or apologetic for having needs? Do I think that the ideal is to be a selfless helper? In my personal life, do I consistently take care of others and put myself second? Can I be genuinely interested in others and still interested in my own growth?"

It is unlikely that any single motive drives you; rather, needs and motivations are intertwined and can change over time. Even though your original motives and needs change, your desire to be a helper may remain unchanged. Because personal growth is an ongoing process, we encourage you to periodically reexamine your motives for being a helper. It can be a valuable tool toward self-awareness.

OUR OWN BEGINNINGS AS HELPERS

This is a personal book in two ways. It is personal in that we encourage you to find ways to apply the book to yourself. In addition, we have written the book in a personal manner, sharing our own views and experiences whenever we think it is appropriate and useful. As a concrete illustration of how personal motives and experiences can affect career choice, we discuss some of our own motivations for becoming helping professionals and remaining in the field.

Beginning a helping career is not always easy and can involve anxiety and uncertainty. Although at this point we feel more confident than when we were beginning our careers, we have not forgotten our own struggles. We, too, had to cope with many of the fears and self-doubts discussed in the previous pages. By sharing our own difficulties with you, we hope to encourage you not to give up too soon. At this point in our professional lives, we still question why we are doing what we do. We reflect on both what we are giving and what we are getting through our varied work projects.

Jerry Corey's Early Experience

When I was in college studying to become a teacher, I hoped to create a different learning climate for students than I was experiencing as a learner. I wanted to help others, and it was important for me to change the world. I recognize now that the need to make a significant difference has been a theme for the more than 30 years I have been in the helping professions. As a child and as an adolescent, I did not feel that my presence made that much difference. In many ways, during my early years, I felt that I did not fit anywhere and that I was unrecognized and useless. There was a good deal of pain attached to feeling ignored, and one of my early decisions was not to let myself be ignored. This took the form of making myself a nuisance, which of course resulted in negative attention. But I assumed that this type of recognition was better than being ignored! In college I experienced some success and found some positive routes to being recognized. Later, when I began my teaching career, I began to see that I could make a difference, at least within the confines of my classroom. In addition to helping students enjoy learning, I also got personal satisfaction from knowing that I was a useful person, which was quite different from my perception of myself during my youth. In fact, I think that I depended (and still do) to a large extent on my professional accomplishments for my sense of identity.

At the beginning of my career as a counseling psychologist, I did not feel confident, and I often wondered whether I was suited for the field. I recall as being particularly difficult the times that I co-led a group with my supervisor. I felt incompetent and inexperienced next to my co-leader, who was an experienced therapist. Much of the time I didn't know what to say or do. It seemed that there was little place for me to intervene, because my co-leader was so effective. I had many doubts about my ability to say anything meaningful to the members. It just seemed that my supervisor was so insightful and so skillful that I would never attain such a level of professionalism. The effect of working with an experienced group leader was to heighten my own sense of insecurity and inadequacy.

Another thing that I found difficult was practicing individual counseling in a university center. When I began as a practicing counselor, I frequently asked myself what I could do for my clients. I remember progress being very slow, and it seemed that I needed an inordinate amount of immediate and positive feedback. When after several weeks a client was still talking about feeling anxious or depressed, I immediately felt my own incompetence as a helper. I frequently found myself thinking: "How would my supervisor say this? What would he do?" I even caught myself copying his gestures, phrases, and mannerisms. Many times I felt that I did not have what it took to be an effective counselor, and I wondered if I had pursued the wrong path.

I often had no idea of what, if anything, my clients were getting from our sessions. Indications of whether clients were getting better, staying the same, or getting worse were typically very subtle. What I didn't know at the time was that clients need to struggle as a part of finding their own answers. My expectation was that they should feel better quickly, for then I would know that I was surely helping them. I also did not appreciate that clients often begin to feel worse as they give up their defenses and open themselves to their pain. When I saw clients expressing their fear and uncertainty about their future, it only brought out my own lack of certainty that I could help them. Because I was concerned about saying "the wrong thing," I often listened a lot but didn't give too many of my own reactions in return.

Even though it is uncomfortable for me to admit this, I was more inclined to accept clients who were bright, verbal, attractive, and willing to talk about their problems than clients who seemed depressed or unmotivated to change. Those whom I considered "good and cooperative clients" I encouraged to come back. As long as they were talking and working, and preferably letting me know that they were getting somewhere with our sessions, I was quick to schedule other appointments. Those clients who seemed to make very few changes were the ones who increased my own anxiety. Rather than seeing their own part in their progress or lack of it, I typically blamed myself for not knowing enough and not being able to solve their problems. I took full responsibility for what they did during the session. It never occurred to me that the fact that they did not return for another session might have said something about them and their unwillingness to change. I had limited tolerance for uncertainty and for their struggle in finding their own direction. My self-doubts grew when they did not show up for following appointments. I was sure that this was a sign that they were dissatisfied with what they were getting from me.

I particularly remember encouraging depressed clients to make an appointment with one of the other counselors on the staff. I learned in my own supervision that working with depressed clients was difficult for me because of my own reluctance to deal with my own fears of depression. If I allowed myself to really enter the world of these depressed clients, I might get in touch with some of my anxiety. This experience taught me the important lesson that I could not take clients in any direction that I had not been willing to explore in my own life.

Although I am not engaged in counseling people individually, I do teach counselors and write textbooks on counseling practice. Had I not challenged my fears and self-doubts, I am quite certain that I would not be a counselor educator and an author today.

Marianne Corey's Early Experience

I was a helper long before I studied counseling in school. From childhood on I responded to the needs of my brothers and sisters. At age 8 I was made almost totally responsible for my newly born brother. I not only took care of him but also attended to other members of an extended family.

My family owned a restaurant in a German village. The restaurant, which was in our home, was the meeting place for many of the local men. These men came mostly to socialize rather than to eat and drink. For hours they would sit and talk, and I was taught that I had better listen attentively. Furthermore, I learned that I should not repeat the personal conversations and gossip to other townspeople. At this early age I learned three very important skills: attentive listening, empathic understanding, and confidentiality. It became apparent to me that a variety of people found it easy to talk to me and tell me about their personal problems.

In my growing-up years I felt liked and respected by most people. I remember feeling compassion, especially for those who had a difficult or unusual life situation. For example, I recall seeing a woman who had a psychotic episode standing naked by an upstairs window. She threw her clothes and furniture out of the window as onlookers baited her. I felt sad and thought that she must be very unhappy. I also had special feelings for two persons in my village who were considered "town drunks." I was curious about why they wanted to drink.

I have always been interested in looking beyond the facade that people present to others. I became convinced that people could be more than they appeared if they were willing to make an effort to change. My belief was atypical in my culture, which conveyed the message that "this is fate, and there is nothing you can do about it."

In my own life I overcame many obstacles and exceeded my dreams. As a result, I am often successful in challenging and encouraging my clients not to give up too soon when limits are imposed on them. Through my work I derive a great sense of satisfaction when I have been instrumental in the lives of individuals who are willing to take risks, to tolerate uncertainty, to dare to be different, and to live a fuller life because of their choices. When clients show appreciation for what I have done for them, I enjoy hearing it. However, I always let them know that their progress stems only partially from my efforts; the rest comes from their hard work.

In my life now I find it easy to give to my friends, family, and community as well as to clients. It seems natural to me to give both personally and professionally. It continues to be a struggle for me to find a good balance between giving to others and taking for myself. Although I am considered a good giver, I realize that I am a slow learner when it comes to making my needs known and asking for what I want.

It is interesting for me to compare my cultural conditioning and early role in my family with my development as a professional caregiver. Although I seemed to assume the role of caring for my brothers and sisters "naturally," I did not feel quite as natural when I began formal helping. In my first practical experiences as part of my undergraduate program in behavioral sciences, I had my share of self-doubt.

In one of my earlier internships I was placed in a college counseling center. I remember how petrified I was when one day a student came in and asked for an appointment, and my supervisor asked me to counsel this client. The feedback that I received later from my supervisor on how confident I had appeared was very incongruent with what I had felt. Some of the thoughts that I remember running through my head as I was walking to my office with this client were: "I'm not ready for this. What am I going to do? What if he doesn't talk? What if I don't know how to help him? I wish I could get out of this!" In my self-absorption I never once considered any of my client's feelings. For instance, how might he be approaching this session? What fears might he be having?

I was much more aware of myself than of my clients. I took far too much responsibility, put much pressure on myself to "do it right," and worried a lot about what harm I could do to them. I did not allow my clients to assume their rightful share of the responsibility for making changes. I often worked much harder than they did, and sometimes it seemed that I wanted more for some of my clients than they wanted for themselves. I think I had a tendency to exaggerate my capacity for causing harm because of my fears and insecurities as a helper. When I shared with my supervisor my concern about feeling so responsible for the outcomes of our sessions and about hurting my clients, she responded "You are assuming more power than you have over your clients."

Another time I told my supervisor that I had doubts about being in my profession, that I was overwhelmed by all the pain I saw around me, and that I was concerned that I was not helping anybody. I remember being very emotional and feeling extremely discouraged. My supervisor's smile surprised me. "I would be very concerned about you as a helper," he said, "if you never asked yourself these kinds of questions and were not willing to confront yourself with these feelings." In retrospect, I think he was telling me that he was encouraged for me because I was acknowledging my struggles and was not pretending to be the all-competent counselor who was without fears.

As a beginning counselor I was acutely aware of my own anxieties. Now I am much better able to be present with my clients and to enter their world. Although I am not anxiety-free, I am not watching myself practicing therapy. Furthermore, although I take responsibility for the counseling process, I don't see myself as totally responsible for what goes on in a session, and I am usually not willing to work harder than my clients.

At one time I wanted to abandon the idea of becoming a counselor and instead considered teaching German. I was very aware of comparing myself with professionals who had years of experience, and I thought I should be as effective as they were. What I eventually realized was that my expectations were extremely unrealistic, because I was demanding that I immediately be as skilled as these very experienced people. I had been giving myself no room for learning and for tolerating my rudimentary beginnings.

One of my professional activities now is working with beginning helpers. I find that they are often in the same predicament I was when I began working with others. These students seem focused on how much I know and how easy interventions seem to come to me. By contrast, they feel discouraged with their lack of knowledge and with how much they have to struggle to find "the right thing to say." They usually sigh with relief when I tell them about some of my beginnings and admit that I do not see myself as an expert but as someone who has a certain amount of expertise in counseling. I want most to convey to them that learning never stops and that beginnings are difficult and, at times, discouraging.

A Helping Career Is Not for Everyone

As is clear from our accounts, both of us had self-doubts, and we still doubt ourselves at times. We certainly do not see it as a disgrace if you wonder whether a helping profession is right for you. If you keep the question of whether you want to pursue a helping career open, you are bound to have periods of self-doubt. At times you may feel excited about the prospects of your career choice, and at other times you may feel hopeless and discouraged. Give yourself room for some of these ambivalent feelings. Don't make the decision whether to pursue a helping career by yourself, based on your initial experiences. We encourage you to be open to the pattern of consistent feedback you receive from faculty members, supervisors, and your peers. In some situations you may hear that you are not suited for a particular field. If people have concerns about your entering that helping profession, be willing to listen and to consider what they have to say. Such feedback is certainly hard to accept. Your first inclination may be to decide that the person does not like you, yet the advice may be in your best interest. If you hear such a recommendation, ask for specific reasons for the judgment and find out what alternatives the person can suggest to you.

You will ultimately have to make the decision of whether the helping profession is for you, but before you decide, consult with supervisors, colleagues, friends, and others who know you best. Give yourself credit for being able to change. If you are willing to remain open and apply the effort needed to change, you may find that your limitations can also be your assets.

The temptation to give up too soon is often greatest when you first have to apply what you have learned in your courses. A most difficult time will be when you step out of the lab and into the real world. The chances are that you will find that what worked in the lab will not work so well in real-life helping situations. In the lab you may have worked with fellow students who role-played clients who were cooperative. Now you are facing some clients who, no matter how hard you try, are not responding to you. Realize that it will take time and experience to learn how to apply your knowledge of theories and techniques to actual situations. At first your attempts at helping may seem artificial and rehearsed. You will probably be more aware of this artificiality than your clients. Again, allow yourself the time to gain a greater sense of ease in applying what you have learned and in functioning in your role as a helper.

Counterproductive Attitudes

Up to this point, we have encouraged you to avoid too quickly giving up pursuing one of the helping professions, even though there may be times when you might feel like abandoning this role. However, we also want you to assess your attitudes and personal characteristics to determine which traits may be assets or liabilities in your quest to provide help to others. This section considers some characteristics or attitudes that we see as counterproductive if you want to make a career of helping others. As you take the following self-inventory, strive to be as honest as you can in assessing these traits in yourself. Use the following scale to respond: 4 = this statement is true of me *most* of the time; 3 = this statement is true of me *much* of the time; 2 = this statement is true of me *some* of the time; and 1 = this statement is true of me *almost none* of the time. Although some of these statements may seem a bit extreme at first reading, do your best to remain open to seeing whether the particular characteristic can be applied to you in any way.

_____ 1. I have few problems in my life and therefore am in a position to help others resolve their problems.

_____ 2. My way is the right way, and if my clients accepted my values, they would be happy.

_____ 3. I have very strong religious convictions, and it is my responsibility to guide others to adopt them.

_____ 4. I have no religious affiliation, do not believe in religion, and consider everyone who has religious convictions to be neurotic.

_____ 5. My vision of helping is telling clients what they should do. For every question they raise, I should be able to provide a definite answer.

_____ 6. I have little tolerance for clients expressing feelings such as sadness, grief, or guilt, because that does little to change their situation and is self-indulgent.

_____ 7. My basic belief about humankind is that people are evil, not to be trusted, and in need of being straightened out.

_____ 8. I've had a rough life, and if I've "made it," I think others should be able to make it too.

_____ 9. At times I am hostile, indirect, and sarcastic.

_____ 10. I have made a minimal effort to expose myself to learning situations and have avoided feedback from fellow students, professors, and supervisors as much as possible.

_____ 11. The goal of getting a degree or a license is foremost in my mind; the process of getting there was seen as a necessary, but unpleasant, means to an end.

_____ 12. I believe that those teaching and supervising me know less than I do.

_____ 13. I tend to be intimidating to people and at times seem to enjoy having others be afraid of me.

_____ 14. I have a difficult time seeing people in pain; I want to quickly take their pain away and turn them to more pleasant thoughts.

_____ 15. Although I sometimes experience pain, I am unwilling to acknowledge this suffering and seek help for it; I think that my pain is being taken care of by attending to the pain of my clients.

_____ 16. I consistently make my needs more important than my clients' needs.

_____ 17. I need my clients more than they need me, and therefore I foster their dependency on me.

_____ 18. I have a difficult time entering a client's world; I tend to perceive reality only through my own eyes.

_____ 19. I am chronically depressed when I listen to the sagas of others. I often overidentify with them, and I tend to make their problems my problems.

_____ 20. I see counseling as something that others need, yet I can't imagine myself seeking this kind of help.

_____ 21. I have a very fragile ego that is easily bruised, and thus I'm overly sensitive to any criticisms from others.

_____ 22. I'm easily defensive and have an aversion to being challenged.

_____ 23. I have lived a very sheltered life and have a limited and fixed vision of the world.

_____ 24. I'm unable to accept those who have values different from mine.

_____ 25. I have an intense need to be in control; when I feel that I'm not in control of myself or others, I feel anxious.

Now that you have finished taking this inventory, go over those items that you identified as characteristic of you most or much of the time. We hope that you will not quickly lose heart but will see this as a challenge for making some changes in yourself. For the duration of the semester, it would be a good idea to work on some of these attitudes and traits that you have identified. For instance, if it is difficult for you to listen to others when they are in pain and if you tend to want to cheer them up quickly, you can make a conscious effort to try behaving in different ways the next time someone close to you is experiencing pain. If you become aware of your limited life experience, you can expose yourself to broader experiences. If you discover that you have been assuming that your values are right for everyone else, you can open yourself to recognizing that others fundamentally different from you live productive lives. You can challenge your notion that help is good for others but not for you by getting for yourself what you offer to others. What is absolutely essential is a high degree of honesty and an openness to being challenged.

ATTRIBUTES OF THE "IDEAL HELPER"

Although it is useful to describe some of the characteristics of the "ideal helper," even the most effective helpers do not meet all of these criteria. If you try to match the ideal picture we are about to paint, you will be needlessly setting yourself up for failure and frustration. But it is surely possible to become a more effective helper if you are aware of those areas that need strengthening. You can hone your existing skills and acquire new ones. You can integrate knowledge that will enhance your abilities. You can make personal changes that will allow you to be more present and powerful as you intervene in the lives of your clients.

Portrait of an Effective Helper

What follows are some characteristics that we consider an integral part of effective helping. With these possibilities in mind, consider the following perspective of the helper who is making a significant difference:

- Ideally, you are committed to an honest assessment of your own strengths and weaknesses. You recognize that who you are as a person is the most important instrument you possess as a helper.

- You realize that you are unable to inspire clients to do in their lives what you are unable or unwilling to do in your own life.
- You are open to learning and have a basic curiosity. You realize what you don't know, and you are willing to take steps to fill the gaps in your knowledge. You recognize that your education is never finished but is something that you are continually acquiring.
- You have the interpersonal skills needed to establish good contact with other people, and you can apply these skills in the helping relationship.
- You genuinely care for the people you help, and this caring is expressed by doing what is in their best interest. You are able to deal with a wide range of your clients' thoughts, feelings, and behaviors. You share your persistent reactions to your clients in appropriate and timely ways.
- You realize that it takes hard work to bring about change, and you are willing to stick with clients as they go through this difficult process. You are able to enter the world of your clients and see the world through their eyes rather than imposing your own vision of reality on them. You offer support when it is needed and confront clients on their unused potential when this is required.
- You realize that clients often limit themselves through a restricted imagination of possibilities for their future. You are able to inspire clients to dream and to take the steps necessary to fulfill their dreams in reality. It is often your faith that enables clients who have little hope to begin to believe that they have the potential for a better future.
- You are willing to draw on a number of resources to enable clients to move toward their goals. You are flexible in applying strategies for change, and you are willing to adapt your techniques to the unique situation of each client.
- In working with clients whose ethnic or cultural background is different from yours, you show your respect for them by not fitting them into a neat mold.
- Even though you wrestle with your own problems, this struggle does not intrude on your helping of others. You do not burden clients with long tales about your own personal problems, but you are willing to draw on your life experiences to deepen clients' self-exploration.
- You take care of yourself physically, mentally, psychologically, socially, and spiritually. You do in your own life what you ask of your clients. If you are confronted with problems, you deal with them.
- You question life and engage in critical self-examination of your beliefs and values. You are aware of your needs and motivations, and you make choices that are congruent with your life goals. Your philosophy of life is your own creation, not one that has been imposed on you.
- You are capable of establishing meaningful relationships with at least a few significant people.
- Although you have a healthy sense of self-love and pride, you are not arrogant.

This is not a complete list, and no one fits the portrait of the ideal helper perfectly. Our intent in presenting this list is not to overwhelm you but to provide you with some characteristics that are worthy of reflection. You might be telling yourself that you lack many of these characteristics. An unskilled helper can become a skilled one, and all of us can become more effective in reaching and touching the lives of the clients we encounter.

Assessing Your Personal Characteristics

In applying to an educational program in the helping professions, you were probably evaluated on both your academic background and your promise for personal and professional development. Most graduate counselor-training programs make use of a formal review at specific points to assess the academic progress of students. At this point we will not discuss the screening out of students who show signs of being impaired. But we do want to challenge you to assess your own personal characteristics that could work either for or against you in your role as a professional helper.

In addressing the question "Are the helping professions for me?" you are encouraged to use this book as a catalyst for honest self-reflection. Below is a list of qualities, traits, attitudes, values, and convictions that one graduate program uses to assess candidates' level of personal development. Assume either that you are applying for admission to such a program or that you are now in a training program that evaluates you on the basis of personal characteristics. As you review the attributes below, reflect on how well you know yourself, and assess your current level of interpersonal functioning.

- *Sensitivity.* How interested are you in others and the personal welfare of others?
- *Personal presence.* How respectful and genuinely involved are you in your interpersonal interactions?
- *Compassion and empathy.* How able are you to respond to the needs of others with concern and understanding?
- *Flexibility and a willingness to receive feedback.* Can you openly consider feedback offered by others and make changes in your attitudes and behavior?
- *Integrity.* How well do you demonstrate self-respect and respect for others in your interactions?
- *Modeling.* Can you model functional human behavior and coping processes?
- *Insight.* What is your capacity for perceiving, understanding, abstracting, and generalizing from professional sources and personal experiences?

Many training programs offer some self-exploration experiences in which students can become more aware of how their personal attributes manifest themselves in relationships. In your practicum and internship seminars, there are typically opportunities to focus on ways in which your personal style influences your ability to establish helping relationships with clients. If your program does not offer formal personal-growth experiences, seek these resources in the community. Much of the rest of this book will deal with the interplay between you as a person and your work as a professional helper. Our underlying assumption is that the best way to prepare for a dynamic career is to come to a fuller appreciation of the richness of your being and to be able to use your own life experiences in your evolution in the helping professions.

SELECTING A PROFESSIONAL PROGRAM AND CAREER PATH

Students planning to enter one of the helping professions sometimes fall into the trap of idealizing the profession. In their minds, they may build up the glory of helping others, seeing only the positives. They may envision themselves as being able to help virtually everyone who comes to them, and even reaching those who do not seek their counsel. Although having ideals and goals to strive for is part of being a helper who makes a difference, it is easy to paint an unrealistic picture of what your career as a helper will be like. You need to engage in ongoing reality testing to maintain a balanced outlook. You can test your vision by talking to various practitioners in many different settings. Ask them to tell you what they do in a typical week. Inquire about their motivations for choosing and remaining in the helping professions. Ask especially about the rewards, challenges, and demands of their work.

When you begin fieldwork, you'll be able to test many of your ideas and expectations against the real world of work. This is a good time to reflect on your motives and needs for considering helping as a career. Observations in various field settings and practical experience working with different client populations will provide a more accurate picture of how your career is likely to satisfy your needs for becoming a helper in the first place.

At this point, you may not even be certain you want to pursue a career in the helping professions. If you are enrolled in a two-year community college program in human services, you may be wondering whether it would be best for you to get a job when you complete your program. A wide range of human-services jobs are available, including skills training, social service assistants, work with the mentally handicapped, outreach workers in the community, work with parolees or in prison settings, and a host of community agency settings. Those who graduate with a substance abuse certificate often find jobs in drug and alcohol treatment centers. It is generally true that the higher your educational level the more career options are open to you. However, you may want to get a job for a time to gain experience once you complete a community college program. Later you may see the need to return to school for a bachelor's or a master's degree in one of the helping professions.

Whether you are an undergraduate or a graduate student, you have probably experienced some anxiety in selecting the right program. We encourage students to be open to new ideas. There are no absolute guidelines or perfect choices. Gather program material from several universities and talk with professors and students. Talking with professionals about their work experience can also broaden your perspective. Ask about the specific educational and practical background that they most value. In selecting a program, ask yourself these questions:

"Will the program give me what I need to do the work I want to do? Does the orientation of the program fit with my values? Am I compatible with the program?"

If you are taking an introductory course on the helping professions as an elective and are undecided about pursuing a career in the field, you can take selected courses and fieldwork classes to explore your interest in continuing. We have met students who remained in a course of study even though they had discovered that they were not enthusiastic about the field. They were hesitant to change because doing so could be interpreted as a failure. Others are reluctant to change majors because they would face added requirements for graduation. It seems to us that such students are likely to fail in the long run if they don't pursue their real interests.

If you find yourself in a program that you really don't like, consider getting out. But be sure you evaluate the overall direction of the program rather than a specific course or requirement that you do not like. One of our graduates complained that some of the classes she had to take were unrelated to her career interests. Specifically, she couldn't understand why research-oriented and grant-writing courses were required. However, she discovered that these courses were valuable in helping her land a job. In hindsight, she found value in a part of her education that she at one time had thought was meaningless.

Deciding Which Professional Route to Take

Students often ask which professional specialty we think is best for them. You can take many routes as a helper in the human services. You might ask: "Should I become a social worker? a psychiatric technician? a marriage and family therapist? a mental-health counselor? a psychologist? a paraprofessional worker?" These professional specialties have different focuses, yet all have in common working with people.

We tell students that they will have to choose a specialty through a process of reading and thinking about the alternatives. Much depends on what you want to do, how much time you are willing to invest in a program, where you want to live, and what your other interests are. Realize that there is no "perfect profession" and that each profession has advantages and drawbacks. In the Appendix we list the addresses of major professional organizations from which you can obtain information on the educational and training background needed for the various professions.

At the undergraduate level, human-services programs train practitioners for community-agency work, especially for drug and alcohol rehabilitation programs. Human-services workers generally carry out specific roles and functions under the supervision of clinical social workers, psychologists, and licensed counselors. At the master's degree level, students can choose among four types of programs: counseling, rehabilitation counseling, marriage and family therapy, and clinical social work. At the doctoral level, there are generally four approved programs for those wanting to become practitioners: social work, counselor education, counseling psychology, and clinical psychology. Each specialization has its own perspective and emphasizes different roles and functions for practitioners.

Regardless of which of the helping professions interests you the most, you are likely to discover that you will occupy many different positions within an area of specialization. For instance, if you pursue a clinical-social-work program, you may eventually hold a variety of jobs. You are likely to provide direct service to clients, including case work, counseling, assessment, and community work. You may also assume a role in formulating social policy, doing advocacy work, and writing grants to fund social programs. At some point your professional services may be more indirect, such as supervising interns, working as a consultant, and designing or managing human-services programs. You may begin by doing a great deal of counseling and case work, and at some point you may find management and administration to be challenging. Be open to the vast range of possibilities before you. Do not fall into the trap of convincing yourself that once you accept a position you are locked into the specific job forever. Too often we find that students are overly anxious about making the "right decision," as though there were only one or two positions they would ever occupy. Instead, allow yourself to consider your professional life in a developmental way, whereby you will see new possibilities as you gain additional work experiences.

Advantages and Disadvantages of Various Specializations

We asked some of our colleagues to identify what they tell students who ask about graduate training in their specialty. We were mainly interested in comparing social work with marital and family therapy, because many of our students raise questions pertaining to choosing one of these two graduate programs after they have completed a bachelor's degree in human services. Below are some of the common threads that we received from our informal survey.

Marital and family counseling. The specialization of marital and family therapy is primarily concerned with relationship counseling. It deals with assessing and treating clients from a family-systems perspective. Students in a master's program in marital and family therapy take a variety of courses in assessment and treatment, as well as theory courses. They also do extensive supervised fieldwork with children and adults, couples, and families. Several of the instructors in our program, who have training and a license in family counseling, offered the following perspectives on this professional route. Their responses have been paraphrased.

- Having a professional license will open many doors, but the type of license is less important than one's academic courses, life experiences, and internship practice. Most programs in marital and family therapy emphasize clinical applications and involve a great deal of experiential work.
- Marital and family therapy, being in its infancy, is still an emerging field. If a student has a pioneer spirit and is interested in being able to influence the direction of the field, this is certainly a road he or she might consider. People who do well in this field are innovative, are self-directed, and

understand themselves, and they are in basic agreement with the tenets of the systems approach.

- Traditionally, only social workers, as well as psychiatric workers, have worked with the aging, dying, and bereaved, but this situation is changing somewhat. The bottom line when it comes to advice for students is to follow your own interests. I recommend going where your heart is.
- A drawback of marital and family therapy is that there is no nationwide licensure. Some states also do not have a specialized license in this field. In addition, the marital and family therapist license is sometimes not considered as prestigious as other licenses.
- The greatest joy for me is to see children and adolescents I helped 20 years ago come back and see me as a group. At such times, the feeling of having made a contribution is overwhelming. There is a sense of having a place in the lives of families and in the history of our civilization.

Social work. This specialization attends not only to the inner workings of a person but also to an understanding of the person in the environment. A master's program in social work (MSW) prepares students broadly in areas such as case work, counseling, community intervention, social policy and planning, research and development, and administration and management. The course work tends to be broader than that in counseling, and it focuses on developing skills to intervene and bring about social change on levels beyond the individual. Although clinical social workers are engaged in assessment and treatment of individuals, couples, families, and groups, they tend to view environmental factors as contributing strongly to an individual's or a family's problems. In addition to academic courses, a two-year supervised internship is part of the social worker's preparation for either direct or indirect social services. Several of our instructors, all of whom are social workers, provided the following input:

- In my own education, I found that my social-work program was broad-based, so less time was devoted to learning specific therapeutic techniques. I was frustrated with this as a student because I was eager to become a therapist. Now I am quite grateful for the background in policy and research.
- The MSW gives tremendous career flexibility because of the range of practice, including administration, planning, and policy areas.
- Because of the range within social work, you can actually change careers without a major retooling. You can go from direct practice to research to teaching to policy and planning.
- Employee assistance programs will become the new mental-health movement of the 1990s. Corporations are discovering that psychologically healthy employees are a better investment, and thus there will be many jobs in this area.
- An advantage of social work is job variety. Social workers are able to use their skills in different areas, such as employment in welfare agencies, industry, community organization, and clinical practice.
- A licensed clinical social worker (LCSW) has many options open for securing a position. I know of many licensed counselors who are struggling as

their job options are decreased. The LCSW degree provides maximum options in regard to specialties. You can specialize in clinical, child, family, group, community, and administration. The LCSW is an old, well-established profession with solid support nationwide. You can move from agency to agency, location to location, and state to state more easily than with certain other professional licenses.

Clinical and counseling psychology.   Although clinical and counseling psychology are different specializations, there are no rigid boundaries separating their professional functions. We briefly consider them together to round out the picture of your options of a career as a professional helper. Although you can be licensed as a social worker, counselor, and marital and family therapist with a master's degree, this is not the case if you wish to refer to yourself as a psychologist. Both counseling and clinical psychology require a doctorate as a basic requisite for licensure. Clinical psychologists focus on assessment, diagnosis, and treatment procedures of mildly to severely disturbed persons. They interview clients and write case studies. Counseling psychologists assist relatively healthy people in solving developmental problems and functioning more effectively. They help clients find and use information to make better personal, educational, and occupational choices. Professional psychologists in both specialties often offer psychotherapy to individuals, couples, families, and groups; they may teach or conduct research. Both specializations focus on evaluation of treatments and programs and help clients develop action plans.

Factors to Consider in Choosing Your Career Path

Making career choices is an ongoing process rather than an isolated event. People generally go through a series of stages when choosing a career path. Information from practitioners and professors can help you define a professional direction. But you cannot rely solely on the advice of others when making your career decisions. In today's world, it is wise to consider the advantages of becoming a generalist. Your chances of gaining employment in a managed care system are greater if you are able to work with a range of client populations in a variety of problem areas. Although you may develop expertise in a specific area, flexibility is often necessary to meet the changing demands in the marketplace.

Ultimately you must decide for yourself which path is likely to best tap your talents and bring you the most fulfillment. Consider the following factors in the career decision-making process: self-concept, interests, abilities, values, occupational attitudes, socioeconomic level, parental influence, ethnic identity, gender, and physical, mental, emotional, and social handicaps. We will discuss five of these factors in more detail—self-concept, motivation and achievement, interests, abilities, and values. Apply these areas to yourself as you consider the range of career possibilities you might want to pursue.

Self-concept.   Some writers in career development contend that a vocational choice is an attempt to fulfill one's self-concept. People with a poor self-concept, for example, are not likely to envision themselves in a meaningful or important job. They are likely to keep their aspirations low; as a result, their achievements will probably be low. They may select and remain in a job that they do not enjoy or derive satisfaction from because they are convinced that such a job is all they are worthy of. In this regard, choosing a vocation can be thought of as a public declaration of the kind of person you see yourself as being. Casey and Vanceburg (1985) capture the notion that how we view ourselves has a great deal to do with how others perceive and treat us: "Our self-perception determines how we present ourselves. The posture we've assumed invites others' praise, interest, or criticism. What others think of us accurately reflects our personal self-assessment, a message we've conveyed directly or subtly."

Motivation and achievement.   Setting goals is at the core of the process of deciding on a vocation. If you have goals but do not have the energy and persistence to pursue them, your goals will not materialize. Your need to achieve, along with your achievements to date, is related to your motivation to translate goals into action plans. In thinking about your career choices, identify those areas where your drive is the greatest. Also, reflect on specific personal achievements. What have you accomplished that you feel particularly proud of? What are you doing now that moves you in the direction of achieving what is important to you? What are some of the things you dream about doing in the future? Thinking about your goals, needs, motivations, and achievements is a good way to get a clearer focus on your career direction.

Interests.   Interest measurement is used extensively in career planning. Once you have determined your areas of vocational interest, you can identify possible positions for which these interests are appropriate. You can then focus your attention on those jobs for which you have the abilities required for satisfactory job performance. Working as a volunteer in a community agency is an excellent way to test your interests and abilities. Going to the career center for information, testing, and vocational counseling can also be helpful. Although interests are a significant element, you must also consider whether you have the ability to perform well on the job.

Abilities.   Ability or aptitude is a significant factor in the career decision-making process, and it is probably used more often than any other factor. *Ability* refers to your competence in an activity; *aptitude* is your ability to learn. Scholastic aptitude is particularly significant if you need to enter a graduate program that will be a gateway to a position you seek in the helping professions. Consider the activities you have engaged in where you think you do especially well. Ask yourself what kind of activities you would find rewarding. To get a clearer sense of your aptitude, review your academic strengths and weaknesses. How open are you to academic learning? How quickly do you grasp concepts, and to what degree are you able to apply and use what you know? How far are you willing to go in your schooling?

Values.   Once you have determined how your interests and abilities match with possible career choices, explore your values. It is important to assess, identify, and clarify your values so that you will be able to match them with your career.

Your *work values* pertain to what you hope to accomplish in an occupation. Work values are an important aspect of your total value system. Recognizing those things that bring meaning to your life is crucial if you hope to find a career that has personal value for you. A few examples of work values include: helping others, influencing people, finding meaning, prestige, status, competition, friendships, creativity, stability, recognition, adventure, physical challenge, change and variety, opportunity for travel, moral fulfillment, and independence. Because certain work values are related to certain occupations, they can be the basis of a good match between you and a position. Take the time to complete the following self-inventory as a way of clarifying some of your values pertaining to work.

Decide how important each of the following values is to you in your work. Write the appropriate number next to each: 4 = most important to me; 3 = important, but not a top priority; 2 = slightly important; and 1 = of little or no importance.

____ 1. *High income:* opportunity for high pay or other financial gain.
____ 2. *Power:* opportunity to influence, lead, and direct others.
____ 3. *Prestige:* opportunity for respect and admiration from others.
____ 4. *Job security:* security from unemployment and economic changes.
____ 5. *Variety:* chances to do many different things in a job.
____ 6. *Achievement:* opportunities to accomplish goals.
____ 7. *Responsibility:* chance to be in charge of myself and others; being able to show trustworthiness.
____ 8. *Independence:* freedom from rigid hours or controls.
____ 9. *Family relationships:* time to be with family in addition to the job.
____ 10. *Interests:* work that matches my field of interest.
____ 11. *Opportunity to serve people:* being able to make a difference in the lives of others; helping others help themselves.
____ 12. *Adventure:* a high level of excitement on the job.
____ 13. *Creativity:* opportunities to come up with new ideas and do things in creative ways.
____ 14. *Inner harmony:* peace and contentment through work.
____ 15. *Teamwork:* opportunities to cooperate with others toward common goals.
____ 16. *Intellectual challenge:* demands at work for a high level of problem solving and creative thinking.
____ 17. *Competition:* the need to compete against others.
____ 18. *Advancement:* opportunities for promotion.
____ 19. *Continued learning:* chances to update learning and knowledge.
____ 20. *Structure and routine:* a predictable routine on the job that requires a certain pattern of responses.

Go over the list again and identify the top three values—the ones you deem to be essential in a job you would accept. What does your list tell you? What other values do you consider to be extremely important in work? To clarify some of these values, ask yourself these questions: "Do I like working with a wide range of people? Am I able to ask for help from others when faced with problematic situations? Do I place a value on doing in my own life what I encourage others to do for themselves? How do I feel about offering help to others with their problems? Am I interested in organizing, coordinating, and leading others in work projects? Do I value working on projects I have designed, or do I tend to look to others to come up with ideas for projects with which I can become involved?" Your values and interests are intertwined; knowing them can help you identify areas of work where you will find the most personal satisfaction.

By Way of Review

Near the end of each chapter we list some of the chapter's highlights. These key points serve as a review of the messages we've attempted to get across. We encourage you to spend a few minutes after you finish each chapter to write down central issues and points that have the most meaning for you.

- A helping career is not for everyone. We hope you will keep open the question of whether it is right for you.
- In deciding whether to pursue one of the helping professions, do not give up too soon. Be prepared for doubts and setbacks.
- Although the "ideal helper" does not exist in reality, a number of behaviors and attitudes characterize effective helpers. Even though you might not reach the ideal, you can progress, especially with the willingness to question what you are doing.
- It is essential that helpers examine their motivations for going into the field. Helpers meet their own needs through their work, and they must recognize these needs. It is possible for both client and helper to benefit from the helping relationship.
- Some of the needs for going into the helping professions include the need to be needed, the need for prestige and status, and the need to make a difference. These needs can work both for you and against you in becoming an effective helper.
- In selecting an educational program, follow your interests. Be willing to experiment by taking classes and by getting experience as a volunteer worker.
- In choosing a career path, consider factors such as self-concept, interests, abilities, values, occupational attitudes, socioeconomic level, parental influence, ethnic identity, gender, and physical, mental, emotional, and social handicaps.
- Be willing to seek information about careers in mental health from others, such as professionals in the field and faculty members, but realize that ultimately you will decide which career path is best for you.
- Do not consider the selection of a career as a one-time event. Instead, allow yourself to entertain many job possibilities over your lifetime.
- Realize that you must have a beginning to your career. Be patient, and allow yourself time to feel comfortable in the role of helper. You don't have to be the perfect person or the perfect helper.

WHAT WILL YOU DO NOW?

After each chapter review we provide concrete suggestions you can put into action. These suggested activities grow out of the major points developed in the chapter. Once you have read the chapter, we hope you will find some way to develop an action program. If you commit yourself to doing even one of these activities for each chapter, you will become more actively involved in the process of reading and reflecting.

1. If you are an undergraduate and if you think you'd like to pursue a graduate program, select at least one graduate school to visit so you can talk with faculty members and students. If you are in a graduate program, contact several community agencies or attend a professional conference to determine what kinds of positions will be available to you. If you have an interest in obtaining a professional license, contact the appropriate board early in your program to obtain information on the requirements.

2. Ask a helper whom you know about his or her motivations for becoming a helper and for remaining in the profession. What does this person get out of helping clients?

3. Conduct an interview with a mental-health professional who works in a position similar to the one you hope to obtain. Before the interview, develop a list of questions that you are interested in exploring. Write up the salient points of your interview, and share the results in your class.

4. The career-guidance center in your college or university probably offers several computer-based programs to help students decide on a career. One popular program is known as the System of Interactive Guidance and Information (SIGI). This program assesses and categorizes your work values. Taking it will aid you in identifying specific occupations that you might want to explore.

5. Create your own activity or project (for this chapter or any of the chapters to follow). Find some ways to get involved by taking action. Think of ways you can apply what you read in each chapter to yourself. Decide on something specific, a step you can take now, that will help you get actively engaged in a positive endeavor. After reading this chapter, for example, you could decide to reflect on your own needs and motives for considering a career in the helping professions. Review some significant turning points in your life that might have contributed to your desire to become a helper.

6. We strongly encourage you to keep a journal as an adjunct to reading this book and taking this course. Write in your journal in a free-flowing and unedited style. Be honest, and use journal writing as an opportunity to get to know yourself better, to clarify your thinking on issues raised in each chapter, and to explore your thoughts and feelings about working in the helping professions. At the end of each chapter, we'll provide a few suggestions of topics for you to reflect on and include in your journal writing. For this chapter, consider these areas:

- Write about your main motives for wanting to become a helper. How do you expect your needs to be satisfied through your work?
- Write about factors that have influenced your conception of what it means to be a helper. Who are your role models? What kind of helping did you receive?

- Spend some time thinking about the attributes of the ideal helper. What are your personal strengths that might help you as a helper? How realistic are your expectations about what you'll be doing as a helper?
- What are your thoughts about selecting an educational and professional route to pursue? Write a bit on factors you will need to consider in choosing your own career path.

7. At the end of each chapter we will provide some suggestions for further reading. For the full bibliographic entry for each of the sources listed below, consult the References and Reading List at the back of the book.

For a discussion on a wide array of issues confronting those in the helping professions, see Kottler (1993, 1997). For comprehensive coverage of topics such as development of a professional identity, ethical standards, basic process skills, approaches to counseling, and the making of a professional counselor, see Kottler and Brown (1996). Consult Hutchins and Cole Vaught (1997) and Doyle (1992) for an overview of strategies for helping and the building blocks of the interview, along with skills in the helping process.

Chapter 2

Getting the Most from Your Education and Training

FOCUS QUESTIONS

1. How would you describe yourself as a learner? Would you like to change your style of learning? If so, how?
2. What can you do to make your educational program more meaningful? How can you derive the maximum benefit from your academic courses?
3. What can you do to maximize your learning from fieldwork placements?
4. How can you better profit from your supervision? If you are not getting the quality of supervision you need, what steps can you take?
5. What are some ways to challenge your self-doubts in both your academic courses and your fieldwork placement? How can you change your fears into assets and opportunities for learning?
6. What are some possible benefits of sticking with a field placement that is not to your liking?
7. In meetings with your supervisor and fellow students, what attitude can you assume that will lead to maximizing your learning? What specific steps can you take to confront any difficulties you are experiencing in your field placement?
8. What are your thoughts about receiving personal counseling as part of your sessions with your supervisor? What advantages and disadvantages do you see with this arrangement?

AIM OF THE CHAPTER

The theme of this chapter is that you will get far more from your program of studies and your fieldwork activities if you assume an *active stance* in your education. So often we hear students passively complaining about their department, their professors, their supervisors, and everything and everybody but themselves. There are faults in any educational system, but it is more useful in the long run to look beyond these faults to see how you can get the most from your education. Rather than concentrating on all that you cannot do, for whatever reasons, take responsibility for your education.

Any system imposes limitations on you. The challenge is to learn how to work creatively within that system to attain your key goals without sacrificing your integrity by "selling out." We often hear both students in college and professionals in a human-services system argue that they could be more creative and productive "it it weren't for . . . ." Below we list some of these common assertions. See how many of them sound familiar to you.

For students: "I would be a good learner if it weren't for . . .

- the dull professors, who really don't care."
- the long hours I work that cut into studying."
- my spouse, who won't support my efforts in going to college."
- my children, who take up so much of my time and interrupt my studies."
- an educational system that kills any creativity."
- so much reading and so many papers to write, leaving me no time to be concerned with what I'm learning."
- the other unmotivated students in my classes."
- the silly requirements and the grading game."
- the unrealistic pressures placed on me by my professors."

For professional helpers: "I would be productive, dynamic, and creative if it weren't for . . .

- my burned-out colleagues, who infect me with their cynicism."
- the director at my agency, who is an unfeeling dictator."
- the managed care system."
- my resistant clients."
- the lack of funding of our community program."
- all the paperwork, bureaucratic demands, and politics."
- my large caseload."
- my family, who make demands on me when I get home."
- supervisors who don't support my ideas."

These lists could easily be extended, but the point we want to make is that you could eternally create reasons outside of yourself to justify why you are not being productive. As long as you focus on "them out there," you are powerless to change your situation until someone or something else changes. We agree that these factors can surely contribute to hampering your efforts to find meaning at school and work, but the challenge is to avoid letting these external barriers block you from attaining your goals.

Exercising a measure of freedom within external demands and restrictions entails accepting responsibility for doing what you can do, rather than focusing on what you can't do. In this chapter we will be encouraging you to assume a more powerful role in choosing an appropriate educational program, working in meaningful fieldwork placements, demanding adequate supervision, and continuing your learning after graduation.

CREATING MEANING IN YOUR EDUCATION
Learning to Cope with the System

There are real problems in working within any system. The reality of an educational program is grades, requirements, courses, and evaluation. Although students often balk at being evaluated and feel that grades are unfair, this system of evaluation does exist. Moreover, it is a mistake to assume that grading stops when you graduate from a university. There are reviews and evaluation practices on all levels in the professional world. In a business, for example, your supervisors rate you and determine whether you get a promotion or a raise. If you are a professional, your clients rate you by the business they bring to you or take away from you.

Students sometimes assume that there are worlds of difference between the roles they play in college and the roles they will assume as professionals. Many of the traits that you have as a student will no doubt carry over into your behavior as a worker. If you have great difficulty in showing up for classes regularly, for example, you are likely to carry this habit into your work appointments. Getting a position in a community agency is a highly competitive effort. If you hope to gain entry into the professional world, it is essential that you be prepared to cope with the realities of the marketplace. You are not being treated kindly if little is expected of you and if you are allowed to get by with minimal effort.

Students in the human services sometimes expect that their professors will make fewer demands on them or give them better grades because of the informal relationships established in the classroom. Many human-services instructors are friendly, care about their students, and interact with them in a personal way. Some students have problems in knowing where to establish boundaries. They mistakenly assume that there should be no limits and that no demands should be placed on them because of this relatively close relationship. From our perspective a humanistic approach to education can be balanced with reasonable standards and expectations. Developing these academic standards is one basic way of preparing students to cope with the demands of the job market.

We asked some human-services practitioners to comment on the degree to which both their undergraduate and graduate programs had prepared them for their jobs. We also asked them to say how much power they had had to provide input or to make meaningful changes in their educational program. Some of these responses are given below:

- "Undergraduate studies prepared me well for counseling and proposal writing. Because I was a student representative to the program I was part of, I had a lot of power to provide input. I felt that my ideas were considered and that I had a voice."
- "I would have liked to have more administrative-type classes that dealt with how to best manage people. I often felt that I had the power to provide input, but I did not exercise this very often."
- "The kind of education and training that I most value is the practical and applied. Some of our professors asked us to relate our own issues with the course work. For example, in my graduate program in social work, we studied our own families. More than just learning material about families, we were encouraged to apply personal issues with the academic. We had a behavior class that consisted of weekly treatment cases. Vignettes on psychosocial problems were presented for us to analyze and discuss. We also talked about our job experiences, which proved to be useful."
- "It [the program] was a challenge! It gave me a wonderful foundation for the helping professions. It made me learn and believe in myself and my abilities."

- "My undergraduate program made me stop and take a look at who I was and what I wanted to do with my life, both personally and professionally. So many times I hear students say that their classes are not relevant to the real world. Fortunately, this was not the case for me with my program."

Investing in Your Education

At the beginning of your educational program you may feel that you'll have to remain in school forever to do what you want professionally. However, if you are enjoying and gaining from the experience, you'll likely be surprised at how soon you complete your program. The key is that you are personally involved in your educational program and that you can see a connection between your formal studies and your personal and professional goals. Think about how much of your time and energy you're prepared to devote to making your education meaningful. It may help to consider your education as an investment, and then decide what you can do to get the most from this investment.

Investments are often evaluated by their cost-benefit ratio. The cost of your educational investment includes not just money but your time and energy too. Look at the potential benefits of this investment, including what you hope you'll gain from your investment. Basically, evaluating the cost-benefit ratio of your investment involves asking yourself if what you are putting in (costs) is worth what you hope to get out of it in return (benefits). What are the benefits of putting a great deal of yourself into your formal studies? What will taking responsibility for your education cost you in terms of time taken away from other facets of your life?

What is most important is that you take responsibility for your own learning. Students who fail to see their own role in the learning process may find others to blame for their failures. If you're dissatisfied with your education, consider how much you're willing to invest to make it more vital. If you were dissatisfied with your earlier education, now is a good time to look at yourself and ask how much you're willing to invest to get more out of this experience. Are you waiting for others to do something for you? How much are you willing to do to change the things you don't like?

Regardless of the structure of the course in which you are using this book, you can find ways to become personally involved in the course. You can decide to be either actively engaged or marginally involved in applying the themes in this book and your course in your life. *You* can make this class different by applying some of the ideas provided in this chapter. Once you become aware of those aspects of your education that you don't like, *you* can decide to change your style of learning.

Becoming an Active Learner for Life

Most of us spend years acquiring information about the world around us. We may even equate learning with absorbing facts that are external to us. Although academic knowledge provides a foundation for becoming a helper, it is equally important to learn about yourself and about how to live fully. What you get from your educational program will depend on the degree to which you become an active agent in your learning. The following guidelines will help you develop this active stance.

1. *Preparing.* Many students have been conditioned to view reading as an unpleasant assignment, and they tolerate textbooks as something to plow through for an examination. As an active learner, however, you can selectively read this book, reflecting on those sections that have special meaning to you. Write brief reactions in the margins as you read, and come to class prepared to share your thoughts on these topics. Taking the time to think about the topics explored in this book and the personal meaning they have for you will enhance your learning experience.

2. *Dealing with anxieties.* Personal learning is not without anxiety. Anxiety is a response to fear. Some of the fears students often express include: the fear of taking an honest look at yourself and discovering terrible things; the fear of the unknown; the fear of looking foolish in front of others, especially your instructor; the fear of being criticized or ridiculed; and the fear of speaking out and expressing your values. How you deal with your fears is more important than trying to eliminate all of your anxieties. Facing your fears takes both courage and a genuine desire to increase your awareness of yourself. In doing so, you take a big step toward becoming the kind of person who can make a significant difference in the lives of others.

3. *Taking risks.* If you make the choice to get personally involved in the course, you should be prepared for the possibility of some disruption in your life. You may find yourself changing certain values, beliefs, and behaviors. You may like many of the changes you make that are an outgrowth of your participation in a program designed to educate and train professional helpers. However, some people may neither like nor appreciate your changes, and, indeed, some may be intimidated by you and stubbornly resist your attempt to step outside of old and familiar patterns.

4. *Establishing trust.* It is up to you to take the initiative in establishing the trust necessary for you to participate in this course in a meaningful way. If you become aware that you hold yourself back from getting verbally active in class discussions, consider seeing the instructor outside of class to talk about this.

5. *Self-disclosing.* Disclosing yourself to others is one way to come to know yourself more fully. It is also a good way to let others in your educational program know you. You can be open and at the same time retain your privacy by deciding how much you will disclose. Although it may be new and uncomfortable for you to express your ideas and share learnings based on your life experiences, we hope you challenge yourself to express your thoughts and feelings to the degree that it is appropriate in all phases of your educational program.

6. *Listening.* One of the basic helping skills is being able to listen fully to others and respond to the core of their messages. To develop this skill, listen to what others are saying without thinking of what you will say in reply. The first step in understanding is to listen carefully without judging what you hear. *Active listening* (really hearing the full message another is sending) requires that you remain open and carefully consider what others say rather than rushing to give reasons and explanations.

7. Practicing outside of class. One way to get the maximum benefit from your educational program is to think about ways of applying what you learn to your everyday life. You can make specific contracts with yourself (or with others) detailing what you're willing to do to experiment with new behavior and work toward the changes you want to make.

Integrating Knowledge, Skills, and Self

In our view you need to integrate what you know, what you can do, and the person who you are. Knowledge alone is not sufficient, yet without it you cannot become an effective helper. If you focus mainly on acquiring skills but neglect theory and knowledge, these skills will be of little use. Furthermore, your ability to use the skills and knowledge you have is very much a function of your being sensitive to the interpersonal dimension of the helping process. You need to know yourself and your client to effectively apply helping skills. The helper who has a low degree of self-awareness is at best a skilled technician, and we doubt that he or she will make a positive difference in clients. Helping is more than technique; it is an art that is an expression of who the helper is.

We asked some practitioners what specialized knowledge and skills they saw as most important in their present job. Their comments were informal, and we did not conduct a comprehensive sample of practitioners. But these reactions do give some idea of what is most useful in education.

Most of these professionals commented on the value of internships and field-work placements. These supervised practical experiences had helped them learn about "the system" and how best to survive in it. The skills most people felt they needed included counseling skills, supervisory skills, communication skills, the ability to interact with different levels of management, the ability to write a proposal, organizational skills, the ability to deal with crisis intervention, and networking skills. A number of the professionals pointed out the value of self-exploratory experiences, especially groups aimed at personal and interpersonal growth. These therapeutic experiences gave them opportunities to look at themselves and to deal with their own feelings and problems, activities that were seen as especially helpful in preparing them to relate to clients. Even those professionals who were primarily engaged in the administration of human-services programs commented on the value of self-awareness and the understanding of interpersonal dynamics as tools they utilized in their managerial functions. Those in management pointed out that they would not be able to develop and coordinate their programs if they did not know how to work effectively with people.

Keeping Current

It is essential that you discover ways to extend your education beyond graduation, for your knowledge and skills will soon be outdated unless you take steps to keep abreast of new developments. Some current issues in the helping professions that are receiving increased attention are methods of dealing with substance abuse; eating disorders; gay and lesbian issues; physical and psychological abuse of children, the elderly, and spouses; AIDS; and legal and ethical issues. Keeping professionally alert implies that you avail yourself of in-service and continuing-education programs. It is important to remember that your education is not completed when you finish school. The challenge is to find ways to go outside the confines of your daily work and not to become encapsulated by its boundaries.

Although many professionals have mandatory continuing-education requirements for the relicensing or recertification of their members, we hope that you develop your own self-directed program and do not merely comply with the minimal requirements. You can do this by taking specialized courses and workshops that deal with particular client groups and newer techniques.

Reading is another good way to keep abreast of developments in your field. In addition to professional journals and books dealing with your specific subject of interest, novels and nonfiction works about other cultures are also of value in your continuing education.

Perhaps one of the best ways of keeping yourself up to date is to be involved in a professional network with colleagues who are willing to learn from one another as well as assume a teaching role (see Kreiser, Domokos-Cheng Ham, Wiggers, & Feldstein, 1991). Colleagues can offer both the challenge and the support for practitioners to adopt a fresh perspective on problems they encounter in professional practice. According to Borders (1991), peer-consultation groups offer skill development, conceptual growth, participation, instructive feedback, and self-monitoring. For students, peer groups provide a supportive atmosphere and help trainees learn that they are not alone with their concerns. For professionals engaged in practice, they provide an opportunity for continued professional growth.

Networking among professionals can also provide a consistent means of identifying and addressing sources of negative feelings and loss of objectivity.

MAKING THE MOST OF YOUR FIELDWORK

In the helping professions of counseling, social work, psychology, and marriage and family therapy, most graduate programs have fieldwork and internship at their core. Most undergraduate programs in human services have a comprehensive fieldwork component, which is often the heart of the program. These activities provide a bridge between theory and practice. Students can compare their expectations of the field with the reality imposed by most agencies. Actual experience in a field placement gives students opportunities to learn first-hand about paperwork, agency policies and procedures, and the challenge of working with a wide range of client populations and problems. The goals of a fieldwork instruction program include:

- Providing students with knowledge of the varied approaches and methods used in human-services programs
- Helping students extend self-awareness and achieve a sense of professional identity

- Broadening students' sociocultural understanding of the individual, the family, the community, and relevant social systems
- Assisting students in recognizing and respecting cultural diversity and offering ways to use this understanding in practice
- Helping students expand their awareness of professional role relationships within their organization as well as the agency's role in the community

Of course, before you can meaningfully participate in fieldwork and internship placements, you need theory courses, specific knowledge, and a range of helping skills. It is the combination of academic course work, fieldwork placement, skills training, and personal development that makes for a sound program. For a variety of reasons, students often do not derive the maximum benefit from fieldwork and supervision. Here are some practical strategies for making the most of these applied experiences.

The Value of Fieldwork Experiences

When we talk with graduates of human-services programs, they typically mention that they found their current job as a result of contacts they established at their fieldwork placement. In fact, most graduates report wishing they had been able to participate in even more fieldwork activities. Some regret not having had a broader range of experience in their internships. We recommend that you visit as many sites as possible before making your selection, if that is allowed in your program. Get job descriptions and arrange interviews with selected agencies.

Here are some other suggestions on how to get the most value out of your field placements:

- Instead of limiting yourself to one kind of population, seek a variety of placements. Stretch your boundaries to help you to discover where your talents lie and the kind of population you would eventually like to work with. Through your internships you may learn what you don't want to do as well as what you would like to do. Some students who initially want to "do counseling" exclusively later find themselves in the role of an administrator or a supervisor.
- Take courses and workshops that will prepare you for the type of work expected of you in your placement. These workshops can be a useful resource for staying on the cutting edge of new developments with specialized populations.
- Let yourself fit into the agency, instead of trying to make it fit you. Be open to learning from the staff and the clients who come to the agency. Attempt to suspend your preconceived judgments about what you should be learning and focus instead on what lessons are available to you. Learn as much as you can about the politics of the agency by talking with people who work there, by attending staff meetings, and by asking questions. All of your learning will not result merely from interacting with clients. You can learn a good deal about an agency by being attentive and by talking with co-workers.
- Be aware of the toll that your work might have on you both emotionally and physically. Certain aspects of your life that you have not been willing to look at may be opened up as you get involved with clients. Know that your increased awareness could lead to more anxiety in your life.

- Recognize the limits of your training, practice only within these boundaries, and put yourself in situations where you will be able to obtain supervised experience. Regardless of your educational level, there is always more to learn. It is essential to learn the delicate balance between being overly confident and doubting yourself.
- Strive to be flexible in applying techniques to the different client populations, but do so under supervision. Avoid falling into the trap of fitting your clients to one particular theory. Use theory as a means of helping you understand the behavior of your clients. Realize that diverse client backgrounds necessitate diverse communication approaches. Although it is essential to learn therapeutic skills and techniques, they should be applied in appropriate ways.
- If you have a placement that you do not particularly like, don't write it off as a waste of time. At least you are learning that working in a drug-rehabilitation center, for example, is not what you want for a career. It helps to realize that none of your decisions need to be cast in concrete. Determine what you don't find productive about the placement, and why. You can also think of ways to make your assignment more meaningful rather than just telling yourself that you'll put in your time and get your credit. There are probably at least a few avenues for creating learning opportunities. Welcome all experiences as resources that can teach you what you will need to know in future situations.
- Make connections in the community. Learn how to use community resources and how to draw on support systems beyond your office. You can do this by talking to other professionals in the field, by asking fellow students about their connections in the community, and by developing a network of contacts. This kind of networking may well lead to a range of job opportunities.
- Keep a journal; record your observations, experiences, concerns, and personal reactions to your work. Your journal is an excellent way to stay focused on yourself as well as to keep track of what you are doing with clients.
- Be open to trying new things. If you have not worked with a family, for example, observe a family session or, if possible, work with a supervisor who is counseling a family. Avoid setting yourself up by thinking that if you do not succeed perfectly in a new endeavor you are a dismal failure. Give yourself room to learn by doing, at the same time gaining supervised experience.
- Look for ways to apply what you are learning in your academic courses to your experiences in the field. For example, one professional recalls having taken abnormal psychology as part of her graduate program and also having served as an intern in a state mental institution. Through this internship she was able to actually see some of the concepts she was studying come to life. One important lesson she learned was that many of the patients did not fit neatly into some diagnostic category.
- Be prepared to adjust your expectations. Don't expect an agency to give you responsibility for providing services to clients before it has a chance to know you. You'll probably start your fieldwork by being in an observing role. Later you may sit in on a counseling group, for example, and function as a co-leader.
- Find ways to work cooperatively with other students and to combine your talents with theirs. Look for means of tapping into your own creativity. If you are talented musically, for example, look for a way in which you might incorporate music into your field placement activities. If a fellow student has talents in dance

and movement, perhaps you can combine forces in an innovative therapeutic intervention.

• Treat your field placement like a job. Approach fieldwork in much the same way as you would if you were employed by the agency. Demonstrate responsibility, be on time for your appointments and meetings, and strive to do your best. Although you may be in an unpaid placement, this does not mean you can be irresponsible on the job. Often an unpaid internship can turn into a paid position.

• Learn as much as you can about the structure of the agency where you are placed. Ask about agency policies, about the way the programs are administered, and about management of the staff. At some point, you may be involved in the administrative aspects of a social program.

• Think and act in a self-directed way by involving yourself in a variety of activities. If you merely wait for a supervisor or other workers to take the initiative and give you meaningful assignments, you may be less than satisfied with your placement.

The Challenge of Diversity

As we have suggested, it is a good idea to seek a placement where you will be challenged to work with a variety of clients and tasks. Your learning will be limited if you attempt to get placements with clients just like yourself or those with whom you already know how to work. If you think you want to work with children, for example, you might consider an internship with the elderly. By working with diverse populations, you can test out your interests and develop new ones. If you focus narrowly on the population or problem you want as a specialization, you are likely to close off many rich avenues of learning and also limit your possibilities of finding a job.

As a part of your fieldwork for internship placement, you usually receive on-the-job training and supervision. Therefore, you might not need expertise in counseling rape victims before being accepted for such a placement. You will learn from co-workers and supervisors some interventions in working with such clients. Thus, more important than knowing how to work with a specific population or a specific problem is having a general background of knowledge and skills and being open to acquiring more specific abilities.

Helping someone different from you.   One of our colleagues told us that her paralyzed client became upset and angry when she said to him "I understand how you feel." His reply was: "How would you know? You can walk out of here, and I can't." On reflection, our colleague thought that she might have said: "You're right, I don't fully understand your situation. I can imagine your frustration and pain over becoming paralyzed at such a young age in a motorcycle accident. But I haven't been in your situation, so I don't know what you're thinking and feeling. I hope you'll help me understand what this is like for you, and I hope I can help you work through your own feelings about being paralyzed."

Some interns make the mistake of clinging to the conviction that to help a person they must have had the same life experience. Thus, a male counselor may doubt his capacity to effectively counsel an adolescent girl who is struggling with what she wants to do about being pregnant. A counselor may doubt that she can work with a client of a different race. Or a counselor who has not experienced trauma may wonder about her ability to empathize with clients who have had pain in their lives. When these counselors are challenged by a client, they often tend to backtrack and become apologetic. We hope that you can see the value of drawing on your own life experience in working with clients who are different from you. You may not have had the same problem, yet you may be able to identify with the feelings of loneliness or rejection of your client. It is more important to be able to understand the client's world than to have had the identical problem. What is crucial is that you realize that some of your clients will view the world from a different perspective than you do. In Chapter 7 we deal with this topic of diverse world views in more detail.

Challenging your self-doubt. Interns are often unsure, apologetic, and unwilling to credit themselves with what they are able to do. Ask yourself how you deal with your own feelings about what you know and don't know.

Consider how you might deal with a client who challenged you. At the initial session your client is surprised at your age. "Who are you to be helping me?" he asks. "You look so young, and I wonder if you have the experience to help me." Assume that this challenge opens up some of your own fears and doubts. Can you imagine saying any of the following things silently to yourself?

- "He's right. There are many years separating us. I wonder if I can understand his situation?"
- "This guy's attitude really makes me mad. He's not giving me a chance, and I feel attacked before I've even had a chance to know him."
- "Well, I don't feel comfortable with this confrontation, but I don't want to back down. I feel like letting him know that even though we differ in age, we might have many similarities in our struggles. I'd like an opportunity to at least explore whether we can form a relationship."
- "He's right. What makes me think I have anything to offer him? Maybe I should have chosen another line of work."

Most professionals have feelings of self-doubt and question their competence at certain times and in certain situations. The purpose of your supervised fieldwork is to provide you with a rich and meaningful learning opportunity. This is a place where you can acquire specific knowledge and where you can develop the skills to translate the theory you have learned into practice. We hope you have the courage to face your feelings of incompetence rather than running from them or pretending that they do not exist.

Selecting a fieldwork placement. If you have some choice in selecting the place where you will be gaining supervised practical experience, take an active role in securing the best placement possible. One way of actively participating in securing a quality fieldwork placement is by asking questions of potential agency settings when you are going through the interviewing process for a field placement. Some of the questions you might ask are:

- What are the goals and purposes of your agency or organization? What services are provided?
- Have you worked with student interns before? If so, what have been some of their activities?
- What internship opportunities are now available at this agency?
- What would be my specific responsibilities?
- Are there any special skills or requirements for the placement?
- To whom would I report? Who would supervise me? How often would I be able to meet with this person for direct supervision?
- Are there training or staff development opportunities at the agency? What kinds of training might I receive prior to and during my placement?
- Is any travel involved? If so, will I be reimbursed for travel?
- Would I be covered by the agency for malpractice liability?

Sometimes students seek placements that are expedient, convenient, and not very challenging. We hope you value your education enough to strive for a placement where you will receive adequate supervision and where you will be exposed to a variety of problems that clients bring to a community agency.

You may be employed at a community agency and want to use your work as your fieldwork placement. We recommend that you branch out to get as much variety as possible in your placements. This does not mean that you cannot use your place of work as a potential internship, but we suggest that you do different tasks, occupy a different role, or work with a different client population. Your fieldwork experience should provide you with a different setting in which to work and also with a different supervising environment. Trying to accomplish double duty by using your work experience as a substitute does not seem to us to be getting the most from your fieldwork.

Although it may be possible to combine some aspects of your employment with an internship, we hope you do not take the easiest and quickest path toward getting your degree. A wide range of opportunities exist within an agency. Secure training in areas new to you so you will be able to acquire new knowledge and skills. The more practical and supervised experience you can get the better. Commit yourself to becoming the most competent practitioner you can be.

PROFITING FROM YOUR SUPERVISION

Be clear in your own mind about what you expect from your supervisors, and discuss your desires with them from the outset. This section suggests how to approach your supervision and actively participate in this process.

Be Open to Learning from Your Supervisors

You will limit your opportunities for learning if you assume a know-it-all stance. Be open to input not only from supervisors but also from teachers, peers, colleagues, and clients. Have the courage to admit your imperfections, and don't become frozen out of fear of making errors. Be willing to make mistakes, and talk openly with your supervisor about them. If you do not have the courage to fail, you won't be willing to try anything new. You will be overly conscious about what you are doing and whether you are doing it "right." Take advantage of your student role; as a student, you are certainly not expected to know everything. Give yourself permission to be a learner. If you can free yourself from the shackles of trying to live up to the unrealistic ideal of perfection, you will allow your clients to be your teachers in some significant ways.

In our training of group leaders we typically find that the students approach workshops with considerable anxiety over looking incompetent in the eyes of their peers and supervisors. Early in the workshop we tell them: "Be active. One sure way not to learn much in this workshop is by being extremely self-conscious and critically judging most of what you want to say or do. No matter what happens, there is something to be learned. If a group session is unproductive, you can explore what specific factors contributed to that outcome."

When we give students these instructions, they usually react with relief and tell us they feel much less anxious. We let them know that we understand and empathize with their difficulty in being observed by their peers and by supervisors. It is not possible to escape from being watched by clients, supervisors, and fellow workers. Talking about our experience of being observed allows us to be in control of this process rather than being controlled by what others might think of us. Students often find it helpful to openly share their fears. Paradoxically, the fears of the students appear to be diminished by this act of acknowledgment.

Be able to say "I don't know."   Being willing to admit your ignorance is important in interactions with both your supervisor and your clients. If you feel intimidated because you have to tell a client that you do not know an answer to her problem, you can say something like this: "You know, I'm not sure what to say about your concerns that you might be pregnant. I'm aware that you're a minor, and I'm somewhat cautious about suggesting a particular course of action. I'm also aware that you're anxious and that you'd very much like me to tell you what you should do. I'd be willing to consult my supervisor and get some ideas that I can bring back to you in a couple of days." In this way you acknowledge your limitations to your client, but you keep the door open to providing her with information she can use in resolving her own problems.

Express your reactions.   In working with both students and professionals, we often find that they have many good reactions that they keep to themselves. We typically encourage our trainees to talk out loud more often rather than engaging in an internal monologue. In a recent workshop a group counselor was quiet throughout the group session. The supervisor asked her what was going on. "Well, I'm very aware that you, my supervisor, are present in this session," she replied. "I feel inhibited in following my hunches, because I'm wondering what you might think of what I'm doing. I'm afraid that you might be judging me and that I might not be measuring up very well." Her supervisor told her that this was what would have been best for her to say aloud.

In another instance one trainee continually suggested one exercise after another during a particular group-training session. Later, when he was asked why he had introduced so many different exercises in such a short session, he replied: "Well, the group seemed to be getting nowhere. People seemed bored, and I felt responsible for making something happen! I was hoping to bring the group alive by trying some interaction exercises." We told the trainee that it would have been good to describe what he saw happening in the group. He could have talked about his feelings of responsibility and about how his perception of boredom affected him. Instead, he ignored expressing his own important reactions in favor of trying some mechanical techniques, which didn't work in the long run. We are not suggesting that you express your every fleeting reaction to your clients, but in your supervision meetings it is wise to talk about unrehearsed material.

Focus on both elements of supervision.   Some approaches to supervision emphasize the client's dynamics and teach you strategies for intervening in specific problems. Others focus on your dynamics as a helper and as a person and on your behavior in relationship to your client. Adequate supervision must take both of these elements into consideration. You need to understand models of helping clients, and you need to understand yourself if you hope to form truly therapeutic alliances. If your supervision is focused solely on what your client is doing or on teaching you specific techniques for what to do next, it will be lacking in a most important dimension. A critical focus for discussion in supervision sessions is the degree to which you are as present as possible for your clients. If you are overly concerned about what to do about a client's problem, this concern will distract you from making connections with the person. A useful focus of supervision is the variables that define the quality of the relationship between you and your clients. In supervision, you can talk about what you are experiencing as you work with different clients. This focus will reveal a good deal about both you and your clients.

Learn, but don't copy.   We have observed that some trainees limit their own development by trying too hard to copy the style of a supervisor or teacher. You are likely to watch carefully supervisors whom you respect, and you may tend to adopt their methods. It is important, however, to be aware of how easy it is to become a carbon copy of another person. To get the most from your supervision, try different styles, but continually evaluate what works for you and what doesn't. You might ask yourself: "What fits my belief system, both personal and theoretical? Do I have any conflicts between the theory or application of my supervisor's way and my own?"

If you pay too much attention to another person, you are likely to blur your own uniqueness. You need to be able to take what is good from your various supervisors and teachers, yet it is important to avoid being a clone. A balance is needed. Be willing to learn from others, but don't feel that you need to *be* them. If you learn to listen to your own inner voice and to respect your inner promptings, you will eventually have less need to look to outside authorities.

Learn to Be Assertive

Define how you want to spend your time in an agency, and get the supervision you need. Don't wait passively to be told what to do. Think about what you would like to learn and what skills you would like to acquire. A placement typically involves a written contract signed by the student and the supervisor of the agency. This contract usually spells out the number of hours to be worked per week, the activities that will be performed, the learning objectives, the opportunities for training, the expectations for the intern, and the expectations for the supervisor. Before agreeing to your contract with your supervisor, you can discuss in some detail the ways in which you think you could be of greatest benefit to the agency. In collaboration with your supervisor, you can spell out what you would like to experience and learn before you leave. Although you may not always get what you want, if you have a clear idea of what that is, you will have a better chance of obtaining it.

The assertion skills you practice in getting adequate supervision will be useful in your relationships with both clients and colleagues. Being assertive does not mean being aggressive, which alienates most people. By bulldozing your way into an agency, you will needlessly put others on the defensive. Being passive-aggressive is not useful either, whether it involves rebelling against all authority, appearing bored, or consistently showing up for appointments or meetings late. Resisting in such passive ways is likely to shut you off from many chances to learn.

It helps to realize that supervisors are people too. They get bogged down with their own burdens. As their client load grows and pressures increase, they may not initiate the regular supervision sessions that they have promised. Furthermore, some practitioners do not volunteer to become supervisors but are told that they should add interns to their already heavy work load. At times their training for being a supervisor is minimal, and they are expected to "learn by doing." If you are able to understand the predicament of supervisors, you are more likely to establish a basis of communication with them. Within a climate of open communication, you can sensitively and assertively let them know that you need help. If you have a difficult case, you can say something like this: "I really feel stuck with Susan. For several weeks now, we've been getting nowhere. Every suggestion I make seems to fall on deaf ears, and she has many reasons why it won't work. I suggested termination, and she got angry with me. Now I don't know what to do. Can I meet with you for a few minutes to talk about some alternatives?" If you merely complain that your supervisor is always too busy or fails to show up for appointments, all you will get is frustration. But by being clear, specific, and persistent, you are likely to have your needs met.

We suggest that you give your supervisors credit for wanting to do their best. If you approach them with a genuine attitude of letting them know what you would like from them, they are more likely to respond positively than if you keep your distance from them and expect them to do all the work. If you learn to be assertive in asking for what you need from your supervisors without being aggressive, you will be going a long way toward creating a positive fieldwork experience and using supervision to its fullest extent.

Unfortunately, many students have negative experiences with fieldwork and with supervisors. At a recent conference of human-service educators, Tricia McClam of the University of Tennessee made a presentation on effective field supervision. She commented that 9 out of 15 students had reported negative first field experiences! The relationship between the field supervisor and the student seems to be a key variable in determining whether the student's reactions are positive or negative. Supervisors certainly play a key role in the student's learning and it is part of the student's responsibility to communicate with them, even if they are less than ideal.

Students with positive reactions to supervisors made comments such as: "She was available." "She was involved in my cases." "My supervisor clearly stated what he expected of me and what I could expect of him." "My supervisor was both supportive and flexible." Students with negative reactions to supervisors observed: "He was too busy to properly supervise." "I had only two meetings with my supervisor during the entire semester." "My supervisor was not organized."

In her presentation, McClam indicated that when students begin their fieldwork activity, they need supervisors who are clear about their expectations and who provide support and guidance. Firmness coupled with flexibility is useful for beginning trainees. When students have gained some fieldwork experience, they still need support and guidance, along with feedback from their supervisors, but they can profit from experiences that will demand more intuition and skill. Most important is establishing regular communication between supervisors and supervisees. Take the initiative to communicate with your supervisor. This is particularly challenging in cases where you perceive your supervision to be inadequate, a topic we explore shortly.

Case example. Picture yourself as an intern in this situation. Your supervisor asks you to counsel a family, consisting of mother, father, and two young boys. The supervisor tells you that the parents are primarily interested in learning how to manage their problem children and want to learn disciplinary techniques. In the supervisor's view a more important problem consists of the conflicts between the wife and husband. You have had very little course work or training in working with families, and you feel lacking in the competencies to do family counseling. Below is a sample of some of the things that might be going on inside your head:

- "Now what am I going to do? I feel overwhelmed, but I don't want to appear like a neophyte, so I'd better take this family on."
- "I'm unprepared to counsel a family. I haven't even had a single course on family dynamics or family therapy. But if I don't agree to see the family, my supervisor might get angry and might think less of me. What should I do?"
- "The thought of dealing with this family terrifies me. I wouldn't know where to begin. I'd like to sit in on some sessions with my supervisor and observe and participate as a co-therapist. Do I dare suggest this?"

This inner dialogue gives some sense of the struggle you might go through in dealing with a supervisor who asks you to go beyond what you consider to be the boundaries of your competence. Let your supervisor know your concerns, and the two of you can talk about alternatives. Consider the following dialogue, and see how you might say some of the same or different things as the trainee.

SUPERVISOR: We are short on personnel in the agency, and we really need you to work with some families.

TRAINEE: My first reaction is to feel flattered that you think enough of me to ask for my help in seeing families. Yet at this stage of my professional development, I am going to have to decline.

SUPERVISOR: Look, one way to learn is by jumping in and getting involved. Most of us have hesitations when we begin working with new populations.

TRAINEE: In my case it is more than feeling anxious and having self-doubts. I have yet to take a single course in family therapy. It just does not seem ethical for me to undertake this task now.

SUPERVISOR: Well, I don't want you to do something that doesn't seem ethical to you. But I would be available for supervision, so you won't be without any guidance.

TRAINEE: I appreciate your offer for supervision. Perhaps I could observe your work with a family, with their permission of course, and then we could talk about your interventions after the session.

SUPERVISOR: If I had the time that would be great, but that would be adding one more thing to an already overbooked schedule.

TRAINEE: After I take the family therapy course next semester, perhaps I'll be in a better position to assist in this kind of work. For now, I need to work within my own limits.

This example is realistic in the sense that most organizations use interns as relatively "free" staff. The problem is not so much using interns to fill critical service needs but being unwilling to provide adequate supervision for trainees. Student interns do need some minimal theoretical foundation and knowledge competencies in working with families before they are able to effectively participate in actual clinical work with families. Certainly, when trainees are moving into a new area, they will need to acquire practical skills that will enable them to work effectively in this new setting. Good supervision allows trainees to apply their knowledge while acquiring these intervention strategies.

If you were the trainee in the situation described above, would you have considered working with a family if you were not qualified to do so? Might you have given in to pressure, especially with the offer of some supervision? How might you have looked for ways on the job to acquire the knowledge base that would allow you to work with a family? How would you like to be able to respond to this supervisor?

Dealing with Inadequate Supervision

Realistically, there are times when you will have to deal with supervision that is far from ideal. How can you recognize substandard supervision? What assertive courses of action are open to you in dealing with it?

Recognizing the effective supervisor.   Although there is no one way of conducting clinical supervision, there are established standards for counseling supervisors. The *Ethical Guidelines for Counseling Supervisors* (Association for Counselor Education and Supervision [ACES], 1993) are designed to help supervisors: (1) observe ethical and legal protection of clients' and supervisees' rights; (2) provide training for supervisees in ways that are consistent with clients' welfare and requirements of the program; and (3) establish policies, procedures, and standards for implementing programs. The supervisor's main functions are to teach trainees, to foster their personal and professional development, and to assist in the provision of the effective delivery of counseling (helping) services. An underlying assumption of the ACES guidelines is that "supervision should be ongoing throughout a counselor's career and not stop when a particular level of education, certification, or membership in a professional organization is attained."

The characteristics of effective supervisors as defined by ACES include:

- Counseling supervisors are themselves effective counselors.
- Professional supervisors demonstrate personal characteristics that enable them to carry out their roles and functions. For instance, supervisors are encouraging and optimistic, sensitive to individual differences, able to demonstrate a sense of humor, comfortable with the authority of their role, and committed to updating their own skills as a counselor and as a supervisor.
- Supervisors are knowledgeable about ethical, legal, and regulatory aspects of the profession.
- Supervisors inform supervisees of the goals, policies, theoretical orientations toward counseling, training, and supervision model on which the supervision is based.
- Supervisors demonstrate knowledge of individual differences with respect to gender, race, ethnicity, culture, sexual orientation, and age and understand the importance of these characteristics in the supervision process.
- Supervisors possess appropriate levels of empathy and respect genuineness, concreteness, and self-disclosure.
- Professional supervisors have training in supervision prior to initiating their role as supervisors.
- Supervisors set clear and explicit goals and use these goals to guide them in using various teaching techniques; they state the purposes of the supervisory relationship and explain the procedures to be used.
- Supervisors demonstrate knowledge and competency in case conceptualization and management.
- Supervisors of counselors meet regularly in face-to-face sessions with their supervisees.
- Supervisors provide supervisees with ongoing and immediate feedback that is closely tied to a supervisee's behavior. This feedback is systematic, objective, accurate, timely, and clearly understood.

You may meet and work with supervisors who demonstrate effectiveness in some of the areas listed above. Other supervisors may feel ill equipped to do what is expected of them, and some may be as insecure in their supervisory role as you are in your new role as an intern. However, it is up to you to get the most from your supervisors, despite any limitations that may exist.

Accepting different styles of supervision. You can benefit from learning how to function under a range of supervisory styles, both now as a student and later as a helping professional. One supervisor may believe that harsh confrontation is a way to cut through a client's stubborn defenses. Another treats clients as victims who are not responsible for their problems. Another provides unlimited advice for clients and promotes a problem-solving orientation for every client problem. There are supervisors who foster a supportive and positive orientation and who give out "warm fuzzies" exclusively. Other supervisors seem to thrive on crises and problems and tend to escalate such situations rather than defuse them. Some supervisors work very hard at becoming friends with their interns, whereas others create a professionally aloof relationship. Be open to supervisors with various orientations, and learn to incorporate their viewpoints into your style of helping. Do not be too quick to criticize a style different from yours, but consider it an opportunity for learning.

If you do have trouble with a supervisor, the answer is not always merely finding a new one. You can learn a great deal by working with supervisors who have perspectives different from yours and from supervisors who may initially appear to be difficult for you to make contact with. When you experience conflicts with a supervisor, it is a good idea to discuss them and do all that you can to work them out. Rather than convincing yourself that your supervisor will not be cooperative, assume that he or she will be open to your suggestions. Later, when you accept a position in an agency, you typically do not have the option of changing supervisors. What is more, you often don't have choices in who your coworkers will be. Thus, it is important to learn the interpersonal skills necessary in working out differences while the stakes are not so high.

At this point you might write down what kind of supervisor you think would be the most difficult for you to work with, and why. What might you do if it were impractical to change positions? What strategies could you use in constructively dealing with this supervisor?

Solving problems in your supervision. You may encounter a number of problems in working with a supervisor. Communication may not be open or encouraged. Some supervisors may poorly define what they expect of you. Some may fail to show up for appointments. Others may delegate their responsibilities to their secretary. There is also the supervisor who is insecure but disguises this insecurity by being overly controlling and autocratic. Some supervisors dump too much on an intern too soon or delegate menial work and unwanted jobs. Supervisors may be guilty of unethical practices. One supervisor had her supervisee do her work and then wrote up the proceedings as though she had seen the client. Some supervisors misuse power through a need to be seen as always right. There are supervisors who do not carry out their responsibility to give feedback. They keep the student intern in the dark and offer very little direction.

These are but a few possible conflicts you are likely to face in your internship. What do you think you might do if your supervisor were to give you very little feedback? Would you be willing to let the supervisor know that you wanted more response? Would you ask for it? Would you insist on it? What might you do if no feedback were forthcoming?

Supervisory roles and functions themselves can be detrimental to efforts to create an open relationship. Supervisors are responsible for and will evaluate the supervisee, so that supervisees are understandably anxious about being observed and evaluated. Interns can challenge themselves by converting their anxiety into productive energy. They can spend time thinking about what they want and begin to find ways to ask directly for it. They need not submit to their anxiety of being evaluated or allow themselves to be frozen by their fears.

Informed consent in supervision. The ACES (1993) *Ethical Guidelines for Counseling Supervisors* indicate that informed consent should be a basic part of the supervisory relationship. McCarthy, Sugden, Koker, Lamendola, Maurer, and Renninger (1995) provide a practical guide to informed consent in clinical supervision. They conclude that informed consent is an essential ingredient of effective supervision and that it should be clearly articulated through written documents and a discussion between the supervisor and supervisee. Accountability can be increased by developing a written contractual agreement for supervision. When expectations are discussed and clarified at the beginning of a supervisory relationship, the relationship will be enhanced, promoting quality client care. McCarthy and her colleagues identified seven topic areas that are significant to informed consent: purpose, professional disclosure, practical issues, supervision process, administrative issues, ethical and legal issues, and statement of agreement. When these issue areas are addressed in the informed consent process in supervision, both supervisors and supervisees have a clearer idea of the nature of their respective roles, rights, and responsibilities. Written informed consent documents, along with a discussion of their contents, are an excellent way for supervisors to model for supervisees an approach they can use with their clients.

The Value of Group Supervision

Although group supervision is widely practiced, it appears to be poorly understood (Prieto, 1996). Group supervision is a time-efficient and unique format that assists trainees in developing skills in conceptualizing cases and in implementing a variety of treatment interventions. In group supervision you learn not only from your supervisor but also from fellow trainees. Trainees learn that they are not alone with their anxiety and concerns surrounding clinical work, and they are exposed to different perspectives of the helping relationship. After reviewing the empirical investigations of group supervision, Prieto (1996) concluded that researchers need to begin building a foundation of knowledge concerning group supervision that will benefit trainees and supervisors in all of the helping professions.

It is important to talk to other interns and to share experiences and struggles. The group supervision model is enhanced when you make the process a personal one. You can do this by focusing on your own reactions and sharing them in your supervision group. What clients seem to trigger you? What clients do you hope won't show up next week? What clients threaten you? What clients do you find yourself especially liking? By focusing on your relationships with your clients and your own dynamics, you can increase your self-awareness through the feedback you get from others in the group.

It is also helpful to explore your values and attitudes in conjunction with your supervision. If you become aware that you have a tendency to seek gratitude from clients, for example, it could be useful to explore your own need for approval and your fear of rejection, either in your own personal therapy or in a group supervision session.

Supervision versus Therapy

Supervisors play multiple roles in the supervision process, functioning as teachers, consultants, mentors, and, at times, counselors. This complexity of roles means that the boundaries are not always clear. The process of supervision has some similarities with the instructor-student and therapist-client relationships, but there are also distinctions. It is essential to keep the primary purpose of supervisory relationships in mind—that is, to ensure that clients receive the best possible services.

The therapeutic role of the supervisor is certainly not the same as the role of the counselor, yet the distinction between these two roles is not well defined. Whiston and Emerson (1989) propose a model of supervision that includes an exploration of a supervisee's personal problems that lead to an impasse in the trainee's counseling work. However, once the personal issues of supervisees are identified in the supervisory relationship, they contend that the trainee must be given the responsibility for resolving these problems. The ACES (1993) ethical guidelines state: "Supervisors should not establish a psychotherapeutic relationship as a substitute for supervision. Personal issues should be addressed in supervision only in terms of the impact of these issues on clients and on professional functioning." One study suggests that exploring supervisees' personal issues in an appropriate manner does not necessarily affect the supervisory relationship negatively. Such supervisors confront their supervisees with personal issues that influence their work with clients, but in a warm and supportive instructional manner. As supervisees gain experience, they may be more able to benefit from identifying and exploring personal issues that affect their relationships with clients (Sumerel & Borders, 1996).

Although the boundaries between supervision and counseling are not always clear, it does help to raise this issue. Corey and Herlihy (1996c) offer the following general guideline on the proper focus of supervision:

> Because supervisory relationships are a complex blend of professional, educational, and therapeutic relationships, supervisors need to work to create and maintain an ethical climate for both skill development and self-exploration. Again, it is the supervisor's responsibility to help trainees identify how their personal dynamics are likely to influence their professional work, but it is not the supervisor's proper role to serve as a personal counselor to supervisees. (p. 277)

We agree that supervision and therapy should not be combined, but we *do* think that the two processes have much in common. Furthermore, good supervision can focus on the problems and blind spots of the intern, and these potential problem areas need to be pointed out. Supervisors are in a good position to recognize some of your blocks and countertransferences. They can help you recognize some of the attitudes, feelings, and behaviors that are likely to interfere with your handling of certain clients.

If further exploration is needed and if your difficulties with certain clients are rooted in your own dynamics, a supervisor may encourage you to get involved in some form of personal therapy. You should not misconstrue such a suggestion as an indication that you are not personally fit for the profession. Getting involved in the lives of clients in a placement is bound to open up some of your own psychological wounds, and unresolved conflicts are likely to surface. Be open to looking at whatever arises in you as you encounter a diversity of clients. Personal therapy along with your supervision can be an ideal combination provided your supervisor and your therapist are not the same person. Receiving supervision from one professional and psychotherapy from another professional can yield the maximum benefit for the supervisee's personal and professional development. This arrangement prevents blurring of boundaries and allows the proper focus to be either on working with clients (in supervision) or on dealing with your personal issues (in personal therapy).

BY WAY OF REVIEW

- Become active in getting the most from your education. No program is perfect, but you can do a lot to bring more meaning to your course of study.
- Just as you are graded in your educational program, you will be evaluated in the professional world. Evaluation creates stresses and strains, but it is still possible to find meaning within the system.
- Skills and knowledge are obviously important in becoming an effective professional. But your quality as a person is an equally important determinant of your success as a helper.
- Graduation from a training program does not signal the end of learning but merely the beginning of a process of professional growth and development. To maintain your effectiveness, continuing education is a necessity. One of the best ways of keeping on the cutting edge of one's profession is to become involved in a peer-consultation group that affords professionals opportunities to share their concerns and learn from one another. Through peer groups, helpers can actively contribute to their own personal and professional development and that of their colleagues.
- Your fieldwork courses are likely to be among the most important experiences you will have in your program. Select these experiences wisely, and arrange for a diversity in your placements. Realize that these placements can help you decide on your professional specialization.
- Treat your field placement like a job, even if you don't get paid for your internship.
- Don't burden yourself with trying to be a perfect intern. Fieldwork experiences are designed to teach you about the skills of helping, and you can learn much from your mistakes.
- In getting the most from supervision, learn how to ask for what you need from your supervisor. It is important that you learn your limits and communicate them to your supervisor.

- Supervisors have different styles, and no one way is right. You can learn a great deal from various supervisors, but be cautious about copying their style.
- The ideal supervisor may be hard to find. Supervisors are sometimes assigned to this role with little preparation or training.
- If your supervision is inadequate, be assertive in doing something about the situation. Persist in identifying what you need by taking an active stance.
- Even though supervision is like therapy in some ways, there are important differences. Personal therapy can be a useful adjunct to supervision, but it is best that the supervisor and the therapist not be the same person.
- Students often experience some period of depression and anxiety when they graduate from a program and enter the world of work. Not only do they need to challenge certain myths about the meaning of a degree but they must also begin the process of establishing a professional sense of identity.

WHAT WILL YOU DO NOW?

1. If you are in a training program, now is an ideal time to begin getting involved in professional organizations. You might join at least one such organization as an active student member. To help you find an organization that fits your needs, we have listed a number of them in the Appendix. By joining an organization, you can take advantage of its workshops and conferences. Membership also puts you in touch with other professionals with similar interests, gives you ideas for updating your skills, and helps you make excellent contacts.

2. If you have a supervisor (for your fieldwork or in your job), make up a short list of questions that you'd like to discuss with him or her. What would you like to gain from supervision? Approach your supervisor before the end of the semester to discuss your desires.

3. Make it a point to visit several community agencies where you might work as an intern. Interview the director of the agency or the supervisors who make decisions about accepting fieldwork students. Learn to ask questions that will help you select a placement that will teach you about various client populations and a range of problems. Each student in your class could visit just one agency and then present the findings to the rest of the class.

4. Reflect on some of the following issues and use this as a basis for your journal writing. Remember to write whatever comes to mind rather than censoring your thoughts and the flow of your writing.

- Write about the kind of learner you see yourself as being. What does the concept of active learning imply to you? In what ways might you want to become a more active learner? How can you do this as you read this book and take this course?
- Write about the ideal kind of fieldwork experience you'd like to obtain. What can you do to get the best possible field placement?
- If you are already in a field placement, write at least briefly about the work you are doing. What are your reactions to the staff at the agency? What is

it like for you to interact with clients? What is this experience teaching you about yourself?

- If you are in supervision currently, what are you doing to get the most from this process? What kind of relationship do you have with your supervisor? Write about any ideas for improving the quality of your supervision sessions. Are any personal issues emerging as a result of your work with clients? (Consider bringing personal issues that pertain to your ability to work effectively with your clients into supervision. At the very least, write in your journal about any personal problems that are surfacing as a result of your field placement and supervision.)

5. The full bibliographic entry for each of the sources listed below can be found in the References and Reading List at the back of the book.

For a good handbook on counseling supervision, see Borders and Leddick (1987). Another useful source that describes a model of supervision is Stoltenberg and Delworth (1987). Useful introductory texts to the human-services field include Neukrug (1994) and Woodside and McClam (1994). For a practical and concise guide to the internship experience, see Faiver, Eisengart, and Colonna (1995). Refer to Baird's (1996) handbook for internship, practicum, and field placements for helpful suggestions on ways to get the most from a fieldwork experience. For a discussion of facilitating personal growth in self and others, see Long (1996).

Chapter 3

Stages in the Helping Process

FOCUS QUESTIONS

1. What beliefs do you hold about the capacity of people to change? How can change best be facilitated? What constitutes effective helping? What is the best way to evaluate the degree of change in clients?

2. How are your views and beliefs about human nature related to your approach to working with people who seek your help?

3. What basic beliefs do you hold about the helping process? If a client asked you how you work or about your orientation to helping, what would you most want to say?

4. Which of your assets and resources can you draw on in establishing helping relationships? What liabilities or limitations do you have that might interfere with forming working relationships with certain clients?

5. What are the advantages and disadvantages of brief models of therapy? How do brief, solution-focused intervention strategies fit the requirements of managed care programs? How do these approaches fit with your beliefs about what constitutes effective helping?

6. How do you determine whether an intervention you are planning to use is for you or for the client?

7. What guidelines would you use in confronting clients? What is the purpose of confrontation? Can you think of anything that might get in the way of effective confrontation on your part?

8. How important is helper self-disclosure in the helping relationship? What guidelines would you use to determine when self-disclosure would be appropriate? Can you think of any difficulties you might have in engaging in self-disclosure?

9. What are your thoughts about working with clients collaboratively to formulate goals that will guide the helping relationship? How might you develop action plans in a collaborative way with your clients?

10. How would you best prepare clients for termination? Can you think of any factors that might make it difficult for you to terminate clients? What guidelines might you use for effective termination?

AIM OF THE CHAPTER

The purpose of this chapter is to help you clarify your role at various stages in the helping process. Your beliefs about the nature of people will influence the helping strategies you employ and the way you define the helper's role in the helping process. We have found that helpers often operate without a clear awareness of their beliefs and attitudes. It is essential to recognize how you came to acquire your beliefs, how they have changed over time, and how they affect what you do with clients.

In this chapter we address the stages in the helping process and the main tasks and strategies at the various stages of helping from the initial session to termination. We look at the skills and knowledge you need at the various stages of helping, along with the personal characteristics that are required to apply your skills. Our basic assumption is that the kind of person you are and the attitudes you bring to the helping relationship are the major determinants of its quality. We also consider the role of theory as a guiding factor for practicing effectively. The model we describe is an integrative approach that emphasizes the role of thinking, feeling, and acting in human behavior. Your theoretical orientation provides you with a map for making interventions, but we stress the importance of developing a personal stance toward helping that fits the person you are and is flexible enough to meet the unique needs of the client population with which you work.

ORIENTATIONS TO HELPING

Your orientation to the helping process is largely a function of your beliefs about human nature and about how people change. There are various approaches to helping. Sometimes an orientation will be imposed on you, especially if you work in an institution that makes extensive use of a particular therapeutic model. You might work in a state facility that employs behavior-modification strategies. The entire program is likely to be geared to behavioral procedures, which may not be suited to you. Or an agency may make extensive use of a system of diagnoses, and you will be expected to conduct interviews and arrive at a specific diagnostic category for each client you see. Before you accept a position in any setting, find out about its theoretical framework. If the methods of intervention are not compatible with your views of helping, you are bound to experience conflict in this institution.

Clarify your thinking with respect to questions such as "Who is responsible for change in the helping relationship? What focus is most likely to lead to change? a focus on feelings? a focus on insight? a focus on behavior? a focus on cognition? What is the best balance between providing a great deal of structure and providing only minimal structure? What is an appropriate balance between confrontation and support?"

At this point consider some of the components of your theoretical orientation to the helping process. From your perspective, who is responsible for change? Do you see yourself as primarily responsible for whether your clients reach their goals? Or do you place the primary responsibility on the clients? To what degree do you share this responsibility with clients? Do you think you have answers to give clients who come to you, or do you believe clients are capable of finding their own solutions with your assistance?

Various Focuses of Helping

Identify your beliefs about what best facilitates change. If you are not clear about what brings about change, your ability to promote it is very limited. Promoting change has a number of specific dimensions. Some helpers focus on feelings. They think that what clients need most is to identify and express feelings that have been bottled up. If this is your focus, you will be doing a lot to get your clients to emote.

Other helpers put emphasis on gaining insight. If this is what you value, much of your time may be spent in exploring the reasons for actions and in interpreting clients' behavior. You will be interested in having them understand the origins of their problem.

There are those who emphasize the behavioral aspects involved in the helping relationship. They are very much oriented to what individuals are doing now and what they will do in the near future. If this is your orientation, you may not be much concerned about having your clients develop insight or express their feelings, because you will be concerned about a specific action plan designed to help them change what they are doing.

Some helpers like to focus clients on examining their beliefs about themselves and about their world. If you have such a cognitive orientation, your interventions will focus clients on what they are thinking and the things that they continue to tell themselves. You will see change as a result of helping your clients eliminate faulty thinking and replace it with constructive thoughts and self-talk.

Some believe in being active and directive in the helping process, and others believe that very little intervention is necessary. If you hold to the notion that little structure is useful, you will probably not give much advice and won't be locked into a problem-solving mode. If you believe in active intervention, you will do much of the talking, will provide a high degree of structure, and will make sure that the sessions keep moving. The chances are that you will provide clients with information.

Some helpers employ a good deal of confrontation, thinking that clients will surrender their defenses only under the pressure of being challenged. Other helpers think that support is far more useful than confrontation. Depending on your beliefs, your techniques will have the effect of either supporting or challenging.

Some helpers employ short-term strategies, and others use long-term ones. Depending on the setting in which you work and on your clientele, the length of treatment will vary. Do you believe that people can be helped by brief interventions? Or do you think that long-term treatment is necessary if effective change is to occur?

Some therapeutic approaches focus on the past, others on the present, and others on the future. Begin to consider whether you see the past, present, or future as being most productive in the helping process. This is more than just a theoretical notion. If your orientation includes the concept that your clients' past is an important focus for exploration, many of your interventions are likely to be designed to assist them in understanding their past. If you think that your clients' goals and strivings are important, your interventions are likely to focus them on the future. Thus, you might ask questions such as "How would you like your life to be different a year from now? What do you see that you can do now to create the kind of future you say you want in ten years?" If you are oriented toward the present, many of your interventions will focus your clients on what they are thinking, feeling, and doing in the moment. Of course, your theory will largely determine the time frame that you emphasize. It is also possible to work with the past, present, and future in an integrated fashion. You can respect how your clients' past experiences influence them today. You can also be concerned about what people are doing now and yet frequently ask them to look to what kind of future they would like to create for themselves.

Your views and beliefs about human nature are very much related to the helping strategies you will employ with your clients. If you see people as basically good, for example, you will trust that your clients can assume responsibility for the direction of their lives. If you see human nature as basically evil, you will adopt a role as a helper who attempts to correct people's flawed nature. Your interventions are likely to be aimed at "straightening people out." For a moment, reflect on the following statements, and begin to clarify your views about human nature:

- People need direction from an authority to resolve their problems.
- People have the capacity to find their answers within themselves.
- People create their own misery.
- People are victims of outside circumstances.
- People are basically good and are therefore trustworthy.
- People have a basic tendency toward evil and therefore need correcting.
- People are the product of their choices; that is, they are the architects of their lives.
- People are shaped by fate.
- People won't change unless they are in pain.
- People are motivated by their goals.
- People are determined by their early childhood experiences.

Your orientation to helping will certainly develop as you gain experience in working with a diversity of clients. It is not essential to establish your orientation before you begin to practice. But it is vital to formulate your views about human nature, because these views have a crucial bearing on the way you work with clients.

The Impact of Your Beliefs on Your Work

If you expect the best in people, they are likely to give you their best. If you treat people as though they have the capacity to understand and resolve their problems, they are more likely to find answers within themselves. By developing a collaborative partnership with your clients, you are telling them that they can use the helping relationship as a pathway to recreating their lives.

Effective helpers hold positive beliefs about people; have a healthy self-concept; ground their interventions in values; are respectful of cultural differences; and possess empathy, congruence, warmth, compassion, genuineness, and unconditional positive regard. They test their beliefs and examine whether their interventions are expressions of their core beliefs and assumptions about how people change.

In contrast, ineffective helpers tend to hold rigid and judgmental beliefs about people. They tend to tell clients how they should think and how to solve their problems. Ineffective helpers do not believe that their clients have the means to assume control of their own destiny. Ineffective helpers are not willing to challenge their own assumptions and tend to look for client behaviors that support their hunches and convictions. We have heard most of the following statements from students or professionals. As you review these examples of helpers' assumptions, ask yourself if you might have made some of these statements. Reflect on how you think your beliefs about people might lead to placing them in a category and judging them.

- "A sociopath is resistant to therapy and will never change."
- "Old people can't change. They should be given support but not challenged."
- "I'm 'color blind'—I can work equally well with any racial or ethnic group."
- "If clients don't change, it's their fault, not mine."
- "People who come to me need help, which means they're not able to direct their own lives. It's my job to provide them with a high degree of structure."
- "People who are on welfare are basically lazy and really don't want to work."
- "Most people don't want to change. They just want to learn how to manipulate people more effectively so they can get what they want."
- "People can't be depended on to follow through with their commitments."
- "The clients in this institution are highly resistant and want to hide their true feelings and thoughts."
- "The best way to get through the client's resistance is to employ very directive and highly confrontive techniques. You have to strip away a client's defenses."
- "If you're empathic and supportive, clients will merely use this against you by manipulating you."

We do not mean to imply that if you hold any one of these beliefs you are necessarily ineffective in helping others. If you worked with a resistant client population over a period of years, for example, you might begin to assume that people generally resist change. But, if you applied this generalization to all the clients you saw, they would be likely to exhibit resistance in response to the messages that they picked up from you. You would be fostering a self-fulfilling prophecy that reinforced your assumptions. A temporary mild cynicism does not mean that you will remain cynical forever. You might ask yourself questions such as "How rigidly do I hold certain assumptions? Am I quick to generalize on the basis of limited experience? Do I tend to form quick judgments about people and make generalizations? Am I willing to seriously examine the assumptions that I make, and am I open to changing some of them?" It is a positive sign if you demonstrate a willingness to question the origin of your assumptions and to modify them.

Learning to Challenge Your Assumptions

We provided a series of in-service training workshops at a state institution for the criminally insane and for mentally disordered sex offenders. Although we had the good fortune to meet and work with some dedicated and effective helpers, we also encountered some ineffective helpers. To us it seemed that they thought their patients could do no right. Certain workers at the institution were quite outspoken in their beliefs that these patients were resistant to therapy, were not motivated to change, and were only putting in their time as ordered by the court. If the clients did not talk during the sessions, they were labeled "resistant"; if they did talk, they were often viewed as "manipulative."

In our training workshops we urged the staff members at least to suspend their judgments during the time they were providing therapy. We encouraged them to give their patients a chance to show something more of themselves than the problem with which they had become identified. Although a child molester does have severe problems, we suggested that he be viewed more broadly than as someone who has committed sexual crimes. If the staff members were open to discovering other facets of the patient's personality, they would discover that he had had pain and struggles in his life with which the helper could identify. We hoped that the helpers would challenge some of their assumptions that seemed nontherapeutic and be open to the possibility that they could begin to see clients and the helping process in a different light.

If you are making some of the assumptions we have described, think about how they are likely to influence the way you approach certain clients. Your beliefs about yourself, the people with whom you work, and the nature of the helping process are often more subtle than the assumptions listed above. Whether your beliefs are subtle or extreme, however, you tend to behave on the basis of them. If you basically do not trust your clients to understand and deal with their problems, for example, you will use strategies to get them to accept your assessment and to follow your prescriptions.

After becoming aware of the attitudes and assumptions you hold, you can decide the degree to which your attitudes are being expressed in your behavior. Then you can assess how well such attitudes and behaviors are working for you and helping your clients. We hope you will examine the source of your beliefs about the good life, an individual's capacity to make substantial change, and the nature of the helper-client relationship. Think through, clarify, and challenge these beliefs, confirming them through a conscious process of self-examination.

You may not have clear beliefs about the helping process. You may have incorporated them in an uncritical and unconscious manner. It is possible that they are narrow and have not been tested to determine if they are valid or functional. If you have lived in a sheltered environment and have rarely stepped outside of your social group, you may not even be aware of your narrow belief system. It is possible to live in an encapsulated environment and thereby "see" only what confirms your existing belief system.

One good way to identify and clarify your beliefs is to put yourself in situations that might prove challenging. If you have limited contact with alcoholics and see them as "weak-willed individuals," for instance, consider attending some Alcoholics Anonymous meetings. If you have limited experience with certain cultural and ethnic groups, seek volunteer experiences or fieldwork placements where you will work with a culturally diverse population. If you are aware that you hold stereotypes about old people, volunteer to work with the elderly. If you have fears about working with people who have AIDS or are HIV-positive, consider challenging your fears by learning more about this disease or working with these people. Direct contact with populations that are unfamiliar to you is the best way to learn about people whom you might have stereotyped. Of course, it is essential that you approach these situations with an open mind and that you avoid simply looking for evidence to support your prior judgments. A stance of openness will enable you to develop a personal orientation to helping that will lend itself to modification as you gain experience.

Some Beliefs We Hold about the Helping Process

It took us some time to learn that there is no one right way to approach clients. Instead of looking for the right thing to do or say, we strive to follow what we think is an interesting path to pursue with a client. In this process we trust our intuitions and develop our own ways of working. If our hunches about a client are incorrect, that quickly becomes apparent if we pay attention to the relationship. What we continually relearn is the importance of talking with clients about what we think is going on between us. At times, when we have trouble relating to a particular client, this person is reflecting some dimension within ourselves that we are reluctant to accept. It can be helpful to consider our clients as mirrors that reflect some aspect of our being. We do not necessarily need to change anything, but it does help to simply recognize patterns that we have in common with our clients.

We do not accept the full responsibility for deciding what the focus of a helping relationship will be. Rather than working very hard to figure out what clients should want, we ask them frequently what it is they want. We often ask: "Is what you are doing working for you? If not, what are you willing to do to change it?" If their current behavior is generally serving them well, they may not feel a strong need to change a particular style. We still encourage them to look at the price they often pay for being the way they are, and then the decision whether to change is up to them. We do not see it as our job to decide for them how they should live their lives.

If clients appear to be getting little from the helping relationship, we still examine our part in this outcome by asking ourselves about our involvement and willingness to risk with this client. Yet we also explore with the client his or her part in the lack of progress. We recognize that we cannot make clients want to change, yet we can create a climate where together we look at the advantages and disadvantages of making changes. We see helping as a mutual endeavor in which both parties share the responsibility for making change happen.

Our Theoretical Orientation

Neither of us subscribes to any single theory in its totality. Rather, we function within an integrative framework that we continue to develop and modify as we practice. We draw on concepts and techniques from most of the contemporary counseling models and adapt them to our own unique personalities. Our conceptual framework takes into account the *thinking, feeling,* and *behaving* dimensions of human experience. Thus, our theoretical orientations and styles of practice are primarily a function of the individuals we are.

We value those approaches that emphasize the *thinking* dimension. We typically challenge clients to think about the decisions they have made about themselves. Some of these decisions may have been necessary for their psychological survival as children but now may be clearly out of date. We hope that clients will eventually be able to make necessary revisions that can lead them to live more fully. One way we do this is by asking clients to pay attention to their "self-talk." Questions we encourage clients to ask themselves are: "How are your problems actually caused by the assumptions you make about yourself, about others, and about life? How do you create your problems by the thoughts and beliefs you cling to? How can you begin to free yourself by critically evaluating the sentences you repeat to yourself?" Many of the techniques we use are designed to tap clients' thinking processes, to help them think about events in their lives and how they have interpreted these events, and to work on a cognitive level to change certain belief systems.

Thinking is only one dimension that we pay attention to in our work with clients. The *feeling* dimension is also extremely important. We emphasize this facet of human experience by encouraging clients to identify and express their feelings. Clients are often stuck due to unexpressed and unresolved emotional concerns. If they allow themselves to experience the range of their feelings and talk about how certain events have affected them, their healing process is facilitated. If individuals feel listened to and understood, they are more likely to express feelings that they have kept to themselves.

Thinking and feeling are vital components in the helping process, but eventually clients must express themselves in the *behaving* or *doing* dimension. Clients can spend countless hours gaining insights and ventilating pent-up feelings, but at some point they need to get involved in an action-oriented program of change. Their feelings and thoughts can then be applied to real-life situations. Examining current behavior is the heart of the helping process. We tend to ask questions such as these: "What are you doing? What do you see for yourself now and in the future? Does your present behavior have a reasonable chance of getting you what you want now, and will it take you in the direction you want to go?" If the focus of the helping process is on what people are doing, there is a greater chance that they will also be able to change their thinking and feeling.

In addition to highlighting the thinking, feeling, and behaving dimensions, we help clients consolidate what they are learning and apply these new behaviors to situations they encounter every day. Some strategies we use are "contracts," "homework assignments," action programs, self-monitoring techniques, support systems, and self-directed programs of change. These approaches all stress the role of commitment on the clients' part to practice new behaviors, to follow through with a realistic plan for change, and to develop practical methods of carrying out this plan in everyday life.

Underlying our integrated focus on thinking, feeling, and behaving is our philosophical leaning toward the existential approach, which places primary emphasis on the role of choice and responsibility in the therapeutic process. We challenge people to look at the choices they *do* have, however limited they may be, and to accept responsibility for choosing for themselves.

Most of what we do in our therapeutic work is based on the assumption that people can exercise their freedom to change situations, even though the range of this freedom may be restricted by external factors. It is important for helpers to do more than assume that clients are capable of changing their internal world. Helpers also have a role in bringing about change in the external environment that is directly contributing to a client's problems.

Individuals cannot be understood without considering the various systems that affect them—family, social groups, community, church, and other cultural forces. For the helping process to be effective, it is critical to understand how individuals influence and are influenced by their social world. Sue, Ivey, and Pedersen (1996) point out that people are not only thinking, feeling, behaving, and social beings but are also biological, cultural, spiritual, and political beings. Ignoring any one of these facets of human experience will limit our understanding of human behavior. Effective helpers need to acquire a holistic approach that encompasses all of human experience.

As we work with an individual, we are not consciously thinking about what theory we are using. We adapt the techniques we use to fit the needs of the individual rather than attempting to fit the client to our techniques. In deciding on techniques to introduce, we take into account an array of factors about the client population. We consider the client's readiness to confront an issue, the client's cultural background, the client's value system, and the client's trust in us as helpers. We have a rationale for using the techniques we employ, and our interventions generally flow from some particular theoretical framework. Our concern is to help clients identify and experience whatever they are feeling, identify ways in which their assumptions influence how they feel and behave, and experiment with alternative modes of behaving.

Theory as a Road Map to Guide Your Practice

Attempting to practice without having an explicit theoretical rationale is like flying a plane without a flight plan. You may eventually get there, but you're equally likely to run out of patience and gas. If you operate in a theoretical vacuum and are unable to draw on theory to support your interventions, you may flounder in your attempts to help people change.

Theory is not a rigid set of structures that prescribes, step by step, what and how you should function as a helper. Rather, we see theory as a general framework that enables you to make sense of the many facets of the helping process, providing you with a map that gives direction to what you do and say. We encourage you to look at all the contemporary theories to determine what concepts and techniques you can incorporate into your approach to practice.

Ultimately, the most meaningful perspective is one that is an extension of your values and personality. A theory is not something divorced from you as a person. At best, it is an integral part of the person you are and an expression of your uniqueness. If you are currently a student in training, it is unrealistic to expect to have integrated a well-defined theoretical model. This will take years of extensive reading and practice. Developing a personalized approach that guides your practice is an ongoing process, and your model will continuously undergo revision.

Throughout this book we refer to your ability to draw on your life experiences and your personal characteristics as one of your most powerful tools as a helper. Particularly important is your willingness to examine how your personality and behavior either hinder or facilitate your work with individuals. Although it is essential to become well grounded in the theories underlying practice, to acquire those needed skills in intervening, and to gain supervised experience as a helper, this is not enough to make you an effective helper. It is also essential that you be willing to take an honest look at your own life to determine if you are willing to do for yourself what you challenge clients to do. It will be hard to inspire clients to seek help when they need it if you are not open to asking for help in your own life. It will be difficult to sell others on that which you aren't buying yourself.

An Integrated Approach to Helping

One reason for the current trend toward an integrated approach to the helping process is the recognition that no single theory is comprehensive enough to account for the complexities of human behavior when the full range of client types and their specific problems are taken into consideration. Practitioners who are open to an integrative perspective may find that several theories play a crucial role in their personal approach. Each theory has its unique contributions and its own domain of expertise. By accepting that each theory has strengths and weaknesses and is, by definition, "different" from the others, practitioners have some basis to begin developing a counseling model that fits them.

We encourage you to remain open to the value inherent in each of the theories of counseling. Our hope is that you will study all the major theories, resist subscribing too quickly to any single point of view, and look for a basis for an integrated perspective that will guide your practice.

Each theory represents a different vantage point from which to look at human behavior, but no one theory has "the truth." Because there is no "correct" theoretical approach, it is well for you to search for an approach that fits who you are and to think in terms of working toward an integrated approach that addresses thinking, feeling, and behaving. To develop this kind of integration, you need to be thoroughly grounded in a number of theories, be open to the idea that these theories can be unified in some ways, and be willing to continually test your hypotheses to determine how well they are working. An integrative perspective is the product of a great deal of study, clinical practice, research, and theorizing. Developing an integrative perspective is a lifelong endeavor that is refined with experience.

Of necessity, this discussion of theoretical orientations has been brief. For a more elaborate discussion of the various theoretical approaches, see *Theory and Practice of Counseling and Psychotherapy* (Corey, 1996b).

OVERVIEW OF THE HELPING RELATIONSHIP

This section is designed to help you determine your assets and liabilities as a potential helper. We use the overall framework of Egan's (1994) helping model, describing the stages in the helping process and the major tasks facing helpers at each of these stages. We also draw from the systematic skills-training approaches of Brammer (1993), Gilliland and James (1997), Ivey (1994), and Okun (1997). The skills-development model offers a general framework of the phases of the helping process and is not linked to any particular theoretical approach. You can apply any of the current theories of counseling (Corey, 1996b) to this model of helping.

Our focus, as always, is on the knowledge, skills, beliefs, and personal characteristics required for being an effective helper. Egan (1994) views helping as a *learning* process consisting of learning, unlearning, and relearning. At each stage in this process, helpers face different challenges that require specific skills. The framework we provide will help you assess your ability to engage others in a helping relationship. The human relations skills we describe are crucial for all helpers.

The Stages of Helping

The model of the helping process we will discuss here has four major stages, each with particular tasks to be accomplished. In the initial stage, the central task is to help clients identify and clarify aspects of their lives that are not working for them. This task may include identifying problem situations or missed opportunities for full development. Typically, people become clients when they recognize that they need outside help to understand and cope with their problems. In the second stage, the helper and the client cooperatively establish goals by determining the specific changes desired. If clients hope to make actual changes, they have to be willing to go beyond talking and planning; they must translate their plans into action. Therefore, the third stage of helping deals with identifying strategies for action, choosing which combination of strategies will best meet the client's goals, and putting these plans into a realistic action program. Termination is the fourth stage, and it is here that clients consolidate their learning and make longer-range plans.

At each of these stages the focus is on *you as a helper*. Assess your own qualities to determine your interest and ability in helping others. Realize that the helping relationship is not a mechanical process but a deeply personal human endeavor. As a helper you will be actively involved with those you are helping by drawing on what you know, by applying skills and interventions in a timely and appropriate manner, and by using yourself as a person in creating meaningful relationships with clients or others you help. This is true whether you are involved in the counseling or the administrative aspects of the human services. If you are unable to apply some basic human relations skills, the chances are slim that you will be able to create and maintain adequate rapport with those whom you are supposed to be helping. Although the focus of our discussion is on these skills as they apply to counseling relationships, you can also apply them to a variety of other interpersonal situations.

There are a number of ways in which you can be fully available for others in this helping relationship. You can be present with your clients as they share their experiences and problem situations. You can help them identify and overcome their own distortions. This is a good time to encourage clients to identify exceptions to their problem-saturated lives. Ask them what they can do and have already done to deal with their problems. You can ask clients to focus on possible solutions rather than having them define themselves in light of their presenting problem. By reconceptualizing a particular problem, you can help clients acquire a new perspective that will lead to action. You can help clients who see very few options to develop a variety of alternatives in coping with a given problem. You can help them distinguish between what they can do and what might be difficult for them to do, and you can challenge them to stretch their boundaries. You can encourage them to make choices for themselves and to develop the courage to accept responsibility for their decisions. By providing clients with support and challenge, you can help them change.

In this era of managed care, you will be challenged to work with clients in very few sessions. You will need to develop interventions tailored to short-term and specific behavioral change. Brief interventions stress time-limited, solution-focused, structured, effective strategies that empower clients by enabling them to make specific behavioral changes they desire. Furthermore, the requirements of managed care impose upon agencies and practitioners the expectation of being accountable. Increasingly, you will be expected to quickly assess the salient problems of your clients, formulate a short-term treatment approach, and then demonstrate the degree to which your interventions are effective. Therefore, the stages of helping will be described primarily from the vantage point of a relatively brief model rather than from the perspective of long-term therapy.

Stage 1: Identifying Clients' Problems

At the first stage of the helping process, the main task is to assist clients in defining and clarifying their problems. Helpers are expected to create a relationship in which clients can reveal their story, focus more clearly on what they want to change, and attain a new perspective in dealing with their problems.

People often seek professional assistance when they realize they are not dealing with problem situations satisfactorily. Some clients seek counseling because they struggle with self-doubt, feel trapped by their fears, and suffer from some form of loss. Others seek help not because they feel plagued by major problems but because they are not living as effectively as they would like. They may feel caught in a meaningless job, experience frustration because they are not living up to their own goals and ideals, or feel dissatisfied in their interpersonal lives. In short, most people who become clients are not managing their lives as well as they might. They are not dealing effectively with life problems, and they are not using the full range of their potentials or taking advantage of opportunities available to them. Two general goals of helping arise from these assumptions: one goal relates to clients' managing their lives more effectively and the other relates to clients' abilities to deal realistically with problems and develop opportunities (Egan, 1994).

Of course, not all clients come to you voluntarily. Involuntary clients will surely have some resistance to seeking help, and they may not even believe that you can help them. Working with nonvoluntary clients is extremely challenging because of the degree of minimization and denial clients bring with them. Your task is to get through the initial intimidation such clients can present and to work in such a way that will increase the chances of their acknowledging their problems. A good place to begin is to ascertain why they are seeking you *now* and what they expect from this relationship. Dealing with their resistance, rather than skirting around it, is one of the best ways to begin with the reluctant client.

In dealing with nonvoluntary clients, it is essential to monitor your responses to their resistance. If you respond in a belligerent tone, the tense situation is likely to worsen. Rather than fighting the initial resistance, it is best to view it as a positive sign of strength and recognize ways you can utilize resistance in the helping process. This is an example of how a perceived weakness can actually be reconceptualized into a strength. After all, your clients' defenses have worked for them to some degree, and at one time they may have enabled them to psychologically survive. Your task is to work cooperatively with resistant clients to accomplish something they consider to be of benefit (Loar, 1995).

Some clients who come to you may have had prior negative encounters with a mental-health agency, which may predispose them to approach you with suspicion. In her article on brief therapy with difficult clients, Loar (1995) offers some practical suggestions for building cooperation with difficult clients:

- Realize that initially many clients are angry and defensive about having to meet with a professional helper to deal with the way they handle their problems.
- If clients need to express their feelings about prior failed attempts in receiving help, allow them to state their objections. Listening to their complaints about past efforts in getting help can reduce potential pitfalls in receiving the assistance they are seeking from you.
- Provide clients with the benefits of brief therapy. Let them know the approximate number of sessions available to them, and inform them about ways they can use the relationship with you to help themselves. Inform them that you will be focusing on behaviors that can be observed and that together you will formulate plans that consist of small and tangible steps.
- Let clients know that learning entails some setbacks. If clients know from the beginning that setbacks are part of learning by trial and error, they are less likely to get stuck in discouraging patterns.
- Enlist the client's help in formulating clear goals that will guide the helping process. Clients are more likely to follow a plan they agree to rather than carrying out someone else's directive of how they should live.
- Focus even initial efforts on working toward solutions of problems as presented by clients. This presupposes that both of you are able to arrive at a clear, specific statement of the problem. As soon as possible, design interventions in small, manageable steps that lead to a satisfactory solution.

Creating a therapeutic climate. In your work with both voluntary and involuntary client populations, your clients' willingness to engage in self-exploration will have a lot to do with the kind of climate you establish during the initial sessions. You can make the mistake of working too hard, asking too many questions and offering quick solutions. Your role is to create a collaborative partnership with your clients, which means that they assume a fair share of the responsibility for what takes place both inside and outside the session. During the early sessions you can greatly assist clients by teaching them how they can assess their own problems and search for their own solutions. In *The Elements of Counseling,* Meier and Davis (1997) suggest the following guidelines for the first session with clients:

- Make personal contact
- Develop a working alliance
- Explain the helping process to the client
- Pace and lead the client
- Speak briefly
- Individualize your helping approach
- When in doubt, focus on feelings
- Plan for termination at the beginning of the helping relationship

Meier and Davis (1997) also identify a number of strategies that are useful in encouraging client self-exploration for the duration of the helping relationship. Some of their guidelines include:

- Avoid advice
- Avoid premature problem solving
- Avoid relying on questions
- Listen closely to what clients say
- Pay attention to nonverbals
- Keep the focus on the client
- Be concrete
- Listen for metaphors
- Summarize

During the early stage of helping, it is crucial to teach clients how to identify and clarify problem areas and how to acquire problem-solving skills they can apply in a variety of difficult situations in everyday living. Your role is not to identify the nature of their problems but to assist clients in doing this themselves. In a sense, from the very first meeting you can be most helpful to clients by encouraging them to look within themselves for resources and strengths they can draw on to better manage their lives. Effective helpers also put clients in touch with external resources within the community that they can utilize in meeting the demands of daily living. The confidence your clients have in you will increase if they are convinced that you appreciate the resources both within themselves and in their external world.

By understanding your client's cultural background, you are doing a great deal to establish a therapeutic working relationship. Although it is not necessary to have an in-depth understanding of your client's culture and worldview, you must know some of your client's basic beliefs and values if you hope to help this person. If you are not aware of the central values that guide your client's behavior and decisions, your client will soon pick up on this and likely not return for further sessions. A more detailed discussion of the importance of understanding clients' cultural values appears in Chapters 6 and 7.

Understanding the context. As you engage your clients in identifying and assessing their problems, it is essential to avoid a stance of "blaming the victim." Clients may come to you not to resolve internal conflicts but to better understand and deal with external stressors in their environment. Some people who seek your services may need your guidance to link them up to resources within their community. They may need legal assistance or your help in coping with day-to-day survival issues such as getting a job, arranging for child care, or taking care of an elderly parent. Clients in a crisis situation will require immediate direction in finding external resources to cope effectively with the crisis.

As you listen to your clients, do not assume that they simply need to adjust to problematic situations. They may feel frustration and anger due to societal factors such as being discriminated against in their workplace because of their age, gender, race, religion, or sexual orientation. You will do them a disservice if you encourage them to settle for injustices in an oppressive environment. Instead of merely solving the presenting problems of your clients, you can begin supporting your clients in their efforts to take action within their community to bring about change. Of course, for you to do this means that you are willing to assume a variety of helping roles—educator, advocate, social change agent, and influencer of policy making. A more detailed discussion of your role in influencing change within the community is presented in Chapter 8.

Establishing the relationship. For clients to feel free to talk about their problems, helpers need to provide attention, active listening, and empathy. Clients must sense your respect for them, which you can demonstrate by your attitudes and behaviors. You reveal an attitude of respect for your clients when you are concerned about their best interests, view them as able to exercise control of their own destiny, and treat them as individuals rather than stereotyping them. You actually show clients that you respect them through your behavior, such as actively listening to and understanding them, suspending critical judgment, expressing appropriate warmth and acceptance, communicating to them that you understand their world as they experience it, providing a combination of support and challenge, assisting them in cultivating their inner resources for change, and helping them take the specific steps needed to bring change about.

In addition to demonstrating respect, you help clients tell their story through your own genuineness. Being genuine does not mean acting on any impulse or saying everything that you think or feel. You can be genuine with your clients when you avoid hiding yourself in a professional role; are open and nondefensive, even if you feel threatened; are willing to share yourself and your experiences with clients; and show a consistency between what you are thinking, feeling, and valuing and what you reveal through your words and actions.

Gilliland and James (1997) describe the early stages involved in crisis intervention under the general framework of being able to listen. In crisis intervention work, the first step is to define and understand the problem from the client's point of view. To do this, helpers must possess listening and attending skills. Their capacity to understand and to respond with empathy, genuineness, respect, acceptance, and caring greatly influences their ability to help their clients clearly identify their problems. The next step involves ensuring the safety of clients who are experiencing a crisis. This involves making an assessment of lethality by determining the seriousness of the threat to the client's physical, emotional, and psychological safety. Another step consists of providing support for clients in crisis. Helpers best demonstrate their support not only by their words but even more so by their voice and body language.

Ask yourself how well you are able to pay attention to others, to fully listen to them, and to empathize with their situation. Assess the qualities you possess that will either help or hinder you in doing what is needed to assume the client's internal and subjective frame of reference. Consider these questions:

- Are you able to attend to what clients are telling you both verbally and nonverbally? Do you pay attention mainly to what people tell you with their mouths, or do you also notice the way they deliver their messages?
- Do you let others tell their story, or do you get impatient and want to talk too soon? Do you encourage clients to tell stories in great detail for the sake of your curiosity? Do you have a tendency to get lost in the details of their story and miss the essence of their struggle?
- Are you able to set aside your own biases for a time and attempt to enter the client's world? For example, if you consider yourself a liberated woman, are you willing to accept the client who tells you that she is satisfied in her traditional role as a housewife?
- As your client speaks, are you able to listen to and detect the core messages? How do you check with your client to make certain that you are understanding him or her?
- Are you able to keep your clients focused on issues they want to explore? Are you able to keep your own centeredness, even when your clients may seem very fragmented or are making demands on you?
- Are you able to communicate your understanding and acceptance to your clients?
- Are you able to work nondefensively with signs of resistance from your clients? Can you use this resistance as a way of helping them explore their issues more deeply?

Although it may seem deceptively simple to merely listen to others, the attempt to understand the world as others see it is demanding. Respect, genuineness, and empathy are best considered as a "way of being," not as mechanical techniques to be used on clients. Consider just a few ways in which you might interfere with allowing clients to express themselves. You could strive too hard to be real and thus, in the process, actually be nongenuine. For example, you may want to prove to clients that you are a real person and that you struggle with your own problems. To demonstrate your "realness," you may take the focus away from your clients and put it on yourself by telling detailed stories about your life experiences. Ask yourself if your clients are getting what they need from their relationship with you.

Establishing a working relationship with clients implies that you are genuine and respectful in behavioral ways, that the relationship is a two-way process, and that the clients' interests are supreme. This means that you avoid doing for clients what they are capable of doing for themselves. For example, assume that an adolescent client tells you that he wants more time with his father but feels intimidated and shy around him. He is afraid to approach his father. You show respect for this client when you encourage him to risk approaching his father and teach him ways of taking this initiative. You demonstrate a lack of trust in his ability if you take it upon yourself to talk to his father, even if your client has asked you to intervene.

Part of creating a working relationship means that you can recognize the signs of resistance, both in your client and in yourself. It is important to understand the many meanings of client resistance and not to interpret it as a sign of your failure as a helper. If you are focused on defending yourself against the various forms of resistance you will encounter with clients, you deprive them of opportunities to explore the meanings of their resistance.

One way of not reacting defensively to a client's resistance and of exploring its meaning is illustrated by the following example. You are seeing an involuntary client for the first time. She is extremely hostile and lets you know that she neither wants nor needs your help. She attacks your abilities as a counselor. As an effective helper you cannot indulge yourself in feelings of rejection. However, in a nondefensive way you can explore with this client her unwillingness and her difficulty in seeing you. If you are patient, you may discover that this client has some very good reasons not to trust a professional like you. She may have felt betrayed by a counselor, and she may fear that the information she gives you will be used against her one more time.

Helping clients gain a focus.   Some people who come for help feel overwhelmed with a number of problems. By trying to talk about everything that is troubling them in one session, they also may manage to overwhelm the helper. A focusing process is necessary to provide a direction for the helping efforts, enabling both the client and the helper to know where to start. To achieve this focus, make an assessment of the major concerns of the client. You could say to a client who presents you with a long list of problems: "We won't be able to deal with all your problems in one session. What was going on in your life when you finally decided to call for help?" Other focusing questions are "At this time in your life, what seems most pressing and troublesome to you?" "You say that you often wake up in the middle of the night. What do you find yourself ruminating over?" "When you don't want to get up in the morning, what is it that you most want to avoid?" "If you could address only one problem today, which one would you pick?"

Once clients determine what concerns they are seriously willing to explore, they can design a contract with the helper. As a helper you can be instrumental in encouraging clients to explore their key issues in terms of their experiences, feelings, and behaviors. By focusing on what is salient in the present and by avoiding dwelling on the past, you can assist clients in clarifying their own problems and opportunities for change.

Confronting clients.   Confrontation is a practice that is often misunderstood. It should not be viewed as aggressive or as destructive of a supportive relationship. Unfortunately, there are many misconceptions about the purpose and value of confrontation. Some helpers see it as producing defensiveness and withdrawal in clients. Or they may view it as an adversarial stance between them and their clients, which can lead to premature termination of the helping relationship. Helpers sometimes see confrontation as a negative act with destructive potential. Because of this connotation, they sometimes avoid it at all costs, when it is the very thing that they need to provide as the impetus for growth. Remember that a lack of confrontation results in stagnation. Without confrontation, clients often remain stuck in self-defeating behavior and do not develop the new perspectives and skills needed to make changes. Some helpers provide plenty of positive support but are reluctant to confront clients. Helpers cease being effective catalysts to others' growth if all they offer is support and empathy. Such an "understanding" attitude, if carried to excess, can be counterproductive. Confrontation can be viewed as "care-frontation" if it is done out of genuine concern and in a responsible way. Constructive and caring confrontation invites individuals to look at the discrepancies, distortions, games, excuses, resistances, and evasions that are keeping them psychologically stuck. Done with sensitivity, confrontation ultimately helps clients develop the capacity for self-confrontation that they will need in working through their problems.

Ask yourself if you're willing to confront others. You may be timid and apologetic when it comes to confronting. If you find that you have a hard time confronting others, it is important to understand what makes it difficult for you. It could be that you very much want to be liked and approved of by your clients. You might fear that they will turn on you or will not return. Even though confronting might not be easy for you, it is a skill that you will need to acquire if you hope to move clients beyond a mere "talking-about" phase of their counseling. It may help to realize that it is not abnormal to feel anxious about confronting others or being confronted ourselves. Yet even though you may be uncomfortable, one of the ways to develop skills in confronting is by doing what is difficult. If you back down when confrontation is required, you are feeding the anxiety that can keep you in a rigid stance with others.

Confronting clients effectively entails focusing on their awareness of what they are thinking, feeling, and doing. If the confrontation is successful, clients are able to overcome blind spots and develop new perspectives on their life situation, and they are also influenced to make changes based on this self-understanding. Thus, confronting aims at enabling clients to participate actively and fully in the process of helping themselves. Ideally, they will learn the art of self-confrontation.

Here are a few suggestions for making your confronting effective. First of all, earn the right to confront. Know your motivations for confronting. Is it because you want to more deeply understand another, or is it because you want to control the other person? Do you care about your relationships with clients? Are you really interested in getting closer to them, and are you aware of what gets in the way of a closer relationship? Challenge clients only if you feel an investment in them and if you have the time and effort to continue building the relationship with them. If you have not established a working relationship with a client, your confrontation is likely to be received defensively. The degree to which you can confront your clients depends on how much they trust and like you and how much you trust and like them.

Be willing to be confronted yourself. If you model a nondefensive stance in the counseling relationship, your clients will be much more willing to consider what you tell them. Before you confront others, imagine being the recipient of what is said. The tone and your general manner of giving your message will have a lot to do with how others receive what you tell them. It is also useful to present your confrontations in a tentative manner, as opposed to issuing a dogmatic pronouncement. Confronting is your chance not to "put down" clients but to inspire them to look at what they most want to change in themselves and what seems to be blocking this change.

Confrontation is not intended to rip away the defenses of clients; rather, it invites them to challenge their defensive ways and keep moving toward more effective behavior. Confrontations should not be dogmatic statements concerning who or what others are. Here is an example of a confrontation that would be certain to arouse a client's defensiveness and evoke resistance: "I'm very tired of hearing you complain every week about how horrible your life is. You're a whiner and a martyr, and I don't know if you'll ever change."

A confrontation that could lead to a more productive exploration of the client's difficulties is as follows: "You have said time and again that most of all you want to be successful, feel good about yourself, and feel proud of your accomplishments. Yet much of what you do and say sets you up to fail and to get what you say you don't want. You've done this for a long time, and you tell me that not feeling good is very familiar to you. Your father has never given you his approval, and around him you feel dumb and insignificant. Let's talk about the possibility that your chronic failures have something to do with your relationship with your father."

Likewise, in a marital-counseling session it would be unhelpful to tell a husband to "Be quiet and listen to what she has to say!" This confrontation might shut him up for good. It would be more helpful to describe what you saw going on between the two of them: "You say you want your wife to tell you how she feels about you, but every time she has tried this in the last ten minutes, you've interrupted her and told her all the reasons she shouldn't feel the way she does. Describe your wife's behavior, rather than labeling her. Talk to her about how you're affected by this behavior. Would you be willing for the next few minutes to let her talk and not think about what you're going to say in return? When she's finished, I'd like you to tell her how you're affected by what she has said. Instead of focusing on how your wife is, focus more on yourself, and tell her about yourself." People who are being confronted are less likely to be defensive if they are told what effect they have on others rather than simply being judged and labeled.

Some clients may be talented at inventing excuses for the way they are. You can confront them to accept responsibility for what they are doing rather than inventing excuses for what they are not doing. Some clients insist on seeing themselves as victims, for example, and spend much of their time blaming outside forces for the misery they experience. With effective confrontation you can assist them in redirecting the focus from others to themselves. Other clients may operate on the assumption that they must have universal approval. Again, your challenge of their belief system can help them see where they picked up such a belief and whether it is now serving them well.

You can also challenge clients on the strengths they possess but are not fully using rather than limiting your confrontation to their weaknesses. It helps to be specific, avoiding sweeping judgments and focusing on concrete behaviors. Remember to describe to clients what you see them doing and how this behavior affects you. It is also useful to encourage a dialogue with clients, and your sensitivity to their responses is a key factor in determining the degree to which they will accept your confrontations.

Here is an example of a helper's challenge to a client who is not making the best use of her strengths: "For several weeks now you've made detailed plans to reach out to a friend. You seem able to be assertive, you say that when you do reach out to people they usually like you, and you have no reason to fear that this friend will reject you. Yet you have not made contact with her, and you have many excuses for not doing so. Let's explore the possibility that you don't want to make this contact. What is stopping you from using your assertive skills?"

To make the issue of confrontation more concrete, we present examples of other styles of confronting. The first statements illustrate ineffective confrontation; they are followed by effective confrontations.

- "You're always so cold and aloof, and you make me feel distant from you." This could be changed to: "I feel uncomfortable with you because I'm afraid of what seems like a coolness about you. Rather than avoiding you, I'd like to see if we can be different with each other."
- "You're a phony! You're always smiling, and that's not real." An effective confrontation is: "I find it difficult to trust you, because often when you say you're angry, you're smiling. I have a hard time knowing what you want. This makes it difficult for me to get close to you."
- "If I were your husband, I'd leave you. You're full of venom, and you'll poison any relationship." A more effective statement is: "I find it difficult to be open with you. Many of the things you say really hurt me and distance me from you, and I want to strike back. It would be hard for me to be involved in an intimate relationship with you."

In the ineffective statements, the people being confronted are being told how they are, and in some way they are being discounted. In the effective statements, the helper doing the confronting is revealing his or her perceptions and feelings about the client and is reporting the effects of the person's behavior.

Using self-disclosure appropriately. Sharing yourself can be a powerful intervention in making contact with clients. We are not encouraging indiscriminately revealing your personal problems to your clients. But it can be therapeutic to talk about yourself if doing so is for a client's benefit. Do your disclosures help clients talk more honestly and specifically about themselves? Do they help them put their problems into a new perspective? Do they help them consider new alternatives for action? Do they help them translate their insights into new behavior?

Some helpers use self-disclosure inappropriately as a way of unburdening themselves. In the process they burden the client, and the client doesn't know what to do with this information. To us, self-disclosure does not mean telling clients detailed stories about your personal past or present problems. At times clients may evoke feelings in you that connect their struggles with your problems. If your feelings are very much in the foreground and inhibit you from fully attending to a client, it may be helpful for you and your client if you share how you are being affected. Depending on your relationship with the client, you might give some detail about your own situation, or you might simply reveal that what the client is struggling with touches you personally.

Perhaps the most important type of self-disclosure is that which focuses on the relationship between you and your client. If you are having a difficult time listening to a client, for example, it could be useful to share this information. You might say: "I've noticed at times that it's very difficult for me to stay tuned in to what you're telling me. I'm able to be with you when you talk about yourself and your own feelings, but I tend to get lost as you go into great detail about all the things your daughter is doing or not doing." In this statement the client is not being labeled or judged, but the helper is giving his reactions about what he hears when his client tells stories about others. An example of an unhelpful response would be "You're boring me!" This response is a judgment of the client, and the helper assumes no responsibility for his own part in his boredom.

How willing are you to engage in appropriate and relevant self-disclosure? Do you find it difficult to talk about yourself and what you are feeling? Admittedly, you are vulnerable when you share your own experiences, feelings, and reactions. Yet can you expect your clients to be willing to be vulnerable in front of you if you rarely show them anything of yourself? It is not necessary to share detailed stories of your past to form a trusting relationship with others. Inappropriate sharing of yourself can easily distract the client from productive self-exploration. Strive to let your clients know how you are perceiving and experiencing them. You are bound to have many reactions to your clients in the therapeutic relationship. Selectively discussing some of these reactions can help the clients, especially if you encourage them to discuss the feedback you give them.

Some helpers seem to have an inordinate need to talk about themselves. They may continue to work through their own problems by addressing similar problems with others. They may make the mistake of pulling the focus away from the clients and directing it to their own concerns. Examine the impact that your disclosures have on others, and develop an honesty about your own motivations and behavior. If you are distracting your clients from exploring their issues, this is the time that you could benefit from your own therapy. In your therapy sessions you can put the focus on yourself and work on your concerns.

Stage 2: Helping Clients Create Goals

Egan (1994) believes that many helpers make the mistake of dwelling too long on helping clients identify, explore, and clarify their problems. Directing too much effort at the initial stage of helping may promote insights, yet it often does not succeed in getting clients to translate these insights into new goals in life.

During the second stage, the aim is to help clients devise alternative approaches to dealing with their problems. This is done by guiding them in a brainstorming process to create perspectives that are in line with their values and can lead to action. It is important that these goals be measurable, be realistic in terms of the resources of the client, be chosen by the client, and be achievable in a realistic period.

If you are engaged in crisis intervention work, it is essential that you help clients explore a wide array of appropriate choices and possibilities. Frequently, clients in crisis feel immobilized and may fail to examine the options available to them. In fact, they may not see any options. Effective helping involves teaching clients to recognize that there are alternatives, some of which are better than others. Gilliland and James (1997) describe the following three strategies designed to help clients in crisis consider the options open to them: (1) *situational supports,* which include people in the client's life from whom they can draw strength during their crisis; (2) *coping mechanisms,* which are the actions, behaviors, or environmental resources that clients can use in getting through a crisis; and (3) *positive and constructive thinking patterns,* which can substantially change a client's perspective on a problem and can lessen stress and anxiety. Crisis workers are in a position to examine a number of possibilities for action, and they can enable their clients to develop a different perspective, especially if such clients feel that their situation is hopeless and that they are victims of fate.

A case example.   Brian, a young worker, comes to you because he wants help in pursuing his goal of getting into college. He has put off applying to colleges for several years, and the thought of actually being accepted scares him. His job dissatisfaction is so great that it has begun to affect his personal life.

In his work with you, Brian discovers that he has accepted some early messages from his parents. They communicated to him that he was ignorant and would never amount to anything, and they attributed his early difficulties in school to laziness. Test results have shown that Brian is performing far below his intellectual abilities. His insight that he unconditionally accepted these early messages has been important. He realizes now that he must acquire better reading and writing skills before he can successfully compete in college. As a helper, you could make a mistake by focusing mainly on his feelings about his parents and himself and by endlessly exploring the reasons why he feels inadequate. At this stage he is aware of what has stopped him so far in accomplishing his goals. He knows specifically what he needs to do to make a change in his life. Now he has clarified a new set of goals, and his task is to identify the specific steps to take in accomplishing them.

A different problem that some helpers have is being too impatient and setting out too quickly to solve clients' problems. The need of helpers to solve problems for others could easily block them from hearing what clients want to communicate. A common mistake we observe with trainees is their tendency to short-circuit the exploration of feelings of clients and provide them too readily with a solution to their presenting problem. This problem-solving focus aborts the struggle of clients in expressing and dealing with feelings and thoughts and eventually coming up with alternatives that are best for them. You need to help clients understand why it is important for them to express feelings that they have bottled up for years. You need to teach them the value of searching for their own solutions.

Again, if you are too intent on providing cures for every problem, it is likely that you are focused on your own needs for being a competent helper who wants to see results. You may be uncomfortable with the client's struggle, and you may push for resolution long before thorough exploration has even begun. If you were the helper in the case of Brian, you would have spent no time listening and exploring his deep feelings of inadequacy. You would not have assisted him in examining what had kept him time and again from succeeding academically. With your problem-solving orientation, you would have urged him to apply prematurely for college. If Brian had not had enough opportunity to express and explore his fears and self-doubts and if he had not acquired any insights into his own part in setting himself up to fail, he would not be likely to succeed in college.

Stage 3: Encouraging Clients to Take Action

Once the goals of the helper-client relationship have been identified, it becomes necessary to decide on the various avenues by which these goals can be accomplished. Knowing *what* you want to change is the first step, and knowing *how* to bring about this change is the next step. Helpers first assist clients in developing and assessing action strategies for making their vision a reality. After an action plan has been formulated, the steps need to be carried out, and then the plan needs to be evaluated. What follows is a description of the major tasks of this stage of the helping process.

Identifying and assessing action strategies.   Clients often do not accomplish their goals because they rush into the first strategy that comes to mind or devise strategies that are unrealistically difficult. One function of helping at this stage is to assist clients in thinking of many possible routes to achieving their goals. Together, helpers and clients can come up with a wide range of alternatives for coping with problems, can assess how practical these strategies are, and can decide on the best plans for action. Helpers guide clients to recognize the skills they need to put their goals into action. If they don't have certain skills, they can acquire them during the helping sessions or learn about resources that are available to them.

Referring back to the case of Brian, assume that he tells you that he intends to sign up for 16 units at a nearby college. It would be appropriate for you to challenge him on how realistic his plans are. Is he taking on too much and setting himself up to fail one more time? You could guide him in creating a more realistic plan and assessing it. Because you know that Brian lacks fundamental skills, you could explore with him some ways to acquire these needed skills: tutoring, remedial classes, or adult-education programs. You could also discuss taking fewer units and less demanding classes as a way of increasing his chances for success.

At this stage of helping, the focus is on asking clients to come up with clear plans for what they will do today, tomorrow, and the next day to bring about change and to anticipate what might get in the way of their plans. In choosing action strategies, clients consider their internal and external resources and limitations and then determine which strategies are best suited to their capabilities. Helpers work with them to ensure that these strategies are specific and realistic, are related to their goals, and are consistent with their value system. This process is especially important in working with clients in crisis situations. In these cases it is helpful to work collaboratively with clients so that they will have some degree of responsibility for their plan. Even in crisis intervention, the critical element in developing a plan is that clients do not feel robbed of their power and independence (Gilliland & James, 1997).

The process of creating and carrying out plans enables people to gain effective control over their lives. This is clearly the teaching phase of the helping process, which is best directed toward providing clients with new information and assisting them in the discovery of more effective ways of getting what they want and need. Throughout this planning phase, the helper continually urges clients to assume responsibility for their own choices and actions. This is done by reminding them that no one in the world will do things for them or live their life for them.

Wubbolding (1988) devotes a chapter in his book on reality therapy to planning and commitment, explaining that clients gain more effective control over their lives with plans that have the following characteristics:

- The plan should be within the limits of the motivation and capacities of each client. Plans should be realistic and attainable. Helpers do well to caution clients about plans that are too ambitious or unrealistic.
- Good plans are simple and easy to understand. Although they need to be concrete and measurable, they should be flexible and open to modification as clients gain a deeper understanding of the specific behaviors that they want to change.
- The plan should involve positive action and should be stated in terms of what the client is willing to do.
- Helpers should encourage clients to develop plans that they can carry out independently. Plans that are contingent on what others will do lead clients to sense that they are not steering their own ship but are at the mercy of others.
- Good plans are specific. Clients can develop specificity when helpers raise questions such as "What?" "Where?" "With whom?" "When?" and "How often?"
- Effective plans are repetitive and ideally are performed daily. For people to overcome symptoms of depression, anxiety, negative thinking, or psychosomatic complaints, it is essential for them to replace these symptoms with new patterns of thinking and behaving. Each day, clients might choose a course that will lead to a sense of being in charge of their lives.
- Plans should be done as soon as possible. Helpers can ask questions such as "What are you willing to do today to begin to change your life?" "You say you'd like to stop depressing yourself. What are you going to do now to attain this goal?"
- Effective planning involves process-centered activities. For example, clients may state that they will do any of the following: apply for a job, write a letter to a friend, take a yoga class, substitute nutritious food for

junk food, devote two hours a week to volunteer work, or take a vacation that they have been wanting.

- Before clients carry out their plan, it is a good idea for them to evaluate it to determine if it is realistic, attainable, and reflective of what they need and want. After the plan has been carried out in real life, it is useful to evaluate it again. Helpers can raise the question to the client "Is your plan helpful?" If the plan does not work, it can be reevaluated and alternatives can be considered.
- For clients to commit themselves to their plan, it is useful for them to firm it up in writing.
- Part of developing a plan for action involves a discussion of the main costs and benefits of each strategy as well as a discussion of the possible risks involved and the chances for success. It is the helper's task to work with clients in constructively dealing with any resistance they might have to formulating plans or carrying them out.

Resolutions and plans are empty unless there is a decision to carry them out. It is crucial that clients commit themselves to a definite plan that they can realistically accomplish. The ultimate responsibility for making plans and following them through rests with the client. It is up to each client to determine ways of carrying these plans outside the helping relationship itself and into the everyday world. Effective helping can be the catalyst that leads to this self-directed, responsible living.

Carrying out an action program.　Clients are encouraged to see the value in actively trying new behavior rather than being passive and leaving action to chance. One way of fostering an active stance by clients is to formulate clear contracts. In this way clients are continually confronted with what they want and what they are willing to do. Contracts are also a useful frame of reference for evaluating the outcomes of helping. Discussion can be focused on how well the contract is being met and what modifications of it are in order.

If certain plans don't work out well, this is a topic for exploration in a subsequent session. For example, if a mother does not follow through with her plan to deal with her unruly son who is getting in trouble in school, the counselor can explore with her what got in her way of carrying it out. Contingency plans are also developed. The counselor might role-play different ways the mother could deal with setbacks or with her son's lack of cooperation. Clients learn how to deal with reverses and how to predict possible roadblocks to their progress. Consider Brian's situation again. After signing up for some skill-building classes, he tells you that he feels overwhelmed in his classes, is very discouraged, and wants to quit. You can explore with him ways in which he can stick to his plan and how he can overcome his self-doubts.

Stage 4: Termination

Just as the initial session sets the tone for the helping relationship, the ending phase enables clients to maximize the benefits from the relationship and decide how they can continue the change process. As a helper, your goal is to work with clients in such a way that they can terminate the professional relationship with you as soon as possible and continue to make changes on their own. In settings where brief therapy is the standard, it is especially important that termination and issues pertaining to restrictions on time be addressed at the initial session. If an agency policy specifies that clients can be seen for only six sessions, for example, they have a right to know this from the onset. Working in a short-term therapy approach, the final phase of the helping process should always be in the background. With brief interventions, the goal is to teach clients, as quickly and efficiently as possible, the coping skills they need to live in self-directed ways. Your overriding goal is to increase the chances that your client will not continue to need you. Kramer (1990) puts this well when he writes: "The therapist must be clear from the first contact, unless there are mitigating circumstances, that the intent of treatment is to help the patient function without the therapist" (p. 166).

In cases of structured, time-limited counseling, both you and your client know from the beginning the approximate number of sessions available. However, while clients may know cognitively that they have only 6 to 12 sessions, they may emotionally deny the reality that counseling will be short term. Not only should termination be discussed at the first session but it should be explored as necessary throughout the course of the helping relationship. In this way, the discussion of termination does not come as a surprise to the client.

The limitation of time can actually assist both you and your clients in establishing short-term, realistic goals of helping. Toward the end of each session, you can ask clients the degree to which they see themselves reaching the goals they have established. By reviewing the course of treatment, clients are in a position to identify what is and is not working for them in the helping process. Each session can be assessed in light of having a specific number of sessions devoted to accomplishing pre-set goals.

Basically, the interventions for endings pertain to assisting clients in consolidating their learning and determining how they can proceed once they stop coming in for treatment. Here are some considerations for effectively accomplishing these tasks:

- Remind clients of the approaching ending of the sessions with you. This should be done a couple of sessions before the final one. You might ask clients to think about any unfinished business they have and what they'd most like to talk about in the final two meetings with you. You could even ask at a session prior to the last one, "If this were our last meeting, how would that be for you?"

- If you are not limited to a specified number of sessions, and both you and your client determine that termination is appropriate, one option is to space out the final few sessions. Instead of meeting weekly, your client might come in every three weeks. This schedule allows more opportunity to practice and to prepare for termination.

- Review the course of treatment. What lessons did clients learn, how did they learn them, and what do they intend to do with what they have learned? What did they find most helpful in the sessions with you? What did they think about their own participation in this process?

- Allow clients to talk about their feelings of separation. Just as they may have had fears about seeking help, they may have different fears about ending the work with you.

• Be clear about your own feelings about endings. Helpers often have ambivalence in letting go of clients. It is possible to hold back clients because of your own reluctance to terminate with a client, for whatever reason. It is essential that you reflect on the degree to which you may need your clients more than they need you. Clients are likely to give you positive feedback by letting you know how influential you've been in their lives. It is critical to remember that if you are a good helper you'll eventually put yourself out of business—at least with your current clients. Your task is to get them moving on their own, not to keep them coming to you for advice. If you can teach them ways of finding their own solutions to problems, they can use what they learn in dealing not only with present concerns but also with any future problems they'll meet.

• It is a good idea to have an open-door policy, meaning that clients might be encouraged to return at a later time should they feel a need for further learning. Although professional helping is best viewed as a terminal process, at a later period of development clients may be ready to deal with a new set of problems or concerns in ways they were not willing to do when they initially began counseling. Clients may need only a session or a few sessions to get refocused.

• Assisting clients to translate their learning into action programs is one of the most important functions during the action phase and the ending phase of helping. If clients have been successful, the ending stage is a *commencement;* they now have some new directions to follow in dealing with problems as they arise. Furthermore, clients acquire some needed tools and resources for continuing the process of personal growth. For this reason, discussing available programs and making referrals are especially timely toward the end of your work with clients. In this way the end leads to new beginnings.

Developing Helping Skills Takes Time

People are not "naturally born" helpers. Helping skills are learned, practiced, and refined. As you consider what is involved in the overall process of encountering and helping clients, you may feel somewhat overwhelmed by all that needs to be done. Just as you might have felt lost when you were learning how to drive a car, how to ski, or how to play the violin, you may be intimidated by all of the variables you are expected to pay attention to, both in your clients and in yourself. You could make the mistake of being so focused on anything that your clients say and do that you forget to pay attention to your reactions. By trying too hard to catch every gesture and to understand every sentence, you can easily distract yourself from being present with clients. One supervisor gave a student sound advice when she said "If you miss something with a client, the person will no doubt bring it up again later."

Conversely, you can be so acutely aware of yourself that you largely forget about your client. If you are so attuned to thinking about what you should do next, about saying the "right" thing, about being sure that you are "helpful," and about making sure that you are seeing results, you are bound to miss some of what a client is telling you. By being overly self-conscious and uncertain about your adequacy as a helper, you are missing making contact with your clients.

We want to offer some assurance that you don't have to be able to focus on all aspects of the helping process at one time and that you can learn these helping skills with practice and supervised feedback. We see the learning of these abilities as an ongoing process rather than a state that is achieved once and for all. You need not be perfect, and it is important to give yourself the latitude to learn from any mistakes you might make.

THE CHANGING ROLE OF HELPERS IN A MANAGED CARE SYSTEM

Much of what we have written about your role as a helper will take on a different perspective if you work in an organization that receives funding from a managed care system. A revolution is transforming the delivery of helping services in the private sector. This revolution, known as managed mental-health care, involves delivering services in ways that are driven more by cost containment than by client needs. The traditional fee-for-service system is being replaced by a system that curbs costs by placing limits on the number and types of helping services, by monitoring services carefully, and by emphasizing short-term interventions (Foos, Ottens, & Hill, 1991). As Cummings (1995) has pointed out, there is a shift in values and a fundamental redefinition of the role of mental-health practitioners in this transition from the traditional fee-for-service model to the managed care model that stresses time-limited interventions, cost-effective methods, and focuses on preventive strategies more than on curative strategies.

Rapidly escalating costs, especially in inpatient care, and associated concerns for quality and client outcome, have led third-party payors and employers to demand more effective cost and quality controls (see Cummings, 1995; Foos, Ottens, & Hill, 1991; Haas & Cummings, 1991; Hersch, 1995; Karon, 1995; Newman & Bricklin, 1991). In large measure, failure within the professional ranks to control rising costs has contributed to external control by the managed care industry. One of the major goals of managed care is to provide services that are as brief as possible to ameliorate presenting problems.

Although managed health care was once a reasoned response to real problems, Karon (1995) asserts that current managed care practice is characterized by an interest more in reducing costs than in quality of service. He contends that owners and managers of the managed care system are primarily interested in cost containment as a route to profitability and are concerned only secondarily with consumer needs and preferences. Foos, Ottens, and Hill (1991) contend that with the time limitations of managed care plans, mental-health practitioners are forced to become more proficient in time-limited approaches to counseling. Treatment plans need to be formulated rapidly, goals must be limited in scope, and the emphasis must be on attaining results.

It is true that the costs of health care have soared, but is managed care the appropriate solution to a problem of escalating costs and restricted availability of helping services? Or does managed care introduce a new set of problems that need to be solved? The debate is far from over. However, this new system will certainly have a profound influence on how you work with your clients.

In a managed care environment the emphasis will be on making relatively quick assessments of clients' problems and designing brief interventions geared more to relief of problematic symptoms than to intensive self-exploration aimed at personal growth. This change in the focus of helping will have an impact on your role as a helper. In addition to short-term interventions aimed at a variety of client problems, you are likely to be expected to participate in prevention programs such as assertiveness training, stress management, parent education, vocational counseling, marital counseling, and a host of wellness programs that teach healthy lifestyle patterns. The stages of helping described here will be accelerated. Because most programs have a cap on the number of sessions allowed in a year, you'll be challenged to design a range of psychoeducational methods that can help clients cope more effectively with specific problems of living.

Delivering mental-health services under a managed care framework compels helpers to work in a restricted environment. Haas and Cummings (1991) identify some of the limitations imposed on a client's treatment. The most severe limitation is time. Managed care guidelines often limit treatment to 20 sessions annually with lifetime cost caps. Clients may be denied the care they need if it extends beyond their benefits and they are unable to pay for additional care. Although this makes financial sense for the provider, it can become ethically problematic. Other ethical issues include competence, informed consent, and division of loyalties.

Practitioners must be proficient in providing time-limited, effective services. Delivering a variety of brief services in a flexible and holistic manner with a diverse range of client populations and client problems requires an eclectic or integrative theoretical orientation. Helpers who are not competent in short-term interventions should probably avoid involvement in a managed care program.

Informed consent assumes particular importance under this system. Practitioners need to give their prospective clients clear information about the benefits and limitations of treatment. Although practitioners are ethically bound to offer the best quality of service available, they also must deliver methods of care that are balanced with cost containment. Helpers have an obligation to educate their clients about the potential benefits and problems inherent in mental-health services rendered through managed care entities. From an ethical perspective, clients have a right to know that the focus on cost containment can have an adverse impact on the quality of care available to them. Prospective clients must be given clear information about the benefits to which they are entitled and clear information about the limits of treatment as the clinician envisions them (Haas & Cummings, 1991).

Helpers in a managed care system clearly have divided loyalties between doing what is best for the client and keeping their commitment to a system that demands cost containment through a reliance on short-term interventions. Many times clients need more than the very brief interventions that are available. Karon (1995) reminds us that competent and ethical therapists are primarily concerned with the well-being of their clients, which is an entirely different criterion from cost-effectiveness. Managed care demands that practitioners adopt a set of values congruent with limited interventions that mainly treat symptoms. This could raise ethical issues for therapists who value growth and actualization more than remedial, short-term, solution-focused strategies.

Because managed care providers take an active role in treatment planning, client confidentiality is compromised. Treatment is monitored by the third-party payor, who may influence decisions pertaining to interventions used, access to assessments, and access to outcomes of treatment. If clients want to protect their confidentiality, they may decide to seek treatment that does not involve third-party reimbursement.

Karon (1995) considers psychotherapy under managed health care to be "a growing crisis and national nightmare." There are legitimate ways to save money without impairing the quality of care, but Karon emphasizes that doing so requires careful thought and adequate research. Managed care companies are largely ignoring such reasonable and reasoned approaches. The aim of managed care is to provide as little psychological care as possible, while seemingly providing adequate mental-health care. Karon contends that ethical therapists are bound to encounter dilemmas in working in a system where the median number of sessions is five or six, no matter what services are offered. He adds that medication is often relied on in managed care systems to obviate the need to provide more than six sessions.

Although managed care appears to be alive and well, the policies of certain managed care companies are vulnerable to legal action. The landmark lawsuit in New Jersey against MCC, one of the largest managed behavioral health care providers in the United States, alleged that MCC terminated therapists, purportedly without cause, when they requested more sessions for their clients than the managed care company was willing to provide. In their lawsuit, the plaintiffs claimed that in limiting the number of sessions provided MCC was substituting its judgment for the therapist's professional judgment, contrary to client welfare and public policy, unlawfully preventing psychologists from exercising appropriate standards of care and clinical judgment (Jones & Higuchi, 1996).

It is clear that managed care presents both ethical and legal issues for professional practice. Ethically, professional helpers must not abandon their clients, and they have a responsibility to render competent services. But under managed care, some decisions are made for the client and the practitioner by the program. The number of sessions, the types of interventions to be used, and the content of treatment are all determined by the program. What if the therapist is clearly aware that these external decisions are not therapeutically sound? What options do a practitioner and a client have under such a plan? What if the agency policy is not in the best interests of the client?

Practitioners employed by managed care units are not exempt from malpractice suits if clients claim that they did not receive the standard of care they required. Professionals cannot use the limitations of the managed care plan as a shield for failing to render crisis intervention services, make appropriate referrals, or request additional services from the plan. Regardless of the structure underlying the delivery of services, ethical practice requires that you put the best interests of your client first. Consider how you can maximize short-term strategies that teach clients problem-solving skills that they can apply to their current and future problems. Ask yourself how you can best balance quality care with cost-containment requirements in the workplace:

- How will your role as a helper be affected by managed care?
- How might your ability to establish a working relationship with your clients be affected under managed care?
- How would you educate your clients about the benefits and limitations inherent in a managed care plan?
- What ideas do you have for keeping the welfare of your clients as your primary concern while at the same time acquiring competence in short-term interventions that are cost effective?

By Way of Review

- Your orientation to the helping process is largely a function of your beliefs about human nature and about how people change. It is essential that you clarify your beliefs about what brings about change.
- Effective helpers hold positive beliefs about people; have a healthy self-concept; ground their interventions in values; and possess empathy, congruence, warmth, compassion, genuineness, and unconditional positive regard.
- Generalizations that helpers make about clients tend to foster a self-fulfilling prophecy within clients. If individuals are viewed by a helper as being highly dependent and unable to find their own way, they will most likely live up to this expectation.
- Examine your assumptions to determine whether they are helpful for clients. Challenge your beliefs and make them your own through this process of self-examination.
- In clarifying your orientation to helping, useful questions to ponder are: "Who is responsible for change? What best facilitates change? Is insight necessary for change to occur? How useful are confrontation and support? What are the values of a focus on the past, the present, and the future? What is the nature of human nature, and what are the implications for practice?"
- A theoretical orientation that integrates thinking, feeling, and behaving provides the basis for developing interventions that can be used flexibly with clients at various stages of the helping process.
- Because there is no one "right" theoretical approach, you would do well to consider adopting an approach that is congruent with your personality and values.
- There are four stages in the helping process. Stage 1 consists of helping clients identify and clarify their problems. In Stage 2, clients create goals. Stage 3 involves encouraging clients to take action. Stage 4 deals with termination, especially assisting clients to translate what they've learned in therapy to everyday life situations. Specific helper strategies are required at each of these stages. Developing these skills takes time and supervised practice. Your own life experiences play a vital role in your ability to be present and to be effective in working with clients.

- Managed behavioral health-care programs have had a major impact on the kinds of psychological and social services that can be delivered and the quality of those services. It is important that helpers do what they can to inform their clients about the services available. At the same time, helpers must work with managed care companies to ensure that cost-effective methods also give helpers the latitude to offer a range of preventive strategies. The helping process itself—therapeutic goals, length of treatment, and intervention options—is influenced by the limitations imposed by managed care programs.

WHAT WILL YOU DO NOW?

1. Identify a few of your key beliefs and assumptions that stand out after you have read this chapter. As a way of examining how you acquired these beliefs and assumptions, talk with someone you know who tends to hold similar beliefs. Then seek out somebody with a different perspective. With both of these people, discuss how you developed your beliefs.

2. Review the section "Overview of the Helping Relationship" and consider the skills needed for effective helping. Select what you consider to be your one major asset and your one major limitation, and write them down. How do you see your main asset enabling you to be an effective helper? How might your main limitation get in the way of working successfully with others? What can you do to work on your weak area? You might ask people you know well to review your statements about yourself. Do they see you as you see yourself?

3. After reflecting on the section "Orientations to Helping," write no more than a one-page response that describes your personal view of what helping is about. You might imagine that a supervisor had asked you to describe your views about counseling or that in a job interview you had been instructed "Tell us briefly how you see the helping process." You could also imagine that someone who is not sophisticated in your field had said to you: "Oh, you're a counselor. What do you do?"

4. After reflecting on your beliefs about people and about the helping process, write some key ideas in your journal pertaining to the role that your beliefs play in the manner in which you might intervene in the lives of clients. How do your beliefs influence the suggestions you make to clients? How are your beliefs the groundwork for the strategies from which you'll draw in dealing with client populations?

As you review the stages of the helping process, ask yourself what you consider to be your most important tasks at each of the different stages. Write in your journal about some of the challenges you expect to face when working with people at each of these stages. For example, might termination be a difficult process for you? Would you have difficulty appropriately sharing your life experiences with your clients? Might you have difficulty confronting clients? What can you do to develop the personal characteristics and skills you'll need to effectively intervene at each of the stages of helping?

5. For the full bibliographic entry for each of the sources listed below, consult the References and Reading List at the back of the book.

For comprehensive overviews of stages in the helping process, descriptions of systematic skill development, and intervention strategies, see Brammer (1993), Doyle (1992), Egan (1994), Hutchins and Cole Vaught (1992), Ivey (1994), Nelson-Jones (1993), and Okun (1997). Consult Gilliland and James (1997) for an excellent survey text on crisis intervention strategies. Purkey and Schmidt (1996) address topics such as integrating approaches to counseling, ingredients of invitational counseling, beliefs about professional counseling, and characteristics of successful counselors.

Chapter 4

COMMON CONCERNS OF BEGINNING HELPERS

FOCUS QUESTIONS

1. How can helpers best deal with resistant clients? angry clients? unmotivated clients? clients who exhibit traits of the helper?
2. How can you handle your fear of angering clients when you confront them about inconsistent behaviors? How would you deal therapeutically with clients' resistance so they are more likely to look at their behavior than defend themselves?
3. How can helpers learn to avoid bringing the problems of clients home with them? How can helpers remain open and sensitive to their clients' struggles yet at the same time acquire some healthy distance from their problems?
4. How can helpers deal with their own reactions as they work with suicidal clients, sex offenders, abusers, people with AIDS, and people with diverse cultural and ethnic backgrounds?
5. What client behaviors do you find most problematic? Why?
6. When you are faced with working with "difficult clients" (or difficult friends), what do you generally do in such situations?
7. Are you aware of any unfinished business from your past that is likely to affect your ability to work with certain types of clients? What have you done to heal your own psychological wounds?
8. What kind of clients would you be most likely to refer to another professional? What might this answer tell you about yourself?
9. What defensive behaviors do you employ when you feel personally threatened? How open are you to recognizing your patterns of resistance? If you had a caseload composed of clients like yourself, what do you think your job would be like?

AIM OF THE CHAPTER

As a helper you will encounter a range of special concerns throughout your career, but some problems will be particularly pressing when you begin helping others. One challenge you will face is learning how to deal effectively with the feelings that some of your clients have toward you and the corresponding feelings that they evoke in you. Even experienced helpers show an interest in learning creative ways to deal with difficult clients, especially those who exhibit great resistance to their interventions. In this chapter we address the important issues of transference, countertransference, resistance, and management of your own feelings as you work with difficult clients.

This chapter will probably raise more questions than it answers. We are not interested in providing simple solutions to the many complex and challenging situations that you will encounter in your helping relationships. Our purpose is to introduce you to a range of common concerns that beginning helpers typically face.

We will be stressing the value of learning to pay attention to yourself at least as much as you do to your client. Too often helpers become riveted on getting resistant clients to change, and they underplay the importance of being aware of their own dynamics and reactions as they interact with difficult clients. Don't overwhelm yourself with the belief that you should know exactly what to do in every helping situation. You are enrolled in a program in which you have many opportunities to learn and practice the skills that can be applied to challenging situations. Your supervised field placement activities and your supervisory sessions will be ideal places to talk about many of the concerns raised in this chapter as well as to practice various intervention skills. If you are beginning your training program, you are certainly not expected to have the knowledge or skills to cope effectively with some of the cases we present. More important at this point is your capacity for being open to what is emerging inside of you as you confront resistant behavior in your clients. As we will show you in this chapter, your willingness to work on yourself is an index of your ability to work with others.

EXPLORING SELF-DOUBTS AND FEARS

Students in human-services programs sometimes bring up fears, resistances, perfectionist strivings, and other personal concerns. For example, many students express their anxiety over the prospect of facing clients. They ask themselves: "What will my clients want? Will I be able to give them what they want? What will I say, and how will I say it? Will they want to come back? If they do, what will I do then?" It is possible to become so anxiety-ridden that an intern or a practitioner is not able to pay attention to the client. Another concern of many students and practitioners is their expectation that they must be the perfect helpers. They often burden themselves with the belief that they cannot afford to be less than perfect, lest they make a mistake, which would have dire consequences for both their clients and themselves. These become ethical concerns when they are dealt with in a manner that reduces the effectiveness of the helper.

At this point, take the time to review the list of statements below to determine if these are things you might say. The questionnaire is drawn from statements we frequently hear in practicum and internship courses; they represent a sampling of the issues faced by those who begin helping others. Apply these statements to yourself, and decide to what degree you see them as your concerns. If a statement is more true than false for you, place a "T" in front of it; if it is more false than true for you, mark it with an "F":

_____ I'm afraid I'll make mistakes.
_____ My clients will really suffer because of my blunders and my failure to know what to do.
_____ I have real doubts about my ability to help people in a crisis situation.

_____ I demand perfection of myself, and I constantly feel I should know more than I do.

_____ I would feel threatened by silences in counseling situations.

_____ It's important to me to know that my clients are making steady improvement.

_____ It would be difficult for me to deal with demanding clients.

_____ I expect to have trouble working with clients who are not motivated to change or who are required to come to me for counseling.

_____ I have trouble deciding how much of the responsibility for the direction of a counseling session is mine and how much is my client's.

_____ I think that I should be successful with all my clients.

_____ I expect to have trouble being myself and trusting my intuition when I'm counseling.

_____ I'm afraid to express feelings of anger to a client.

_____ I worry that my clients will see that I'm a beginner and wonder if I'm competent.

_____ I'm concerned about looking and acting like an ethical professional.

_____ Sometimes I'm concerned about how honest I should be with clients.

_____ I'm concerned about how much of my personal reactions and my private life I should reveal in counseling sessions.

_____ I tend to worry about whether I'm making the proper intervention.

_____ I sometimes worry that I may overidentify with my client's problems to the extent that they become _my_ problems.

_____ During a counseling session, I would frequently find myself wanting to give advice.

_____ I'm afraid that I might say or do something that would greatly disturb a client.

_____ I'm concerned about working with clients whose values and culture are different from my own.

_____ I would be apprehensive about whether my clients liked and approved of me and whether they would want to come back.

_____ I'm concerned about being mechanical in my work, as though I were following a book.

Now go back and select the issues that represent your greatest concerns. You can then begin to challenge some of the assumptions behind these statements.

TRANSFERENCE AND COUNTERTRANSFERENCE

In the questionnaire that you just took, you may have pinpointed several concerns and fears that could influence your ability to work effectively with clients. Certainly, a major concern of many helpers, both personally and professionally, is being able to deal therapeutically with clients' reactions to them. A central challenge you'll face is identifying when your reactions are the result of your own internal conflicts that surface as you offer services to a range of clients. Recognizing and dealing therapeutically with both transference and countertransference are major concerns for most practitioners.

Dealing with Transference Issues

Transference is the unconscious process whereby clients project onto a helper past feelings or attitudes they had toward significant people in their lives. Transference typically has its origins in the client's early childhood, and it constitutes a repetition of past conflicts. Because of unfinished business, the client perceives you as a helper in a distorted way. A client may view you with a mixture of positive and negative feelings, and at different times the same individual may express love, affection, resentment, rage, dependency, and ambivalence. You are likely to experience transference feelings from clients even if you limit your practice to brief counseling. It is essential that you understand what transference means and that you know how to deal with it skillfully.

Transference tends to evoke reactions in you as a helper. These reactions can become problematic if they result in countertransference. Your unconscious emotional responses to a client may result in a distorted perception of the client's behavior. It is important to be alert to the possibility of countertransference.

In our training workshops for students and mental-health practitioners, we explore examples of difficult client behavior that participants present to us. We stress the importance of understanding the functions that resistive and defensive behaviors serve for individuals, examining the payoffs of a client's defensive style and understanding how resistance is an attempt at coping with anxiety. Rather than focusing on the dynamics of difficult clients and ways of dealing with them, we devote attention to assisting helpers in becoming aware of, understanding, and exploring their own countertransference. We focus on the helper's reactions to resistance and encourage those whom we teach to approach resistance with interest and respect rather than with impatience.

Here are some examples of transference situations that you are likely to encounter. Ask yourself what your response might be to a client's feelings toward you and what feelings are likely to be evoked in you.

Clients who make you into something you are not.   Some clients will want you to be the mother or father they never had but always wanted. These clients may have visions that you will take care of them and solve all their problems. They see you as an all-knowing being who can pull them out of the quandary they are stuck in. In considering clients who make you into a parent and want you to adopt them, ask yourself these questions: "Do I look to others to be the parents I never had? How comfortable or uncomfortable am I with clients who attribute to me traits such as being all-knowing and all-wise? How do I feel when clients expect me to make decisions for them? To what degree do I make it my responsibility to pull clients out of stuck places? What needs of mine could I be satisfying by assuming the role of parent for such clients?"

Other clients may immediately distrust you because you remind them of a former spouse, a critical parent, or some other important figure in their life. For example, consider the female client who is assigned to a male therapist and lets him know that she has no regard for men. All the men in her life have been untrustworthy, and because her therapist is male, he, too, will betray her. If you had a client who prejudged you on the basis of earlier experiences, how might you react? Are you able to recognize your client's behavior as transference reactions, and are you able to deal with them nondefensively? How might you go about showing this client that you are a different person from people in her past? How do you think you might react if your client insisted on treating you as she treated her father? How might you respond if no matter how you treated her, she deeply believed that you would eventually be "just like every other man"?

Some clients will not let themselves get emotionally close to you because they feel that as children they were abandoned by people they cared for. They are taking past experiences and superimposing them on the relationship with you. Assume that a client of yours comes from a divorced family. She is somehow convinced that a fault of hers caused her parents to separate. Because she was abandoned in the past and remembers the pain of that time in her life, she is leery of letting you into her life. She fears that if she gets too close to you, you, too, will abandon her. In working with such a client, consider these questions: "Is there much I can do to convince her that I do not intend to abandon her? What are my reactions to being told that I am going to be like her parents? What might I do in such a situation?"

Clients who see you as a superperson.   Consider having this man as a client: He uses only superlative adjectives to describe you. He sees you as always understanding and supportive and as perfect in all areas of living. He cannot imagine that you might have personal difficulties. He is sure that you have the ideal marriage, that your children are ideally happy, and that you have the ideal career. He tells you that he would be devastated if he ever found out that you were not all that he sees you as being. Furthermore, this client gives you full credit for any changes that he has made. Might you be inclined to believe some of what such a client tells you about yourself? To what degree might you feel burdened by his perception? What do you think you might have to do to live up to his ideal? How would you deal with his giving you total credit for his improvement?

Clients who make unrealistic demands on you.   Some clients make no decisions without first finding out what you think. They want to know if they can call you at any time. These are the clients who time and again want to run over the allotted time for their session. They want you to see them for no fee, with only the promise of paying later when they are in a better financial position. They feel close to you and would like to include you in their social life. They demand that you always be patient with them even when they do little to change. They expect you to accept them no matter what their behavior is during the session. They want you to affirm them and convince them that they are special in your eyes. If you fail to give them what they want, they are likely to be resentful and to react toward you with hostility. Even though you may intellectually understand the nature of these unrealistic demands on you, how do you imagine such demands would affect you emotionally? In what ways could you help such clients see the connection between how they are treating you and how they treated some significant person in their past? In what ways would you want to react to them differently than did significant persons in their past?

Clients who are not able to accept boundaries.   Related to clients who consistently make unrealistic demands on you are those who have problems understanding or accepting appropriate boundaries. As they were growing up, their home environment lacked boundaries, so they never learned the importance of not encroaching on the territory of others. The discipline in their home probably was inconsistent. One of their parents might have pampered and protected them from the other parent, who was overly severe in administering discipline. In their professional relationship with you, such individuals may treat you sometimes as an overprotective parent and at other times as an unduly harsh and punitive parent. Much of their behavior within the helping relationship may be aimed at testing you so that they know how far they can go with you. They will probably give you many excuses for why they fail to follow through on their commitments in the helping relationship. Again, as children they knew no boundaries, and now they are likely to be lost and to feel anxious because they are not certain where they stand with you. In working with such clients, it is essential that you do not fall into the trap of allowing them to treat you as they did a parent.

Clients who displace anger onto you.   Some clients lash out at you with displaced anger. They will be annoyed with you if you dare to become impatient. These clients are basically telling you that because you are supposed to be helping them, you have no right to express your own feelings. It is again the matter of clients who act as if they are unaware of boundaries between them and other people. It is important that you not deny your own feelings by swallowing them or trying too hard to "remain objective." It will help you to recognize that you are probably getting more of this client's anger than you deserve, and you will want to avoid getting into a debate with the person. If you take what you are getting too personally, you are bound to begin to react defensively. With this kind of client, you may need to ventilate some of your own feelings in the safety of a supervised session or with a colleague whom you trust. As a helper, do you give yourself room to have and to express your feelings toward a person who behaves in this way? How do you react to clients who project anger onto you that you do not think you have earned? How can you express your reactions to clients in a way that is therapeutic and does not cause them to become closed?

Clients who easily fall in love with you.   Some clients will make you the object of all of their verbal affection. They may tell you that there is nobody in the world whom they feel as much affection for as you. They may see you as the ideal person and want very much to become the person they see you as being. They are convinced that they could find a resolution to their problems if only they found a person like you who would love and accept them. How might you respond to being the object of adulation? Could you be tempted to solicit such ego-gratifying feedback? Could your client's reactions distort or enhance your self-perceptions?

Working with Transference Therapeutically

These illustrations of transference behaviors demonstrate how essential it is for you to gain awareness of your own needs and motivations. If you are unaware of your own dynamics, you will tie into your clients' projections and get lost in their distortions. You are likely to avoid focusing on key therapeutic issues and instead focus on defending yourself. If you understand your own reactions to a client, you'll have a better frame of reference for understanding others' reactions to this client. Paying attention to your own feelings about a client who imposes on you and makes unreasonable demands of you will give you a sense of how significant people in this client's life are affected by his or her behavior.

When clients appear to work very hard at getting the counselor to push them away, it can be therapeutically useful to explore what they are getting from this self-defeating behavior or how what they are doing serves them. Handled properly in the therapeutic relationship, clients can experience and express feelings toward you that more properly belong to others who have been significant in their lives. When these feelings are productively explored, clients become aware of how they are keeping old patterns functional in many of their present relationships. By paying attention to how your clients behave and react in the helping relationship itself, you can begin to understand how they might react to others.

It is a mistake to think that all feelings your clients have toward you are simply signs of transference. At times clients may be realistically angry with you because of something you have done or said. Their anger does not have to be an irrational response triggered from past situations. If you answer your phone continually during a session with a client, for example, she may become angry with you over the interruptions and your lack of presence. Her anger could be a justifiable reaction and not one that should be "explained away" as a mere expression of transference.

Likewise, clients' affection toward you does not always indicate transference. It could be that they genuinely like some of your traits and enjoy being with you. Of course, many helpers are quick to interpret positive feelings as realistic and negative feelings as distortions. You can err both by being too willing to accept unconditionally whatever clients tell you and by interpreting everything they tell you as a sign of transference.

In a group setting we have found it useful to have the participants recognize their transference reactions to one another and to the group leaders. At the beginning of a group we ask members to pay particular attention to people in the room whom they notice most. We facilitate the process of members' increasing their awareness of others by asking questions such as the following:

- "Whom in this group are you most aware of?"
- "Are you finding yourself drawn to some people more than to others? Are there some people with whom you quickly identify?"
- "Are there some people who seem especially threatening to you?"
- "Are you finding yourself making quick assumptions about others and forming hasty impressions? For example, 'He looks judgmental.' 'She's intimidating me.' 'I think I can trust him and will like him.' 'I definitely want to stay away from her.' 'It looks as if these three people are in a clique.'"

We pay particular attention to members who have strong reactions to another person whom they hardly know. It is common for people to "see" in others some of the very traits that they are disowning in themselves. This process of projection forms the basis of transference. Although we ask the participants to become aware of their first reactions to others, we do not ask them to reveal these thoughts or to respond to others too quickly. Instead, we suggest that participants share their reactions after they have had some chances for interaction. By disclosing such persistent positive or negative responses, they have rich opportunities to come to a deeper understanding of aspects of themselves that they are disowning. Through this process, participants often gain insight into their behaviors outside the group. This insight includes coming to an understanding of how they reacted to important figures in their childhood and how they now act around people who are important to them. With this new insight, people are able to catch themselves when they are triggered by characteristics that others manifest and can adjust their behavior. Thus, an individual who treats most men in authority roles with deference can stop himself from making them into representations of his father. He can then respond to different men more as they really are, rather than indiscriminately making each of them into his father.

Dealing with Countertransference Issues

The other side of transference is countertransference, or unrealistic reactions helpers have toward their clients that may interfere with their objectivity. If you hope to be effective in your helping efforts, it is essential that you consider countertransference as a potential source of difficulties that may develop between you and a person with whom you are working. You do not have to be problem free, but it is crucial that you be aware of how your own problems or countertransference can affect the quality of your working relationships with clients.

Although your countertransference has the potential for getting in the way of working effectively with certain clients, we are not suggesting that countertransference is "evil" or necessarily harmful. You can use all of your reactions in therapeutic ways, assuming that you eventually become aware of the sources of your countertransference. Remember that we are considering countertransference from a broader perspective than the psychoanalytic view of countertransference as being merely a reflection of an individual's unresolved internal conflicts that need to be overcome as a prerequisite to working effectively with a client. Brockett and Gleckman (1991) conceptualize countertransference broadly to encompass all of the counselor's thoughts and feelings in reaction to clients, whether prompted by the clients themselves or by events in the counselor's own life.

The counselor's task is to attend to the feelings he or she is experiencing in relationship to the client and then to identify the sources of these emotional reactions. When counselors' personal issues are brought into awareness, the chances are increased that their countertransference will be managed appropriately, which means that these reactions are less likely to interfere with the therapeutic relationship. Brockett and Gleckman believe that supervision, honest introspection, and involvement in one's own therapy as a client are particularly useful ways of achieving awareness of countertransference phenomena.

Simply having feelings toward a client does not automatically mean that you are having countertransference reactions. You may feel deep empathy and compassion for some of your clients as a function of their life situations. Countertransference occurs when your needs become too much a part of the relationship or when your clients trigger old wounds of yours that may not have healed. Just as your clients will have some unrealistic reactions to you and will project onto you some of their unfinished business, so will you have some unrealistic reactions to them. Your own vulnerabilities will be opened up as you are drawn into some of the transference reactions of those you help.

As you reflect on ways that you may be emotionally triggered in working with certain clients, think about how you are affected by those clients you perceive as being especially difficult. How do you respond to the different forms of transference? What kind of transference tends to elicit your countertransference? Do you take the resistance of a client in a personal way? Do you blame yourself for not being skillful enough? Do you tend to become combative with clients whom you view as problematic?

We encourage you to look at how your own attitudes, behaviors, and reactions to clients may, at times, actually foster resistance in clients. Without blaming yourself, it is useful to examine your reactions to those with whom you work to determine how what you are doing can either decrease or escalate the resistances your clients manifest. As a helper, it is crucial that you be willing to look at your own part in contributing to the problems associated with resistive behaviors in clients.

Countertransference can have both positive and negative effects on the helping process. If your own needs or unresolved personal conflicts become entangled in your professional relationships and blur your sense of objectivity, your countertransference reactions will probably interfere with the client's capacity to change. If you use your own feelings as a way of understanding yourself, your client, and the relationship between the two of you, these feelings can be a positive and healing force. Even though you may be insightful and self-aware, the demands of the helping profession are great. The emotionally intense relationships that develop with your clients can be expected to bring your unresolved conflicts to the surface. Because countertransference may be a form of identification with your client, you can easily get lost in the client's world, and thus your ability to be helpful is limited. Below are some illustrations of countertransference:

- *"Let me help you."* Your client has gotten a raw deal from life. No matter how hard he tries, things typically go sour in spite of his best efforts. You find yourself going out of your way to be helpful to this client and even consider having him move in with a relative of yours.
- *"I hope he cancels."* You are intimidated by a client's anger directed at you or others. When you are in the presence of this client, you are not yourself but are self-conscious and guarded. When he cancels a session, you find yourself relieved.
- *"You remind me of someone I know."* Your clients will often remind you of a significant person in your own life. Put yourself in each of these situations, and imagine how you would respond:
  1. You are a middle-aged therapist, and your husband has left you for a 20-year-old woman. You are faced with a female client who is having an affair with a middle-aged married man. Next, consider that your client is the middle-aged man who is having an affair with the much younger woman.

2. You have been a rape victim, and your client discloses that she has been raped. Or your client informs you that he has raped someone.
3. You were abused as a child, and your client tells you that he has abused some of his own children.
4. You have just dealt at home with a rebellious teenage daughter, and your first client for the day is a hostile, acting-out boy.
5. You lost a grandfather, but you have never really gone through a mourning process and come to terms with his death. One of your elderly male clients is in poor health and almost dies. As he talks about his feelings, you are extremely uncomfortable and find yourself unable to respond to him. You attempt to reassure him that he will be all right.

- *"You are too much like me."* Some of your clients are bound to remind you of some of the traits that you would rather not acknowledge in yourself. Even if you do recognize certain traits, you may find it disconcerting to work with clients who talk about problems and situations that are very much like your own. A client may be a compulsive workaholic, for example, and you may see yourself as working too hard. You might find yourself spending a lot of energy getting this client to slow down and take it easy.
- *"My own reactions are getting in my way."* Sometimes your clients will express pain and show tears. This anguish may make you anxious, because it reminds you of some past or present situation in your life that you would rather avoid. You may intervene by attempting to stop the client's feelings. It is important to realize that such interventions are motivated by bringing comfort to the helper, not by doing what is in the best interest of the client.

No one is immune to countertransference. It is therefore crucial that you be alert to its subtle signs and that you not be too quick to pin the blame for your reactions on your clients. For example, you may find that certain clients evoke a parental response in you. Their behavior can bring out your own critical responses to them. Knowing this about yourself enables you to work through some of your own projections or places where you get stuck.

Among the most vulnerable to the effects of countertransference may be those caregivers who work with the seriously ill or dying. These caregivers are continually confronted with the reality of mortality. In their work they watch others around them die; they may become consumed with stress and grief, but then they are expected to revitalize and once again become effective helpers (Smith & Maher, 1991). Unless helpers have come to terms with their own feelings about death, loss, and separation, their own unfinished business will continue to be activated as they work with clients who trigger their fears. In our experience in training students, we find that many of them have difficulty working with the terminally ill or the elderly because of the constant reminder of their own mortality. Thus, working with the elderly can be anxiety-provoking and stressful (Brockett & Gleckman, 1991).

You will probably not be able to eliminate countertransference altogether. But you can learn to recognize it and deal nondefensively with whatever your clients evoke in you. Here are some signs to watch for in recognizing your own countertransference:

- You become easily irritated by certain clients.
- You feel intense anger toward a person you hardly know.
- With some clients you continually run overtime.
- You find yourself wanting to lend money to some unfortunate clients.
- You feel like adopting an abused child.
- You quickly take away pain from a grieving client.
- You regularly feel depressed after seeing a particular client.
- You feel excited knowing that a certain client is soon to arrive.
- You tend to become very bored with a certain client.
- You are aware of typically working much harder than your client.
- You get highly emotional and get lost in the client's world.
- You become aware of giving a great deal of advice and wanting to have clients do what you think they should do.
- You are quick not to accept a certain type of client, or you suggest a referral with little data.
- You find yourself lecturing or debating with certain clients.

This list is not all-inclusive, but it illustrates how your own reactions as a helper can be activated by different clients. What are some strategies for recognizing and managing your countertransference? To manage countertransference you must have a receptive attitude and welcome self-awareness, be self-disciplined, and be willing to share your responses in a timely and therapeutic manner (Brockett & Gleckman, 1991). A receptive attitude entails accepting whatever feelings you are experiencing without getting stuck in guilt and without criticizing yourself.

Your own supervision will be a central factor in learning how to deal effectively with both transference and countertransference reactions. Your blind spots can easily hamper your ability to deal with "difficult clients" or with your own old wounds. You can become more aware of your own manifestations of countertransference by focusing on yourself in your supervision sessions. Rather than talking exclusively about a client's problem, spend some time talking about how you feel when you are in a session with a client. A good way to expand your awareness of potential countertransference is by talking with colleagues and supervisors about your feelings toward clients. This can be especially helpful if you feel stuck and don't quite know what to do in some of your sessions. Part of what could be stalling you is some feeling that you are reluctant to acknowledge.

Ongoing supervision will enable you to accept responsibility for your reactions and at the same time prevent you from taking full responsibility for directions that your clients take. Self-knowledge is your most basic tool in dealing effectively with transference and countertransference. It is well to remember that helping others change will certainly also have the effect of changing you. If you are unwilling to resolve your own issues, you'll not have much leverage when you challenge your clients to overcome their resistance.

DEALING WITH DIFFICULT CLIENTS

Professional helpers and students alike are concerned with how to handle difficult clients. They hope to learn techniques for making these clients less troublesome, for such clients tax them personally and professionally. There are no simple techniques, however—no tricks that you can pull out of a bag. In our workshops we help students or helpers become aware of and understand their own reactions to resistance, and we teach them ways of constructively sharing their reactions with clients.

The theme of Kottler's *Compassionate Therapy: Working with Difficult Clients* (1992) is that helpers can learn a great deal about themselves by dealing with difficult clients. He believes that by openly discussing those clients with whom they struggle the most, helpers put themselves in a better position to differentiate the dysfunctional behavior of clients from their own dynamics. Although he admits that some of his clients were extremely trying, he thinks that they have taught him more than any supervisor or instructor. The truly difficult clients

> force us to be more flexible, creative, and innovative than we ever thought possible. And they require us to look deep inside ourselves to examine every one of our own unresolved issues that get in the way of our being compassionate and effective—both as professionals and as human beings. (p. xi)

Handling Resistance with Understanding and Respect

Clients can be creative in demonstrating a variety of resistances. Although dealing with client resistance is sometimes painful, this is often the best route to establishing an effective and genuine relationship. It is useful to think of resistance as the very material that can productively be explored in the helping relationship. A degree of resistance is to be expected in many helping situations. It is a normal process and should not be thought of as something that needs to be "gotten around quickly" or bypassed. Learn to respect resistance and understand its meaning. It serves a purpose, and it will help both you and your client if you can understand its context. Realize that some resistance in clients is perfectly normal and makes good sense. Why should your clients automatically trust you? Chances are that many of them have had negative encounters with helpers, and as they approach you, they wonder whether you will be trustworthy. You don't get clients' respect immediately, nor do credentials on your office wall really earn genuine regard. Instead, your clients will come to trust you, and thus let down some of their walls, if you also let some of your barriers down. Part of respecting resistance means that you appreciate that the defenses your clients have created serve a function in their life. If they give up their defenses, what will be left? If you succeed in enabling them to surrender much of their resistance, are you willing to stick with them to create new resources for coping? Sometimes your interventions will take the form of helping clients block out some aspects of reality. People need certain defenses to survive psychologically. Uncovering a client's defenses is often inappropriate, and supportive interventions are called for. This is especially true in crisis intervention situations, when you are expected to deal with an immediate problem in a relatively short time.

In addition to understanding the context that surrounds the client's various forms of defensive behavior, pay attention to your countertransference that is evoked by this resistance. Avoid labeling your clients and thus entrenching their resistant styles. Don't assume that your client merely wants to annoy you. You cannot afford to have a fragile ego as a professional helper. Give your clients some rope, and don't respond to their resistance with resistance of your own. Be patient with your clients; remember that they are coming to you for help.

Resistant clients often make you feel incompetent, thus bringing out feelings of inadequacy and anger. If you too quickly become annoyed with difficult clients, you are likely to cut off avenues of reaching them. You can reframe any pattern of resistance that your clients manifest. Instead of viewing their resistance as behavior that is designed to make your work impossible, approach such behavior with a genuine sense of interest. If a client exhibits hostile behavior, for instance, you might consider reframing this experience by saying to yourself: "It's interesting how hard this client is trying to get me to be angry with her. I wonder how her behavior is serving a purpose and whether she could find another way to get what she wants more directly." Again, we suggest that you describe how you see your clients behaving toward you and how they are affecting you. After this declaration of your personal reactions, you could invite them to explore the meaning their behavior has for them and help them determine if there are alternative ways of getting what they want from you and from others.

Attitude Questionnaire on Understanding and Working with Resistance and Difficult Clients

Before you read the next section on dealing with difficult clients, take a few moments to complete this self-inventory to discover what your attitudes are toward resistance and difficult behaviors exhibited by clients. Indicate your position on each statement using the following scale: 1 = strongly agree; 2 = slightly agree; 3 = slightly disagree; and 4 = strongly disagree.

_____ 1. Difficult clients force me to look deep inside myself and explore my own unresolved issues that get in the way of being an effective helper.

_____ 2. Resistance is best approached with a sense of interest.

_____ 3. Resistance on the part of clients generally leads to ineffective results in the helping process.

_____ 4. When I encounter clients' resistance, it generally gets me to thinking about my own part in contributing to this resistance.

_____ 5. Involuntary clients will rarely benefit from professional helping relationships.

_____ 6. When clients are silent, this is almost always a sign of resistance and lack of willingness to cooperate with treatment.

_____ 7. Resistance is often a sign of handling a transference relationship poorly.

_____ 8. The most effective way of dealing with resistance is to be highly confrontive with clients.

_____ 9. One way of working with difficult clients is to pay attention to my own countertransference.

_____ 10. Labeling or judging clients who exhibit difficult behavior tends to entrench the resistance.

Now look over your responses and try to identify patterns in your perceptions of resistance. At this point, how does resistance from clients generally affect you? What are some ways you can think of to deal with resistance thera-peutically?

Common Forms of Resistance

Some of your clients may have had negative experiences with professional helpers and with community agencies. They are likely to approach you with a "show me" attitude. By taking their resistance seriously and exploring its sources, you are demonstrating respect for them. You are beginning to establish the foun-dations of trust, which is essential for any form of helping.

Albert Ellis (1985, 1986) has described many forms that resistance takes as counselors work with what he calls "difficult customers." Rational emotive behavior therapy (REBT) acknowledges that some resistance is a normal reaction, because fears are attached to the process of change. It also recognizes that resis-tance is caused by a variety of factors within the client (such as irrational think-ing) but that the counselor's attitudes and behavior can also produce much client resistance. What follows is an adapted description of the common forms of resis-tance as detailed by Ellis (1985, 1986):

- *Healthy resistance.* All forms of resistance are not to be considered dys-functional, and some resistance to personality change and therapy is a nor-mal reaction that serves some useful purposes for clients.
- *Resistance motivated by a client/therapist mismatch.* At times clients and ther-apists are not compatible. Clients may simply not like a therapist, for any number of reasons.
- *Resistance caused by counselors' relationship problems.* Counselors are not immune to relationship difficulties. They may not like some of their clients; they may have countertransference difficulties and therefore be biased against some clients; and they may be insensitive to their clients' feelings and may not know how to maintain a good therapeutic relationship. The resistance that clients show in these cases is largely brought about by the counselors' difficulties.
- *Resistance related to counselors' moralistic attitudes.* Some counselors assume a moralistic stance, condemning both themselves and others for "evil" acts. These helpers who damn their clients for their wrongdoings manage to help their clients to damn themselves. Such clients will typically resist any attempts at helping.
- *Resistance created by fear of discomfort.* One of the most stubborn forms of resistance stems from low frustration tolerance, or what REBT calls dis-comfort anxiety. Some clients demand that they achieve pleasure immedi-ately. They have irrational beliefs, which lead to discomfort anxiety: "It's *too hard* to change, and it *must* not be that hard. It's *awful* that I have to go through pain to experience therapeutic gain. I *can't tolerate* the discomfort of working hard. The world is a *horrible place* when it forces me to work so hard. Life *should be* easier." REBT shows clients ways to substitute long-range hedonism for short-range hedonism. It teaches that there is rarely any gain without pain.

- *Resistance due to secondary gain.* Many clients resist change because the payoffs that they get from their problems seem considerable. When clients improve, they sometimes discover hidden penalties. Some men learn to express their emotions, for example, only to be ill rewarded by society. They may then relapse into their old and familiar stoical ways.
- *Resistance stemming from feelings of hopelessness.* Some clients resist because they are convinced that they cannot change their dysfunctional behavior. Although they may make good progress in their counseling, if they show any regression, they are likely to irrationally conclude that they are indeed hopeless.
- *Resistance motivated by fear of change or fear of success.* Some symptoms, such as shyness or fear of public speaking, protect clients against possible failure. Their shyness keeps them from being rejected, and their fear of speaking in public keeps them from making a fool of themselves in front of others. If they gave up their symptoms, they would open themselves to the chance of failure and disapproval. Some clients tell themselves that this would be so "catastrophic" or "awful" that they want to cling to their symptoms.

The foregoing description of some of the common kinds of resistance shows that although clients come to counseling for help because they are plagued with a variety of symptoms of emotional disturbance, they often stubbornly resist efforts on the helper's part. This resistance is at least partly due to what the helper does or does not do. More often, however, clients have their own reasons for resisting the help that they have sought.

Types of Difficult Clients

Ellis (1985) has written about how to deal with the resistance of your most difficult client—you. His main point is that therapists rarely function at an ideal level; rather, they are human and very fallible. Therapists, like their clients, all too often fall prey to irrational beliefs and accept assumptions that they have not questioned. When counselors encounter resistant clients, for example, they often assume that it is their own fault and that if they were the perfect counselors that they should be, their clients would be cooperative.

In many respects we agree with Ellis when he contends that dealing with your resistance (and your countertransference) is likely to be your greatest challenge as a helper. Rather than constantly paying attention to what your clients do or fail to do, occasionally focus on your reactions to your clients. See what these reactions tell you, both about yourself and about your client. You make resistance all the more difficult to deal with in clients when you demand perfection of yourself and labor under irrational beliefs about how the world must be fair.

If you want to be therapeutic with difficult clients, you need to develop patience and give such clients room to maneuver. Regardless of which specific behavior a client exhibits, it is essential that you understand your own countertransference. Certain clients are more difficult for you because they evoke countertransference reactions. Keep this in mind as you review the list of difficult clients below. The list is not all-inclusive, but it does present a sample of the major concerns that helpers discuss with us.

Involuntary clients. You may not have the luxury of seeing clients who freely come to you for your help. Some will be sent by the court, others will be sent by their parents, others will come in under duress with a spouse, and others will be referred by another helper. The point is that involuntary clients are likely to have little motivation for change and to see little value in the help that you offer. For example, Herman attends a class for those found guilty of driving under the influence. His main motivation in coming to this class is to satisfy the judge's order. He figures that attending class is better than going to jail. Although he is willing to come to the sessions, he tells you that he doesn't believe that he has a problem. Rather, his intoxication was due to a series of unfortunate circumstances. He does not see much that he wants to change.

In your role as a helper, you could become either defensive or apologetic. We see it as a mistake to apologize for the fact that an involuntary client is sitting in your office. In Herman's case, he is responsible for being in his situation. It is *he* who needs to accept the consequences of his decisions and behavior. If you work harder than he does, there is little left for him to do. We see nothing wrong with your making some stipulations about how the two of you will spend your time. It helps to remember that when you have an involuntary client, you often have an involuntary helper. With some exploration of his resistance and willingness on your part to provide information about the services you offer, it is possible to melt resistance. Sometimes clients are reluctant to seek help because of their misconceptions about what the helping process entails. You can confront him with the reality that no one dragged him in to see you. Ultimately, he decided that it would be a better deal to come to see you than to accept the consequences if he did not. Together you can make a contract setting out how you are willing to spend your time with him.

Clients who are typically silent and withdrawn. Clients who say very little are bound to evoke your anxiety. Imagine the following client sitting in your office. He looks down at the floor much of the time, responds politely and briefly to your questions, and does not volunteer any information. For you the session drags on, and you feel as though you are a dentist pulling teeth. You might ask "Do you want to be here?" He will reply curtly "Sure, why not?" If you ask him what is going on in his life and what he wants to talk about, he will tell you that he doesn't know.

Do you feel that you need to do something to make this client talk? Are you taking his silence personally? Are you thinking of all sorts of ways to draw him out? Before your ego becomes too involved and you are unable to see his problem, it is useful to attempt to put his silence in some context. You might ask yourself, and even at times your client, what the silence means. His silence could have any one of the following meanings: He is frightened. He sees you as the expert and is waiting for you to ask a question or tell him what to do. He feels dumb; he may be rehearsing every thought and critically judging his every reaction. He is responding to past conditioning of "being seen but not heard." His culture may put a value on silence. He may have been taught to listen respectfully and merely to answer questions. Furthermore, your client may be quiet and invisible because this pattern served to protect him as a child. In other words, all forms of silence should not be interpreted as stubborn resistance and a refusal to cooperate with your attempts to help.

Silent clients can affect you in many ways. You may begin to judge yourself, thinking that if you knew the right things to say and do, your client would open up and talk fully. You could make a mistake by doing the talking for your client or by constantly drawing him out. It might be helpful to say something such as this: "I notice that you are very quiet in this group. You seem to pay attention to what other group members are saying, yet I very rarely hear from you. I'd like to know more about how it is for you to be in this group. Is your silence something that bothers you, or is it OK with you?" If this client does not interpret his silence as a problem, maybe you will be working in vain if you try to change him. This silent group member will have many reasons for being quiet. If he sees his silence as a problem, you can explore with him the ways in which this behavior is problematic. It could be a mistake to continually draw him out by asking him what he is thinking and feeling. If you assume the responsibility for bringing him out, he never has to struggle with the forces that are keeping him quiet.

Clients who talk excessively. The opposite of the client who says nothing is the one who seems never to stop talking. Some clients tend to get lost in telling stories. They jump from one topic to another. They take great care in providing you with every detail so they won't be misunderstood. They often get lost in relating their stories, and you wonder what the point of the story is. Instead of talking about how they are affected by a particular situation, they give you much irrelevant information.

Consider the case of Bertha. When she is in your office, she goes on and on and on. Any attempt you make to stop her results in her telling you that she wants to be sure that you know what she is saying. She gets very involved in "he-said" and "she-said" monologues. Bertha's defense is to keep talking, for then she doesn't have to stay long enough to experience any feelings or insights. If she slows down and experiences some of the things she is talking about, she is likely to feel anxiety.

In working with Bertha, you might feel intimidated. Although she is talking about painful situations, she is doing so in a very detached and rehearsed style. You might have reservations about interrupting her, out of fear of cutting her off. One of your functions is to help Bertha gain awareness into how her behavior serves as a defense. A few examples of some helpful comments are:

- "I notice that when you speak of your relationship with your mother you have tears in your eyes. Yet you quickly move away from your tears when you start talking *about* her instead of how you feel when you are with her."
- "I have trouble following what you're saying, and I wonder why you're telling me all of this."
- "Let's stop right here, and you tell me what you're feeling at this moment."
- "You're making a real effort to give me a lot of details so that I can understand you better. I'm getting lost, and I'm not understanding you. I want

you to know that I do want to understand you, and I can't when you go into so many details."
- "If you had to express in one sentence all that you've been trying to tell me, what would you say?"

If you are having reactions to a client like Bertha who overwhelms you with words, such as noticing that you have a hard time staying with her, it could be therapeutic to deal with your own reactions. Chances are that Bertha is affecting many people in her life in much the same way as she is affecting you. This is an opportunity for her to get feedback on how she comes across and for her to determine if she wants to do anything different. If you chronically suppress your reactions and pretend that you are listening with unconditional positive regard, she will soon pick up that you are not present for her. Also, by not dealing with her, you are reinforcing her talkativeness.

Clients who overwhelm themselves. Some of your clients have so many problems that they feel chronically overwhelmed. Not only that, they may overwhelm you as well. Disaster seems to lurk constantly around the corner. Such clients often have an endless reserve of problems, as if they thrived on having and creating problems. They come in each week and excitedly begin with "Just wait until I tell you what happened to me this week." Although some of the situations they describe are terrible, you suspect that they get some sense of excitement out of reporting these incidents. A sample of the way some clients continue to overwhelm themselves can be seen from Ruth's statements:

"I've just got to tell you everything that happened this week. I got an 'F' on one of my term papers, I'm having trouble getting financial aid, and if I don't get this aid, I can't stay in college. My daughter is having all sorts of problems with her boyfriend, and she comes to me late at night and wants to talk. Of course I listen, and then I get up in the morning feeling like a dishrag. Then I don't have the energy to get through the day. My son is having problems at school. His counselor called me to tell me that he is truant much of the time. I had to go down to the school, and I surely didn't have time for that with all the things that went wrong last week. The toilet got stopped up, and of course I was the one who had to take care of that. Oh, by the way, the garbage disposal broke again, and there was a flood in the kitchen. I feel I have to handle everything, and all by myself. When my husband comes home, all he does is plop himself in front of the TV, watch the sports, and drink beer. I just don't see how I can hold up everything. I've got to be a terrific student, the one who repairs leaks, the counselor to my kids, and on top of that I should be understanding of my husband who doesn't want any more pressure when he comes home. Oh, I don't know where to begin. Everything seems to be pulling at me at once."

Although this may seem a bit dramatic and exaggerated, some of your clients will sound like this. As you listen, you may have a hard time making an impact. If you don't intervene actively and forcefully, yet sensitively, Ruth not only will overwhelm herself but you, too, will be at your wit's end. You will not know where to begin, and you are likely to feel burdened with all of her problems and think that you must solve them.

As with other forms of resistance, you need to explore with Ruth the ways in which she contributes to her problems by overwhelming herself. It can be helpful to tell her something like this: "Ruth, I know there are many things that you feel are pressing on you today. But we have only an hour, and we realistically can't attend to everything that has gone on with you all week. Why don't you sit quietly for a moment and reflect on what it is that you most want from this session? Select the one concern that is most pressing to you at this time." By focusing her, you are a catalyst in helping her to avoid being lost, being drowned in a sea of problems.

Clients who often say "Yes, but . . . ." You will encounter clients who are exceptionally talented at inventing reasons why your interventions just won't work. As a helper faced with such clients, you quickly feel deenergized. No matter what insights or hunches you share or what suggestions you make, the end result is the same: the client quickly retorts with an objection. Some illustrations of the "yes, but" syndrome follow:

HELPER: "Have you considered telling your wife some of what you've told me?"
CLIENT: "Yes, but you don't know my wife." "I agree that it might help, but my wife would be very threatened." "But my wife will never change!" "I'm willing to talk to her, but I don't think it would help."
HELPER: "Every time I suggest something, you come back with plenty of reasons why my suggestion wouldn't work. I wonder if you really do want to change."
CLIENT: "Yes, but you just don't understand my situation." "You expect so much of me. I try, but things just don't work out." "Of course I want to change, but there are just so many things that keep me from changing. Only God knows how hard I try!"

When you are trying to help such clients, there is a danger of becoming too easily discouraged. It doesn't take much to get irritated with them. Even though you are willing to help this client, he is determined to prove to you that he cannot be helped. Eventually you are bound to feel helpless and to be inclined to give up. When you sense that you are working harder than your client is working, it may be time to renegotiate with him what he wants.

Clients who blame others. Some clients assume a stance of being a victim and a martyr. They chronically blame circumstances and other people for everything that happens to them. Carrie is a good illustration of a client who is quick to find fault in the universe for her unhappiness but slow to recognize her part in contributing to her misery. She views herself as having no control over her life. She seems to refuse to consider her role in creating her own unhappiness, largely because she is so attuned to finding fault outside of herself. Just a few of the outside factors that she sees as being responsible for her misery are these: her husband does not understand her; her children are selfish and inconsiderate; she always feels miserable a few days before her period; she feels terrible when there is a full moon; she has severe allergies, which keep her from doing what she wants; she really can't lose weight, because she is too depressed. And on and on it goes.

As long as Carrie puts the focus of her problems outside of herself, no change is possible in her life unless others change. If you allow her to talk continually about these others "out there," you have no power as a helper, because most of what she talks about is not in the room. It is possible for you to work with her to change, but you cannot work with all of the variables apart from her. You cannot control the moon, nor can you change some of the people in her life.

It would not be surprising if Carrie were to annoy you. You might engage in a lot of argumentation with her, challenging her on all of the ways in which she makes herself a martyr. If she continually refused to look at her own role, you might be tempted to refer her. As with most of these forms of resistance, it is important to keep clear within yourself and not get lost in the attempt to sway her. You can challenge her, share your reactions with her, listen to her, and ask her what she is willing to do to get what she says she wants.

Clients who deny needing help. Difficult clients in another category do not see that they have a problem. Such clients may come to a marital counseling session to help their spouse but be unwilling to see their part in the troubled marriage. In fact, they may well deny that a problem even exists in the marriage. You can waste much valuable time by trying to convince these clients that they indeed have a problem when they insist otherwise. The denial of these clients is serving a function, for as long as they don't admit the problem, they don't have to cope with it.

Take Roy. If you ask him what he wants from you, he will probably reply: "My wife wanted me to come to counseling, and I'm here for her sake." You may be better able to get through his resistance if you take his word for it and accept his view that he is problem-free. By asking him how he is being affected by his wife's problems, you may eventually get to problems that he wants to deny. Another alternative is to ask him how it is for him to come to your office. If he replies by saying "Oh, it's fine," you could respond "What were you thinking as you approached the office?" Or you could ask: "You say you're here to help your wife. What are some of the areas that you think she needs help with?" Or you could say: "You tell me that you don't have any problems and that your wife made you come here today. Could *that* be a problem for you?"

Some of the students we work with in a counseling program are quick to say how much they want to help others but not so quick to identify issues in their own lives. We have heard such students talk about their problems in the past tense. They are ready to admit that they had problems, but they maintain that they have dealt with and solved these problems. In some of your classes you have probably had opportunities for experiential and personal-growth activities. Think about how open you were to exploring any facets of your life with others. Were you willing to look at your own life in an honest fashion? How much did you resist? How motivated were you to listen to and reflect on feedback that others gave you? If you find it difficult to own up to potential problems in your life, do you think you will be able to effectively challenge clients to make an honest assessment of what troubles them?

Clients who moralize and judge. Some of your clients will appear to be self-righteous and judgmental. Such clients question you continuously about your interventions. They have a view of the world that they believe is absolutely right, and they wish that everyone else believed as they do.

Consider this illustration of a father who is in a family-therapy session with you. He has views and convictions about everything. In the session he has comments for each family member. To his wife he says: "The trouble with you is that you're trying to do too much. How can you make meals, take care of the kids, pay the bills, go to school, and work part time? Why don't you knock off all this other stuff and stay home where you belong? What the hell good is going to college anyway?" To his son he says: "You wouldn't have half the problems you do if you put your nose to the grindstone. The idle mind is the devil's workshop. You surely have plenty of free time, and you waste most of it." To his daughter he says: "Why don't you go to church more often? You're not living the way I brought you up. Besides, what will the neighbors think?"

Of course, many judgmental individuals are far more subtle than the father depicted here. Even though their proclamations may not be as sharp as his, they may be thinking very much as he does. When we work with clients who seem self-righteous and tend to judge others harshly, we sometimes ask them to give in to their tendency to lecture and provide a very stern lecture. This gives us some material to work with therapeutically. We sometimes ask such clients to reflect on what or whom their statements remind them of. They have often unconsciously incorporated a critical parent whom they now carry around inside of themselves. The therapeutic challenge is to help these clients see what their judgments of others do to their relationships. Such moralism usually has the effect of distancing them from others. If they can come to see this, they can then assess whether any modification of their behavior is necessary.

Clients who are overly dependent on you. Client dependency comes in many forms. There are clients who don't make any move without first checking it with you; those who continuously want you to tell them what you think of them; those who would like to call you at all hours of the day and night; those who want to become your friend; and those who want you to tell them what to do, how to do it, and when to do it.

If you have many clients whom you perceive as dependent, look at your possible role in fostering and maintaining their dependency on you. You might encourage clients to call you at any time, for example, without thinking that they will take you at your word. You might encourage them to call you before a job interview or right after the interview, so they can let you know how it went. It is important that you look at the ego gratification that you get from their dependence. These clients usually fear making decisions. For them, choices represent a threat. If they make the "wrong" choice, they are stuck with the responsibility. Along with accepting that we have choices comes the anxiety of using our freedom constructively and responsibly. Many clients want to escape from their freedom by making you responsible for choosing for them. In some ways they expect you to fill their parents' shoes. They are likely to develop transference reactions toward you and treat you as an authority. If you buy into their manipulations and nurture their dependent tendencies, you are merely reinforcing their vision of themselves as helpless. They are bound to resent you if they consistently put you "up there" and themselves "down there."

Clients who manifest passive-aggressive behavior. Certain clients have learned to defend themselves from hurt by dealing with people indirectly. They use hostility and sarcasm as a part of their style of resistance. Whenever they do or say anything, they are highly evasive. If you want to give your reactions, they are likely to retort: "Well, you really shouldn't feel this way. When I made that remark, I was just kidding. You take me too seriously."

Some common signs of clients who exhibit passive-aggressive behavior are as follows: They often arrive late. They say little. You see reactions on their faces, yet they assure you that everything is fine. They giggle when you talk. They raise eyebrows, frown, sigh, shake their head, look bored, and show other nonverbal reactions but deny that anything is going on with them. They chronically draw attention to themselves, and when they have the attention, they do little with it. They tend to be seductive in many ways.

Clients who behave in passive-aggressive ways may be hard to deal with. You may feel that you have been hit, but you won't know what hit you. It is hard to deal directly with this kind of behavior because of its elusive quality. However, you will certainly have reactions to clients who make hostile remarks, who offer much sarcasm, and who seem to engage in hit-and-run behavior. One way of cutting through this indirect behavior is to be aware of what it brings up in you and to give your reactions. What is important in dealing with this behavior is to avoid making judgments about it. You are more likely to avoid further hostility when you describe the behavior you see and tell the clients how their behavior is affecting you. It is also useful to ask them if they are aware of their behavior and to tell you what it means.

Some possible questions to consider are "Do certain clients who display hostility remind me of any people in my life? What do I feel like when people are not direct and I sense that there are some things they are not telling me? Is it timely and appropriate for me to give my reactions to the hostility I perceive in my clients?"

Clients who rely primarily on their intellect. Individuals who block out any feelings and present themselves in highly detached ways are another type of difficult client. Any time they get close to an emotion, they give a minilecture. They constantly try to figure out why they have a problem. They are adept at self-diagnosis and theorizing abstractly about the nature of their dysfunctions. They have learned that as long as they "stay in their head" they are safe. If they allow themselves to feel jealousy, pain, depression, anger, or any other emotion, they are not safe. To avoid experiencing anxiety, they have learned to insulate themselves from feelings.

Don't attack such clients and insist that they get to a feeling level. You can let them know how it is for you to be with them when they show little affect, but it is not helpful to try to strip away their defense. When they feel ready to let go of it, they will do so. Think about the ways in which you are affected in dealing with a man who remains very cerebral. If you are successful in getting him to give up his protection, will you be able to help him? Will you be able to be present for this person when his resistance melts and he gets in touch with years of bottled-up feelings? Will you be overwhelmed with his pain and run from it? If you are not there when he expresses his fear, will this prove to him that people will let him down when he releases his emotions?

Clients who use emotions as a defense.   The opposite of the client who uses his or her intellect as a defense is the client who thrives on displaying emotions. Such people are quick to weep, have no trouble "getting into feelings," and seem to enjoy catharsis. Their behavior may put you in a bind. You may have trouble trusting their emotions. You may become annoyed, feel manipulated by them, or somehow feel that they are not sincere.

We are not suggesting that clients who genuinely express emotions are resisting. We are talking about the difficult clients who have made a defense out of getting stuck in emotional material. When you are with such clients, reflect on what they bring out in you. It is possible that some of your highly emotional clients could remind you of people in your life who manipulated you with their emotions. For example, a sister might have succeeded in making you feel guilty when she cried and stormed out of the room. Now, as you work with clients who exhibit some of these behaviors, you may feel a lack of compassion for them and, in turn, wonder whether you have a problem with empathy.

Dealing Effectively with Resistance

Think about ways you can intervene when clients seem to make helping them extremely challenging. Some characteristics that we see as being part of an effective helper's behavioral style include these attributes. Effective helpers:

- Express their reactions to clients without putting them down in any way
- Avoid responding to sarcastic remarks with sarcasm; do not meet hostility with hostility
- Provide clients with necessary information so they can get the most from the helping process
- Encourage clients to explore any form of resistance rather than demanding they give up their resistance
- Avoid judging a client; instead, they describe the behavior they are observing that may be self-defeating
- Share with a client how they are personally affected by his or her behavior
- State observations and hunches in a tentative way as opposed to being dogmatic
- Are sensitive to clients who are culturally different from them, without stereotyping a client because of his or her culture
- Let clients who are difficult know how they are affecting them in a non-blaming way
- Are able to detect their own countertransference reactions
- Avoid using their power as a helper to intimidate those seeking help
- Do not take clients' reactions in an overly personal way

- Facilitate a more focused exploration of a problem rather than giving solutions

When we talk about dealing with difficult client behaviors in workshops, participants are always interested in learning specific strategies for dealing with the type of client behavior they find most frustrating. In our discussion here, we have avoided suggesting simple ways to change clients. Instead, we have put the focus on you, as a person and as a helper. You cannot directly change clients who are manifesting resistive and defensive behaviors, but you can learn significant lessons about the dynamics of their behavior as well as better understanding your own defenses.

Focus on why your clients have come to you, what they hope to get, and how you can teach them better ways of fulfilling their needs. If you resist the temptation to attack their defenses, and if you avoid labeling or judging them, the chances of their defenses melting increase. If you are able to retain your own centeredness and be clear within yourself about your reactions to these clients, then avenues open up as you explore with your clients the meaning of their behavior. The point cannot be made too often, however, that your resistance to their resistance will simply entrench their ways of responding.

BY WAY OF REVIEW

- Effective helpers must become aware of clients' transference and of their own countertransference. Neither of these factors is to be eliminated but is to be understood and dealt with therapeutically.
- Countertransference refers to the unrealistic reactions that therapists have toward their clients, which are likely to interfere with their objectivity. One way of becoming more aware of your potential for countertransference is by experiencing your own therapy. Another way is by focusing in your supervisory sessions on yourself and your reactions to clients.
- Resistance takes many forms, and it is necessary to understand the ways in which it serves as a protection for clients. Not all resistance stems from stubbornness on the part of the client. Some is caused, or at least contributed to, by the attitudes and behaviors of helpers.
- The goal in a helping relationship is not to eliminate resistance but to understand what functions it serves and to use it as a focus for exploration.
- There are many types of difficult clients. Some of them will evoke your own countertransference reactions. It is important to avoid reducing clients to a label.

WHAT WILL YOU DO NOW?

1. Select the most difficult client whom you can imagine working with, and reflect on the reasons that this client would present problems for you. What makes this client a difficult one? What do you think you'd do if you actually had

this person as a client? What might you do if you felt that you could not work with him or her?

2. Reflect on the kinds of resistance that you see within yourself. How open are you to accepting your faults and your limitations? If you were a client in counseling, what resistances do you imagine that you might develop to changing? What do you think it would be like if your clients were very much like you? Talk with a friend about this subject as a way of confirming (or contradicting) your views.

3. Look over the descriptive list of difficult client behaviors and identity specific kinds of client behaviors you would find most difficult to deal with in a therapeutic manner. In your journal write down what you can learn about yourself from your reactions to certain behaviors displayed by clients.

Look again at the inventory at the beginning of the chapter that helped you identify your self-doubts and fears pertaining to your role as a helper. Select one or two of these concerns and write about them. What are some steps you might take in dealing with your greatest concerns?

Review the attitude questionnaire on working with resistance and difficult clients. Write down your ideas about how you might become more therapeutic in dealing with resistance and difficult clients.

4. For the full bibliographic entry for each of the sources listed here, consult the References and Reading List at the back of the book.

See Ellis (1985) for a discussion of cognitive, emotive, and behavioral approaches in dealing with resistance. For ways of confronting and dealing with resistances, see Kottler (1991), and for an excellent treatment of what makes clients difficult and how to manage difficult cases, see Kottler (1992). May (1983) provides insightful material on transference and resistance in the therapeutic process.

Chapter 5

Ethical Issues Facing Helpers

FOCUS QUESTIONS

1. What ethical issues most concern you at this stage in your professional development?

2. When you are faced with an ethical dilemma, what route do you take in attempting to resolve the conflicts involved, and how do you make an ethical decision?

3. When would you be inclined to refer a client? On what grounds might you make the referral, and how would you go about it?

4. There are limits to confidentiality in any helping relationship. What would you want your clients to know about the purposes and limitations of confidentiality?

5. If a client were interested in a social relationship with you, what would you say? What are your thoughts about forming social relationships with clients? with former clients?

6. If a client expressed sexual attraction to you, what would you be likely to do or say? What would you do if you experienced sexual attraction to a client?

7. Dual relationships exist when professionals assume two roles simultaneously or sequentially with a person seeking help. Although some contend that dual relationships are fundamentally unethical, others argue that such relationships are inevitable and that they are not always problematic. What are your thoughts about dual relationships?

8. What are your thoughts about dual relationships (social, sexual, business, professional) with *former* clients and students? What do you see as being the ethical, legal, and clinical considerations in deciding about the appropriateness of any of these forms of relationships?

9. What is the role of ethical codes in guiding professionals to practice ethically? What value do you find in ethical codes?

10. Malpractice litigation is becoming more common. What are your concerns about the prospects of being involved in a malpractice suit? What steps can you take to lessen the chances of such an action being taken against you?

AIM OF THE CHAPTER

Regardless of what helping profession you decide on, you will be faced with learning to make ethical decisions. As will become clear in this chapter, part of becoming a professional involves being able to apply ethical codes to practical situations. In this chapter we introduce you to an array of ethical concerns that helpers encounter.

There has been an increased interest in ethical matters in recent years. Articles pertaining to ethical, legal, and professional issues in the helping field are common in professional journals. A number of books have been written on ethical and professional concerns, and many undergraduate and graduate programs include a discussion of these topics in various courses. Separate courses in ethical and professional issues are now being required in most graduate programs. Although we don't want to be cynical about the motivations for the rising interest in ethics, we suspect that some of this trend is a response to the rising tide of malpractice actions against those in the helping professions. How to lessen the chances of a malpractice suit is one topic of this chapter. In addition to the realities of legal constraints, we hope you will become increasingly sensitive to the ethical dimensions of your professional practice by focusing on what is best for your clients.

The chapter will not provide you with an in-depth knowledge of ethical issues, but we hope it will stimulate you to read some of the books listed at the end of the chapter. We encourage you to take an ethics course or, at the very least, to attend professional conferences and workshops dealing with ethical, legal, and professional concerns.

INVENTORY OF ETHICAL ISSUES

What are some of your major concerns about ethical practices? Perhaps at this point you have not even raised this question. We hope you will broaden your awareness of the significant ethical issues that you may face. Read each statement, and decide whether the statement is more TRUE or FALSE as it applies to you. Place a "T" or an "F" in the space provided.

_____ 1. I'm not sure how I would respond to a *current* client who asked me for a date or wanted some other social involvement with me.

_____ 2. I might be willing to consider a social relationship with a *former* client if both of us were interested in meeting on a social basis.

_____ 3. When an ethical concern arises, the best way to deal with it is to refer to the code of ethics.

_____ 4. If I were faced with an ethical dilemma in one of my cases, I would take the initiative in seeking guidance from one of my professors or supervisors.

_____ 5. It would be hard for me to refer a client to another professional, even if I felt this was in the client's best interest.

_____ 6. If I felt that I lacked the competency to work with a certain client, but he or she refused to accept a referral to another professional, I would continue seeing this person.

_____ 7. It would be difficult for me to decide when I had to break confidentiality.

_____ 8. If I were uncertain about keeping a client's confidence, I would want to discuss this with my client.

_____ 9. I would have trouble terminating a client even if it were clear that the client was no longer benefiting.

_____ 10. I am uncertain about how to go about resolving many ethical dilemmas.

_____ 11. I often doubt whether I know enough or possess the skills needed to effectively help others.

_____ 12. I am not at all certain what I might do if I felt that one of my clients posed a danger either to him- or herself or to others.

_____ 13. At times I'm concerned about my ability to keep relationships with my clients professional.

_____ 14. I don't think my training has prepared me to deal with sexual attractions in the helping relationship.

_____ 15. Striking up business relationships with former clients might be appropriate at times.

_____ 16. I am likely to promote dependency on the part of my clients by being too ready to offer advice or too quick to find solutions to their problems.

_____ 17. The obligation to warn and protect others is an area where I am uncertain about taking the appropriate action.

_____ 18. What constitutes ethical practice is very much a concern of mine.

_____ 19. I know the steps I am likely to take in cases where I become aware of unethical behavior on the part of my colleagues.

_____ 20. I'm concerned about the possibility of becoming involved in a malpractice suit as a result of something I do or don't do as a helper.

Once you have finished this inventory, spend a few minutes reflecting on any ethical concerns you have at this time. This reflection can help you read the chapter more actively and formulate ethical questions. Identify a few of the areas where you are uncertain about your position, and bring this ambiguity up in class discussions.

ETHICAL DECISION MAKING

Ethical practice involves far more than merely knowing and following professional groups' codes of ethics. In dealing with ethical dilemmas, you will rarely find clear-cut answers. Most of the problems are complex and defy simple solution. Making ethical decisions involves acquiring a tolerance for dealing with gray areas and for coping with ambiguity. Although knowing the ethical standards of your profession is important, this knowledge alone is not sufficient. Ethical codes are not dogma but are guidelines to assist you in making the best possible decisions for the benefit of your clients and yourself. Standards vary among agencies. It is essential that you become aware of the specific guidelines of the agency in which you are working.

In our teaching we find that students often begin an ethics course with the expectation of getting concrete answers to some of the questions raised in their fieldwork. They do not expect to have to engage in personal and professional self-exploration to find the best course of action. At times, readers of our ethics book (G. Corey, M. Corey, & Callanan, 1998) comment that it raises many more questions than it answers. We tell them that the book's purpose is to challenge them to develop the resources to deal intelligently with ethical dilemmas.

Consider the example of Susan, who became aware of unethical practices in a community agency where she was participating as an intern. She and other interns were expected to take on some difficult clients. She realized that doing so would mean that she was clearly practicing beyond the boundaries of her competence. To make the situation worse, supervision at the agency left much to be desired. Her superior was not willing to offer regular supervision and was often "too busy" to keep appointments to talk about her cases. In her fieldwork seminar on campus she learned that supervisors are ethically and legally responsible for what interns do. Susan had some trouble deciding what to do. She did not want to change placements in the middle of the semester, yet she was struggling with the appropriateness of confronting her supervisor about the situation. Unclear about how to proceed, she made an appointment with her fieldwork professor on campus, who shared responsibility with the agency supervisor.

In consultation with her professor, Susan explored a number of alternatives. She might approach her agency supervisor herself and be more assertive in getting an appointment. Another option could be a meeting of Susan, her agency supervisor, and her professor to explore the situation. It might be decided that this particular agency was inappropriate for students. What was important was that Susan knew she could get help in dealing with her problem. Sometimes students who are in similar predicaments arrive too quickly at the conclusion that they will merely tolerate things as they are rather than stirring up a hornet's nest and also making themselves uncomfortable in the process.

At the beginning of the course, Susan thought that clear answers were available for the variety of situations that would surface. By the end of the semester, she was learning to appreciate that codes and standards provide general guidelines but that she would have to apply these guidelines to specific cases. She had also learned the value of initiating the consultation process in ethical decision making.

Another example involves interpreting the ethical guideline that the client's welfare should be the primary consideration in the therapeutic relationship. Consider the case of a client who is talking about his struggles in an alcoholic family. As the therapist listens, his own pain over having alcoholic parents is triggered. He wonders whether he should tell his client about his personal reactions. Will his disclosure meet his own needs or the needs of the client? How is the therapist to judge whether the disclosure will help or hinder the client in working through places where he is stuck?

Responsible practice requires that you base your actions on informed, sound, and responsible judgment. For us, this means that you must be willing to consult with colleagues, keep your knowledge and skills current, and engage in a continuing process of self-examination. Thinking about ethical issues and learning to make wise decisions is an evolutionary process that requires an always open mind.

Professional Codes and Making Ethical Decisions

Various professional organizations have established codes of ethics that provide broad guidelines for professional helpers. Some of the professional mental-health organizations that have formulated codes of ethics are the National Association of Social Workers ([NASW], 1996), the American Psychological Association ([APA], 1995), the American Counseling Association ([ACA], 1995), the American Association for Marriage and Family Therapy ([AAMFT], 1991), and the National Organization for Human Service Education ([NOHSE], 1995).* Herlihy and Corey (1997b) identify several purposes that codes of ethics serve:

- Codes of ethics educate helpers as to the nature of sound ethical practice. The application of ethical guidelines to particular situations demands a keen ethical sensitivity.
- They provide a mechanism for professional accountability. The ultimate end of a code of ethics is to protect the consumers of psychological services.
- Codes of ethics serve as catalysts for improving practice. Codes can get us to critically examine both the letter and the spirit of ethical principles.

Ethical codes are necessary, but not sufficient, for the exercise of ethical responsibility. Although you have or will become familiar with the ethical guidelines of your specialization, you must still develop your own personal ethical stance that will govern your practice. You have the ongoing challenge of examining your own practices to determine whether you are acting as ethically as you might. The ethical guidelines offered by most professional organizations are general and rarely provide specific answers to the variety of ethical problems you may face. Although ethics codes offer guidance, they do not make decisions for you. Each of us is responsible for our own actions. You will be challenged to grapple with the gray areas, raise questions, discuss your ethical concerns with colleagues, and monitor your behavior (Herlihy & Corey, 1996a).

Ethics codes are a vital part of ethical awakening, but formal ethical principles can never be substituted for an active, deliberative, and creative approach to meeting ethical responsibilities. Although codes may define essential tasks to be addressed, these codes cannot tell us how we can accomplish these tasks when we are dealing with the uniqueness of each client. It is the helper's task to apply ethical guidelines to specific situations and to engage in a process of ethical decision making in determining the best course of action.

Ethics codes are partially designed to protect practitioners in cases of malpractice. Helpers who conscientiously practice in accordance with accepted professional codes have some measure of protection in case of litigation. Compliance with or violation of ethical codes of conduct may be admissible as evidence in some legal proceedings. In a lawsuit, a helper's conduct would probably be judged in comparison with that of other professionals with similar qualifications and duties.

The NASW *Code of Ethics* (1996) states that an ethics code cannot guarantee ethical behavior, nor can it resolve all ethical issues or disputes, nor can it capture

---

*NOHSE standards were approved in 1995. In 1996 they were published in Ethical Standards of Human Service Professionals, *Human Service Education*, Fall 1996, 16(1), 11–17.

the complexity involved in making responsible choices within a moral community. Instead, the code identifies ethical principles and standards to which professionals should aspire and by which their actions can be judged. Indeed, the NASW document reinforces the idea that ethical decision making is a process:

> Reasonable differences of opinion can and do exist among social workers with respect to the ways in which values, ethical principles, and ethical standards should be rank-ordered when they conflict. Ethical decision making in a given situation must apply the informed judgment of the individual social worker and should also consider how the issues would be judged in a peer review process where the ethical standards of the profession would be applied.
>
> Ethical decision making is a process. There are many instances in social work where simple answers are not available to resolve complex ethical issues. Social workers should take into consideration all the values, principles, and standards in this code that are relevant to any situation in which ethical judgment is warranted. Social workers' decisions and actions should be consistent with the spirit as well as the letter of this code.

We suggest that you devote some time to reviewing the code of ethics of your intended professional specialization. Examine the assets and limitations of these codes. As you think about these codes of ethics, identify any areas of possible disagreement that you might have with a particular standard. Be aware that if your practice goes against a specific ethical code, you surely need a rationale for your course of action. Realize also that there are consequences for violating the codes of your profession.

Must you follow all the ethical codes of your profession to be considered an ethical practitioner? If you agree with and follow all the ethical codes of your profession, does this necessarily mean that you are an ethical professional? Practical application of codes and guidelines is often difficult. The complex issues you will encounter as a helper will require not only an understanding of the guidelines for your profession but also knowledgeable interpretations of those guidelines to the real-life situations you face. Understanding the ethical codes of your profession is a good place to start, but remember that it is not your destination.

An Ethical Decision-Making Model

Along with the code of ethics of your professional organization, having a systematic way of examining a difficult ethical dilemma increases your chances of making sound ethical decisions. We cannot overemphasize the importance of seeking consultation when deciding on the best course of action. It is a good idea to consult with more than one colleague or supervisor; doing so can help you see various dimensions of a problem. What follows is an adaptation of a model for ethical decision making that was formulated by Forester-Miller and Davis (1995), which is described in the *ACA Ethical Standards Casebook* (Herlihy & Corey, 1996a).

1. Identify the problem. Gather as much information as you can to clarify the situation you are facing. You might ask yourself these questions: "Is this an ethical, legal, professional, or clinical problem? Is it a combination of more than one of these?" If there are legal dimensions to the problem, get legal consultation.

Remember that many ethical dilemmas are complex, which means that it is best to examine the problem from various perspectives and avoid looking for a simplistic solution. It may be helpful to seek consultation to determine whether there actually is an ethical concern—or to identify the exact nature of the problem.

2. Apply the ethical guidelines. Once you have a clearer picture of the nature of the problem, consult the code of ethics to see if the issue is addressed. If there are specific and clear guidelines, following them may resolve the problem. However, if the problem is more complex and a resolution is not apparent, you may need to employ the steps listed below.

3. Determine the nature and dimensions of the dilemma, and seek consultation. Ask yourself these questions: "How can I best promote client independence and self-determination? What actions have the least chance of bringing harm to a client? What decision will best safeguard the welfare of the client? How can I create a trusting and therapeutic climate where clients can find their own solutions?" At this point it is wise to consult with experienced professional colleagues or supervisors. Your state or national professional association may be able to provide you with guidance in resolving the dilemma.

4. Generate possible courses of action. Brainstorm as many possible courses of action as you can. In doing so, ask colleagues to help you generate possible courses of action.

5. Consider the possible consequences of all options and determine a course of action. After you have followed the steps listed here, evaluate each option with reference to the potential consequences for all parties involved. Eliminate those options that do not promise to give the desired results or that may have problematic consequences. Determine which of the remaining options or combination of options is best suited to the situation.

6. Evaluate the selected course of action. Review the selected course of action to determine if it presents any new ethical problems. If it does, you will need to go back to the beginning and reevaluate each step of the process. Once you have selected a sound course of action, you are ready to implement the plan.

7. Implement the course of action. In carrying out your plan, realize that other professionals might choose different courses of action in the same situation. However, you can only act in accordance with the best information you have. After you carry out your course of action, it is wise to follow up on the situation to evaluate whether your actions had the anticipated effect and consequences.

Even if you follow a systematic model such as the one we have described, you may still experience some anxiety about whether you made the best decision possible in a given case. Rarely is ethical thinking simply a matter of black-or-white categorization. Clear solutions may not be evident, as many ethical issues are controversial. Others involve a blending of ethics and the law. An important sign of your good faith is your willingness to share concerns or struggles with colleagues, supervisors, and fellow students. It is essential that you keep informed about laws that affect your practice, maintain awareness of new developments in your field, reflect on ways that your values will influence your practice, and be willing to engage in an ongoing process of self-reflection. Developing a sense of professional and ethical responsibility is a task never completely finished.

RECOGNIZING COMPETENCE AND LEARNING TO REFER

Virtually all of the professional codes spell out that you should not practice beyond the limits of your competence. In thinking about this matter, you may range from one extreme to the other. At one extreme you may be plagued with self-doubts, fearing that you will never have enough knowledge or skills to help people effectively. At the other extreme you may be overly confident, thinking that you can tackle any problem a client presents.

Knowing When and How to Make Referrals

The ethical standards of most professional organizations stipulate that making referrals is one of the main responsibilities of the professional helper. How do you know when and how to refer? Why would you want to refer? What kind of referral might be the most appropriate? What if few referral resources are available? It is crucial for you to refer clients to other resources when working with them is beyond your ability or when personal factors are likely to interfere with a productive working relationship. A client's failure to make progress with you is another reason to consider a referral.

Learn to assess your ability to work with a range of clients. If you followed the practice of referring all clients with whom you had difficulty, you might have very few left! It is a good idea to think about the reasons you'd be inclined to suggest a referral. In cases where you have limited experience, it is especially important to be open to consulting another professional. We hope that you will always be willing to say to a client "I don't know what to do, but I know where we can get some help." Beginning helpers sometimes believe that they must have all the answers, and they hesitate to let their clients know that they might not be sure how best to proceed. Although we do not expect you to know everything, we certainly expect that you can learn much under supervision.

Referral resources are sometimes limited. This is particularly true in some less-populated areas where mental-health facilities are scant. One helper told us: "I realize that I may not be much to some of my clients, but then again, I'm all they have! The nearest referral agency is over a hundred miles away, so what are they to do?" To make good referrals, it is necessary that you first know of the possibilities that might be best for your clients.

Imagine that you are an intern at a community mental-health center. This is your first experience in this type of setting. One of your first clients presents himself with much confusion about his sexual identity. He is unclear about how to proceed. Should he follow through on his homosexual inclinations or remain in his marriage? You feel overwhelmed, you are very uncomfortable with his choice, and you don't know quite how to handle this situation. What might you say or do? The following are a few approaches you might take:

- You could deny your discomfort and not express any of your feelings or reactions.

- You could share your negative reactions about homosexuality and attempt to persuade the client to remain in his marriage.
- You might let your client know that you feel both uncomfortable and overwhelmed but that you would like to challenge yourself by working with him. You could also tell him that you will seek supervision to help you avoid imposing your values on him.
- You could tell this client that you are very new in this work, that you are uncertain about how to proceed, and that you would like to refer him.

What are your thoughts about this situation and how might you proceed?

Deciding Whether to Terminate

Ethical standards usually imply that it is improper to continue a professional relationship if it is clear that a client is not benefiting. The tricky problem is to assess whether the client is really being helped. What if you are convinced that a client is not making significant gains, yet she assures you that she is growing from the experience? Consider the issues in the following case example, and think about what you would do if you were confronted with a similar situation.

You have been seeing a client for some time. She is very consistent, yet she typically reports that she really has nothing to discuss. You have confronted her on her unwillingness to invest much of herself in the counseling sessions. The client agrees yet continues to return. Finally, you suggest termination, because in your opinion she is not benefiting from the relationship. The client is quite resistant to your suggestion, despite her lack of involvement in the sessions. How would you handle this resistance?

CLIENT RIGHTS

What should you know about the rights of your clients? How can you teach your clients about their rights and responsibilities from the outset of the helping relationship? Clients are often unaware that they have rights. For most clients, asking for formal or professional help is a new experience. They are often unclear about what is expected of them and what they should expect from the helper. The ethical codes of most professional organizations require that clients be given adequate information to make informed choices about entering and continuing in the therapeutic relationship. The ethics codes of both the National Association of Social Workers and the American Counseling Association codify the nature of informed consent:

> Social workers should provide services to clients only in the context of a professional relationship based, when appropriate, on valid informed consent. Social workers should use clear and understandable language to inform clients of the purpose of the service, risks related to the service, limits to service because of the requirements of a third-party payor, relevant costs, reasonable alternatives, clients' right to refuse or withdraw consent, and the time frame covered by the

consent. Social workers should provide clients with an opportunity to ask questions. (NASW, 1996, 1.03.a.)

When counseling is initiated, and throughout the counseling process as necessary, counselors inform clients of the purposes, goals, techniques, procedures, limitations, potential risks, and benefits of services to be performed, and other pertinent information. Counselors take steps to ensure that clients understand the implications of diagnosis, the intended use of tests and reports, fees, and billing arrangements. Clients have a right to expect confidentiality and to be provided with an explanation of its limitations, including supervision and/or treatment team professionals; to obtain clear information about their case records; to participate in the ongoing counseling plans; and to refuse any recommended services and be advised of the consequences of such refusal. (ACA, 1995, A.3.a.)

Informed Consent

Perhaps the best way to safeguard the rights of clients is to develop procedures to help them make informed choices. Informed consent involves the right of clients to be informed about what their relationship with you will entail and to make autonomous decisions pertaining to it. This process of providing clients with information they need to become active participants in the helping relationship begins with the intake interview and continues for the duration of the relationship. Getting their informed consent involves a delicate balance between telling them too little and overwhelming them with too much information too soon.

According to Bednar, Bednar, Lambert, and Waite (1991), informed consent is a relatively new and developing legal doctrine that is rooted in the law's growing recognition of the importance of self-determination. Bednar and his colleagues write that the informed-consent doctrine is gradually becoming a standard part of mental-health practices. Although most professionals agree on the ethical duty to provide clients with relevant information about the helping process, there is not much consensus about what should be revealed and in what manner. In deciding what you would most want to tell a client, consider the following questions:

- What are the goals of the helping relationship?
- What services are you willing to provide?
- What do you expect of your client? What can your client expect of you?
- What are the risks and benefits of helping strategies that are likely to be employed?
- What do you want to tell your client about yourself?
- What are the qualifications of the provider of the services?
- What are the financial considerations?
- What is the estimated duration of the professional relationship? How will termination be handled?
- What are the limitations of confidentiality? When does the law require mandatory reporting?
- Are you likely to consult with a supervisor or other colleagues about the case?
- Are there any alternatives to the approaches you might suggest?

- If you are part of a managed behavioral health-care program, what kind of information would you give your clients about the number of sessions allowed? limitations of confidentiality? focus of treatment? appropriate treatment goals? use of short-term interventions?

Although some mental-health workers use written informed-consent procedures, you will need to decide which approach works best for you and your clients. We suggest that you develop comprehensive written statements that you give to clients at the first session so that they can take the materials home and read them before the next session. In this way they have a basis for asking questions, and valuable time is saved. After all, when clients finally make an appointment, they are often anxious to get help on some pressing problem. It is a mistake to overwhelm them with too much detailed information at once. Talking about the process in great detail can dampen the client's inclination to return for further sessions. Yet it is a mistake to withhold important information that clients need if they are to make wise choices. *What* and *how much* to tell clients are determined in part by the clientele. It is a good practice for helpers to employ an educational approach by encouraging clients' questions about evaluation or treatment and by offering useful feedback as the helping process progresses. Dealing with questions that clients have is especially critical during the initial stages of helping; educating clients about the helping process is not something that must be completed at the intake session.

Professionals have a responsibility to their clients to make reasonable disclosure of all significant facts and of the nature of the helping strategies that might be used. We have found that one of the best ways of building trust with clients is by being open and above board with them from the outset. From our perspective, the more that clients know about how helping relationships work, the more they will benefit from this experience. It is not a good idea to have hidden agendas for clients. By providing your clients with adequate information, you are also increasing the chances that they will become active participants and carry their share of the responsibilities in the helping relationship.

Confidentiality

The helping relationship is built on a foundation of trust. If clients do not trust their helper, it is not likely that they will engage in significant self-disclosure and self-exploration. Trust is largely measured by the degree to which clients feel assured that what they share will be kept confidential.

Although your clients have every right to expect that their relationship with you will remain confidential, there are limits to your responsibility to them. Because your obligation to safeguard your clients' disclosures is not absolute, you need to develop an ethical sense for when you must break confidentiality.

The ethics of confidentiality rest on the assumption that the client-helper relationship is deeply personal and that clients have a right to expect that what they reveal will be kept private. If trust is to be established, clients need some assurance that they will be protected from unauthorized disclosures. As a helper, therefore, you are expected ethically and legally to discuss with your clients the circumstances that might affect the confidential relationship.

State laws spell out special circumstances under which confidentiality must be compromised. One general guideline is that you may have to reveal information when there is clear and imminent danger that clients will bring harm to others or to themselves. There may be options other than breaking confidentiality, because not all states have the same laws.

In cases such as incest and child abuse, there are mandatory reporting laws. You have an ethical and legal obligation to report suspected child abuse and neglect, which implies that you know how to assess signs of abuse. Once you suspect child abuse, you are expected to know the procedures for making an appropriate report. All states require reporting of child abuse or neglect if it results in physical injury. However, mandatory reporting laws for child abuse, and the circumstances under which mandatory reporting is required, differ from state to state.

In addition to cases pertaining to child abuse and clients who pose a serious danger to others, you are expected to take action when clients are likely to harm themselves. For instance, if clients are suicidal, you cannot merely ignore this situation, even if they ask you not to report it. Human-services professionals are vulnerable to lawsuits if they improperly handle confidentiality issues, so it behooves you to know the laws, to follow them, and to be aware of the ethical principles of your profession. Most of the professional organizations can provide you with information leading to assistance in dealing with some thorny ethical dilemmas.

As a way to sharpen your thinking about issues surrounding confidentiality, think about the following cases:

1. **Child abuse.** Two young girls are brought to a community agency by their aunt, who has gained custody of them in the last few months. One girl, age 11, is quite verbal, but the other, 13, is not. As they begin to talk and you ask about their history, they tell you of aunts and uncles who attempted to touch one of them and of an aunt who severely beat them. The 11-year-old tells of a suicide attempt by her sister after one such beating. If you were working with these girls, what action would you take, and why? Would you have available the telephone number of the Child Protective Service for the area in which you are working?

2. **Runaway plan.** A student intern works with pupils in an elementary school. She says to the children in a group "Everything you say in here will stay in here." Then a boy reveals a detailed plan to run away from home. The counselor, who has not talked about the exceptions to confidentiality with the children, does not know what to do. If she reports the boy, he may feel betrayed. If she does not report him, she may face a malpractice action for having failed to notify the parents. What might you suggest to her if she came to you for advice in this situation?

3. **Students' violation of confidentiality.** You are a counselor intern in a local agency. You are part of a training group of students that meets weekly to discuss cases. One day, while you are having lunch in a restaurant with some of the students, they begin to discuss their cases in detail, mentioning names and details

of the clients loudly enough for others in the restaurant to overhear. What would you do in this situation?

The ethics codes of the various professional organizations all specify the importance of preserving the confidential character of the helping relationship. These codes also specify conditions that restrict confidentiality:

> Human service professionals protect the client's right to privacy and confidentiality except when such confidentiality would cause harm to the client or to others, when agency guidelines state otherwise, or under other stated conditions (e.g., local, state, or federal laws). Professionals inform clients of the limits of confidentiality prior to the onset of the helping relationship. (NOHSE, 1995)

> If it is suspected that danger or harm may occur to the client or to others as a result of a client's behavior, the human service professional acts in an appropriate and professional manner to protect the safety of those individuals. This may involve seeking consultation, supervision, and/or breaking the confidentiality of the relationship. (NOHSE, 1995)

> Social workers should protect the confidentiality of all information obtained in the course of professional service, except for compelling professional reasons. The general expectation that social workers will keep information confidential does not apply when disclosure is necessary to prevent serious, foreseeable, and imminent harm to a client or other identifiable person or when laws or regulations require disclosure without a client's consent. In all instances, social workers should disclose the least amount of confidential information necessary to achieve the desired purpose; only information that is directly relevant to the purpose for which the disclosure is made should be revealed. (NASW, 1996, 1.07.c.)

> When counseling is initiated and throughout the counseling process as necessary, counselors inform clients of the limitations of confidentiality and identify foreseeable situations in which confidentiality must be breached. (ACA, 1995, B.1.g.)

Although there are limits to confidentiality, it is clear that professionals are obliged to treat what their clients tell them in a respectful way, using this information for the benefit of their clients. It is tempting to talk about your clients and their stories, especially as others are usually curious about what you do. It may give you a sense of importance to be able to tell interesting anecdotes. You may talk more than you should when you feel overwhelmed by your clients and need to unburden yourself. As a professional helper, you must learn how to talk about clients and how to report without breaking confidentiality. Clients should know that confidentiality cannot be guaranteed absolutely, but they should have your sincere assurance that you will avoid talking about them except when the law requires you to disclose information or it is professionally necessary to do so.

Confidentiality needs to be discussed with clients from the onset of a professional relationship and throughout the helping process as necessary. According to Herlihy and Corey (1996b), it is a good idea to discuss the following points with your clients:

- The helping relationship will be kept confidential, except in certain circumstances. At times it is permissible to share information with others in the interest of providing the best possible services to the client.
- Confidential information may also be shared with other helping professionals when the client requests it or gives permission.

- Confidentiality is not an absolute, and other obligations may override the helper's pledge. For example, it is required that confidentiality be breached to protect someone who is in danger.
- Confidentiality cannot be guaranteed when the client is a minor, or when counseling families or groups.

Confidentiality in Marital and Family Therapy

If you are working with couples or families, confidentiality takes on a special meaning. Some helpers contend that whatever information they get from one family member should never be divulged to the other members. By contrast, other therapists have a policy of refusing to keep any information private within the family. Their assumption is that secrets are counterproductive in the attempt to help family members be open with one another. These helpers encourage bringing all secrets out into the open. It is essential that you be clear in your own mind about how you will deal with disclosures obtained from family members and that you let your clients know your policy before they enter a relationship with you.

Case example.   Owen is involved in individual therapy and later has his wife, Flora, attend some of the sessions so they can receive marriage counseling. Owen discloses to the therapist that he became involved in a gay relationship a few months previously. He doesn't want his wife to know for fear that she will divorce him. In a later session in which the therapist is seeing the couple, Flora complains that she feels neglected and wonders if her husband is really committed to working on their marriage. She says that she is willing to continue marital counseling as long as she is sure that he wants to stay in the marriage and devote his efforts to working through their difficulties. The therapist knows about this gay relationship that is causing Owen a great deal of difficulty. She decides to say nothing about it in the joint session and maintains that it is the husband's decision whether to mention it.

- What do you think of the therapist's ethical decision in this situation?
- If you were involved in a somewhat similar situation, what might you do differently?
- Suppose Owen confided that he was concerned that he had contracted AIDS and was very worried. What action might you take? Are you concerned about the ethics of his withholding this information from Flora? Can a case be made for the duty to warn and protect an innocent party?

Confidentiality in Group Counseling

If you ever lead a group, you will have to consider some special ethical, legal, and professional aspects of confidentiality. In a group setting, as is true for individual counseling, you must disclose the limitations of confidentiality. You must also make it clear that you cannot guarantee confidentiality, because so many more people are privy to information shared in the group. Even if you continually emphasize to the members how essential it is to maintain confidentiality, there is still the possibility that some of them will talk inappropriately to others about what has been shared in the group. Leaders need to encourage members to bring up any of their reservations about possible breaches of confidentiality. If members see it as their responsibility to talk about these concerns, this topic can be openly explored in the group.

Assume that members of a group you were co-leading brought up their reluctance to participate because they were concerned about the need for a firm commitment to keep in the group whatever was discussed. How would you deal with their concerns?

Your Obligation to Warn and Protect

Courts have created an exception to confidentiality when the mental-health professional has a reasonable basis for believing that clients pose a danger either to themselves or to others. Despite your ethical duty to maintain your client's confidentiality, you are legally bound to breach confidentiality when it becomes necessary to protect your client or others.

Put yourself in this situation: A new client visits you at a college counseling center. He says he was severely abused by his father as a child and is now extremely angry. He is making threats to kill his father and tells you he has a gun. How do you proceed?

In light of recent court cases, mental-health professionals are becoming increasingly conscious of a double duty—to protect other people from potentially dangerous clients and to protect clients from themselves. The responsibility to protect the public from potentially violent clients entails liability for civil damages when professionals neglect this duty by failing to diagnose or predict dangerousness, failing to warn potential victims of violent behavior, failing to commit dangerous individuals, and prematurely discharging dangerous clients from a hospital.

HIV issues.   One of the more controversial ethical dilemmas pertaining to a helper's duty to warn and protect others involves working with HIV-positive clients. As a helper, you may need to balance your client's right to confidentiality against the right of a third party to know about your client's HIV status. In the ACA's *Code of Ethics* (1995), a new standard was added pertaining to the helper's role in dealing with contagious, fatal diseases:

> A counselor who receives information confirming that a client has a disease commonly known to be both communicable and fatal is justified in disclosing information to an identifiable third party, who by his or her relationship with the client is at a high risk of contracting the disease. Prior to making a disclosure the counselor should ascertain that the client has not already informed the third party about his or her disease and that the client is not intending to inform the third party in the immediate future. (B.1.d.)

At this time, there is not a *legal* duty to warn, and it will take a court decision to resolve the legal obligation. In the meantime, practitioners who work with HIV-positive clients will have to wrestle with the *ethical* course of action to take in certain situations. It is difficult to identify who in particular is at risk and to assess the degree to which individuals who have intimate relationships with persons with HIV are in imminent danger. Disclosure requires a careful decision and should be made only when the client has not informed the third party and has no intentions of doing so in the immediate future. Although the ACA's guideline for contagious, fatal diseases gives practitioners *permission* to breach confidentiality, it does not state that they have a *duty* to warn, for such a provision would make them vulnerable to a malpractice suit (Herlihy & Corey, 1996b). This example illustrates a situation that could represent a conflict for the helper regarding following a legal versus an ethical course of action.

Case example.   One of your male clients discloses to you that he is HIV-positive, but he says nothing about his sexual practices with a partner or partners. At a later session he discloses that he is not monogamous and that one of his partners is unaware of his condition. Since he has been engaging in unprotected sex with this person for some time, he sees no point in either disclosing his condition or changing his sexual practices.

Consider these questions: What might you do in this case? How useful is the ACA guideline in determining your course of action? Would you initially address possible disclosure of information with others as part of the informed consent process? Why or why not? What do you see as your ethical and legal duty in situations similar to this case? How might you resolve potential conflicts between ethical and legal actions? How would you go about making the best decision?

Harm-to-self issues.   In addition to the duty to warn and to protect others from harm, helpers also have a duty to protect clients who are likely to harm themselves. Many therapists inform their clients that they have an ethical and legal responsibility to break confidentiality when they have good reason to suspect suicidal behavior. Even if clients take the position that they are free to do with their lives what they want, therapists have a legal duty to protect them. The problem is to determine when a client is serious about committing suicide.

Cases have been made both for and against suicide prevention. Fujimura, Weis, and Cochran (1985) contend that most suicides can be prevented if those who work with suicidal clients learn to recognize, evaluate, and intervene effectively in crisis situations. Many clients who are in crisis may feel temporary hopelessness, yet if they are given help in learning to cope with the immediate problem, their potential for suicide can be greatly reduced. It is generally held that once mental-health professionals determine that a significant risk does exist, appropriate action is necessary. Practitioners who fail to act in such a way as to prevent suicide can be held liable.

Szasz (1986) argues the case against suicide prevention. He presents the thesis that suicide is an act of a moral agent who is ultimately responsible. Therefore, he opposes coercive methods of preventing suicide, such as forced hospitalization. He further contends that by attempting to prevent suicide, practitioners basically ally themselves with the police power of the state and resort to coercion. Clients are thus deprived of assuming responsibility for their own actions. Szasz agrees that helpers have an ethical and legal obligation to provide help to those clients who seek this professional assistance for their suicidal tendencies. For those clients who do not ask for this help or who actively reject it, however, he takes the position that professionals have a duty either to persuade them to accept help or to leave them alone.

Although some have argued in favor of the right of clients to decide when and in what manner to end their lives, the codes of ethics of professional associations are in agreement that helpers must actively attempt to prevent suicide. In his article on working with suicidal clients, Wubbolding (1996) contends that counselors need to know how to handle suicide threats. They need practical skills that represent the highest level of ethical practice. He raises the following six questions as a way to assess the lethality of a threat and to determine whether further intervention is necessary:

1. Are you thinking about killing yourself?
2. Have you attempted suicide in the past?
3. Do you have a plan?
4. Do you have the means available to you?
5. Will you make a unilateral no-suicide agreement to stay alive—that is, to not kill yourself accidentally or on purpose—for a specified amount of time?
6. Is there anyone close to you who could prevent you from killing yourself and to whom you could speak when you feel the need to commit suicide?

Wubbolding (1996) contends that if clients say they are not seriously considering suicide, have not made prior suicide attempts, have neither a plan nor the means available, and are willing to make a no-suicide contract, the lethality of the threat is lessened and further intervention may not be necessary. If clients refuse to make plans to stay alive for a specified amount of time, then it is the helper's ethical responsibility to take action outside the session. Possible interventions might include informing the parents, spouse, physician, or another significant person in the client's life.

Case example.   A client is depressed and talks about putting an end to everything. He tells you that he is bringing this topic up only because he trusts you, and he insists that you not mention the conversation to anyone. He wants to talk about how desperate he feels, and he wants you to understand him and ultimately to accept whatever decision he makes. What would you say to him? How would you proceed?

Respecting the Client's Autonomy

Perhaps one of the most basic rights of clients is to have their autonomy safeguarded by the helper. Helpers can foster clients' dependent attitudes and behaviors in many subtle ways. Instead of helping clients find their own direction, helpers sometimes do too much for them, which results in their assuming too little responsibility for action and change. Most professional codes warn about creating a dependent relationship with clients. Although your clients may temporarily become dependent on you, an ethical issue arises if you foster their dependency and actually prevent their growth. You might ask yourself these questions as a way of determining the degree to which you encourage either dependent or independent behavior:

- Do I have a hard time terminating a case? Do I have trouble "losing" a client? Am I concerned about a reduction in my income?
- Might I need some clients more than they need me? Do I have a need to be needed? On some level do I feel a sense of power when clients express dependency on me?
- Do I challenge clients to do for themselves what they are able to do? Am I unwilling to provide clients with quick resolutions or easy answers, even when they press me for such solutions?
- To what degree do I encourage clients to look within themselves for their own answers?
- Do I keep the helping process mysterious as a way of maintaining power, or do I do as much as possible to teach my clients what the therapeutic process is about?

Some helpers foster dependence in their clients as a way of feeling important. They convince themselves that they are all-wise and that they can direct a client's life. They may feed off the dependent needs of clients to derive a sense of significance. When clients play a helpless role and beg for answers, these helpers respond all too quickly with problem-solving solutions. Such actions may not be helpful in the long run, for clients are being reinforced for their lack of willingness to support themselves. Your main job as a helper is to eventually put yourself out of business, which is done by encouraging clients to rely on their own resources rather than yours. By reinforcing the dependency of your clients, you are telling them that you do not trust that they can help themselves or that they can function independently from you.

KEEPING RELATIONSHIPS WITH CLIENTS PROFESSIONAL
The Dual Relationship Controversy

Codes of ethics caution against forming dual or multiple relationships with clients, which are defined as any relationships that might interfere with the effective maintenance of the professional relationship. Such relationships occur when professionals assume two or more roles simultaneously or sequentially with a person seeking their help. Helpers establish a dual relationship in cases where they have another, significantly different relationship with one of their clients, students, or supervisees. In these situations, the potential for a conflict of interest and for exploiting those seeking help cannot be ignored. Consider these examples of ethical guidelines on dual relationships:

> Counselors are aware of their influential positions with respect to clients, and they avoid exploiting the trust and dependency of clients. Counselors make every effort to avoid dual relationships with clients that could impair professional judgment or increase the risk of harm to clients. (Examples of such relationships

include, but are not limited to, familial, social, financial, business, or close personal relationships with clients.) When a dual relationship cannot be avoided, counselors take appropriate professional precautions such as informed consent, consultation, supervision, and documentation to ensure that judgment is not impaired and no exploitation occurs. (ACA, 1995, A.6.a.)

NASW's *Code of Ethics* (1996) focuses on factors of risk of exploitation or potential harm to clients:

> Social workers should not engage in dual or multiple relationships with clients or former clients in which there is a risk of exploitation or potential harm to the client. In instances when dual or multiple relationships are unavoidable, social workers should take steps to protect clients and are responsible for setting clear, appropriate, and culturally sensitive boundaries. (NASW, 1996, 1.06.c.)

NOHSE's *Ethical Standards* (1995) highlights the power and status differential between helper and client:

> Human service professionals are aware that in their relationships with clients power and status are unequal. Therefore they recognize that dual or multiple relationships may increase the risk of harm to, or exploitation of, clients, and may impair their professional judgment. However, in some communities and situations it may not be feasible to avoid social or other nonprofessional contact with clients. Human service professionals support the trust implicit in the helping relationship by avoiding dual relationships that may impair professional judgment, increase the risk of harm to clients or lead to exploitation. (NOHSE, 1995)

The helping professions have become increasingly concerned about the ethics of dual relationships. During the 1980s, the issue of sexual dual relationships was given considerable attention in the professional literature. It is now clear that sexual dual relationships are unethical, and the various professional organizations have prohibitions against them in their ethical codes. In the 1990s, nonsexual dual and multiple relationships have been the subject of increased attention. However, for a variety of nonsexual dual relationships, little consensus has been reached with regard to a determination of ethical practice.

Nonsexual dual or multiple relationships tend to be complex; they cannot be settled with simple and absolute answers. Helpers cannot always perform a singular role when working with clients or in the community, nor is it always desirable that they limit themselves to one role. Many times, helpers will be challenged to balance multiple roles in their professional relationships. Examples of dual relationships include: accepting clients who are family members or friends, dating clients or students, engaging in sexual intimacies with clients, bartering of services, combining roles of supervisor and therapist, forming business arrangements with therapy clients, combining personal counseling with consultation, or any other combination of roles where objectivity will be difficult to maintain.

As Herlihy and Corey (1997a) indicate, some behaviors that helpers may engage in have a potential for creating a dual relationship, but they are not, by themselves, dual relationships. Examples of these behaviors include accepting a small gift from a client, accepting a client's invitation to a graduation ceremony, accepting goods rather than money as payment, or engaging in nonerotic touching when this is appropriate. Some writers (Gabbard, 1995; Smith & Fitzpatrick,

1995) suggest that these incidents might be considered boundary *crossings* rather than boundary *violations*. A crossing is a departure from standard practice, while a violation is a serious breach that causes harm to the client. Interpersonal boundaries are not static and may be redefined over time in the professional relationship. It is important to keep in mind that even though boundary crossings may not be harmful to clients, these crossings can lead to blurring of professional boundaries and can result in dual relationships that do have a potential to be harmful.

Recent revisions of codes of ethics deal more specifically and extensively with setting appropriate boundaries, recognizing potential conflicts of interest, and taking ethical approaches in managing dual or multiple relationships. Codes of ethics that address these issues include those of the American Counseling Association (1995), the American Psychological Association (1995), the National Association of Social Workers (1996), the American Association for Marriage and Family Therapy (1991), and the National Organization for Human Service Education (1995). In addition, governing boards for professional licenses are developing regulatory language that attempts to address this problem. Although codes may serve a function, dual relationships are frequently not a clear-cut matter as ethical reasoning and judgment come into play when ethical codes are applied to specific situations.

As we mentioned, there is considerable disagreement about dual relationships. Some in the profession want to see tighter laws and ethical codes prohibiting dual relationships, whereas others see this trend as eroding confidence in individual practitioners. Many professionals assert that not all dual relationships can be avoided, nor are they necessarily harmful, unethical, or unprofessional (Herlihy & Corey, 1997a). This is particularly true in small, isolated communities. In many rural communities there is a high likelihood that helpers will be involved in multiple relationships (Sleek, 1994). The local pharmacist, physician, mechanic, banker, carpenter, or beautician might be a client of a particular helper. Furthermore, rural professionals see clients in the local store and ponder whether to acknowledge the person in the presence of others. If they are in local organizations such as the Chamber of Commerce or if they attend the same church, they may worry about conflicts with some fellow members who are also clients. In rural settings, helpers typically play multiple roles and are likely to experience more difficulties maintaining clear boundaries than do their colleagues who practice in urban areas. Practicing in an urban versus a rural setting must be taken into account in assessing ethical practices pertaining to multiple relationships.

Granted that there are divergent viewpoints on dual relationships, most professionals will agree that blending the roles of counselor and employee or counselor and lover is not appropriate. Whenever helpers play multiple roles, there is a potential for conflict of interest, loss of objectivity, and exploitation of persons who have sought help. Some multiple relationships can be avoided, and some cannot. In either case, ethical practitioners must take appropriate precautions to ensure that the best interests of their clients are maintained. Herlihy and Corey (1997a) provide the following guidelines in cases where professionals are operating in more than one role:

- Set healthy boundaries from the outset. In your informed-consent document, it is wise to state your policy pertaining to professional versus social or business relationships.
- Involve the client in setting the boundaries of the professional relationship. Discuss with clients what you expect of them and what they can expect of you.
- Informed consent is essential in circumstances where you are playing more than one role with a client. Clients have a right to know about any potential risks associated with dual relationships. Informed consent and discussion of unforeseen problems and conflicts need to be an ongoing process.
- Consultation with colleagues is most useful in obtaining an objective perspective and identifying unanticipated difficulties. If you are functioning in more than one role or engaging in dual relationships, it is a good policy to consult on a regular basis.
- When dual relationships are particularly problematic, or when there is a high degree of risk for harm, it is wise to work under supervision.
- It is essential that counselor educators and supervisors discuss with students and supervisees topics dealing with balance of power issues, boundary concerns, appropriate limits, purposes of the relationship, potential for abusing power, and subtle ways in which harm can result from engaging in multiple and sometimes conflicting roles.
- From a legal perspective, it is good practice to document any discussions about dual relationships with your clients in their records. Include in your notes any actions you have taken to minimize the risk of harm.
- If necessary, refer the client to another professional.

The controversy surrounding nonsexual dual relationships is likely to continue to be discussed and debated. As Herlihy and Corey (1997a) point out:

> As with any complex ethical issue, complete agreement may never be reached nor would it necessarily be desirable. However, as conscientious professionals we need to strive to clarify our own stance and develop our own guidelines for practice, within the limits of the codes of ethics and current knowledge.

Herlihy and Corey (1997a) present a decision-making model that can be applied when helpers are confronted with dual relationship issues. If the potential dual relationship is *unavoidable*, the model suggest that helpers: (1) secure informed consent of clients, (2) seek consultation, (3) document and monitor their practices, and (4) obtain supervision. If the potential dual relationship is *avoidable*, the model suggests that helpers first assess the potential benefits and risks in the case. If the benefits outweigh the risks, the relationship may be justified. However, if the risks outweigh the benefits, helpers might decline to enter the relationship, explain the rationale to the client, and offer a referral to another professional. Another alternative is for helpers to use the same procedures as suggested in dealing with unavoidable dual relationships.

As you read further about specific dual relationship issues, think about these general themes and guidelines and apply them to each situation. Ask yourself how you would proceed in resolving any ethical dilemmas over conflicting roles you may be faced with playing with the same client. What are your guidelines in these situations?

Combining Professional and Personal Relationships

You may be tempted to form social relationships with clients who admire you excessively and who invite you to develop a friendship. This lure can be especially strong if you like your client and if you have a limited circle of friends. It is easy to make the mistake of becoming socially involved with clients, for you may not have had the experience of setting limits. You may also be afraid to deal with your clients' potential feelings of rejection if you tell them that a personal or social relationship is not possible.

Certainly, attempting to balance a professional and a personal relationship with a client is a tricky business. As a helper you may not be inclined to challenge clients, lest you endanger your personal relationship with them. Or you may experience difficulty in separating yourself from your clients. Even if you are able to maintain your objectivity, provide an optimal balance between confrontation and support, and still be a therapeutic agent, your clients may have difficulty keeping the two relationships separate. One factor to consider is that no matter how you look at this issue, the relationship is bound to be unequal. The client/friend pays you for your time and attention. Even if you don't charge a fee, the relationship is still unequal, because you are likely to be doing more of the listening, giving, and challenging. In an equal friendship, both partners are giving and receiving.

Social relationships and, at times, friendships between professionals and their clients do occur. A number of factors need to be weighed in assessing whether such relationships are appropriate and ethical. Some questions to ponder are "Does the social relationship get in the way of working effectively with the client?" "Does the friendship get in the client's way of working with me?" "Am I retaining enough objectivity to determine any possible negative effects?" We do have concerns about helpers who rely on their circle of clients to make social and personal contacts. If most of their social acquaintances are people whom they serve professionally, we wonder if they are relying on their role to meet their needs.

Case example.   A client whom you have been seeing for some time asks whether you would be willing to meet for lunch. When you ask about the reason for the out-of-office meeting, your client tells you that he (she) would like to get to know you better in an informal setting and would like to treat you to lunch as an expression of appreciation for the help you have provided. To make matters a bit more difficult, one of your client's personal issues is the fear of being rejected. The client tells you that he (she) is taking a chance and a risk by asking you for lunch. How would you handle this situation? Would it make a difference whether the client was of the same or the opposite sex? Would your own feelings toward your client influence your decision?

Becoming Friends with Former Clients

Although combining personal and professional relationships with current clients is problematic at best, at least one study suggests that friendships between counselors and clients may be acceptable after termination of counseling (Salisbury &

Kinnier, 1996). A minority (33%) of counselors surveyed believed that sexual relationships with former clients might be acceptable five years after termination. In contrast, 70% of the counselors believed that friendships with former clients were acceptable two years after termination, and 33% reported that they had engaged in such friendships. The most important concern expressed by counselors in determining the circumstances under which posttermination friendships would be appropriate related to avoiding potential harm to the client. Salisbury and Kinnier state that the present ethical codes offer little guidance about friendships with former clients. They recommend that further research be conducted to delineate what constitutes friendship and to investigate how such friendships affect former clients.

In their study of nonromantic, nonsexual posttherapy relationships between psychologists and former clients, Anderson and Kitchener (1996) found little consensus regarding how ethical these contacts are. Some therapists believe that the client-therapist relationship continues in perpetuity. However, many of the participants in Anderson and Kitchener's study did not hold to the concept of "once a client, always a client" when it comes to nonsexual posttherapy relationships. The majority of therapists in this study described nonsexual relationships with former clients as being ethical, especially if there were a certain period of time since termination. Others proposed that such relationships were ethical if the former client decided not to return to therapy with the former therapist and the posttherapy relationship did not seem to hinder later therapy with different therapists.

Although making friends with former clients may not be unethical, the practice may be unwise. In the long run, former clients may need you more as a therapist at some future time than as a friend. If you develop a friendship with a former client, he or she is no longer eligible to use your professional services.

What are your thoughts about developing friendships with present or former clients? Why might you be willing to form such personal or social relationships with clients? What issues would you want to discuss with a current or former client before entering a personal relationship?

Bartering

The practice of bartering psychotherapy for goods or other services has the potential for conflicts. Glosoff, Corey, and Herlihy (1996) identify several potential pitfalls in bartering, even though the helper may have good intentions when forming this dual relationship. When clients are unable to afford the professional services of a counselor, they may suggest a barter arrangement—for example, cleaning house for the helper, performing secretarial services, or doing other personal work. Clients can easily be put in a bind when they are in a position to learn personal information about their helper. This can interfere with the helper-client relationship.

Bartering is an accepted practice in many cultures, but bartering for counseling services is especially problematic. Clients may believe that their counseling is not progressing well, implying that the helper is not following through on his or her agreement. Likewise, helpers may be dissatisfied with the lack of timeliness or the quality of goods and services delivered by clients, which can lead to resentment and ultimately interfere with efforts to provide quality help.

At the present time, most professional ethics codes have a guideline pertaining to bartering. While bartering is not prohibited outright, there are stipulations to the practice, as is clear by reviewing the following codes:

> Counselors ordinarily refrain from accepting goods or services from clients in return for counseling services because such arrangements create inherent potential for conflicts, exploitation, and distortion of the professional relationship. Counselors may participate in bartering only if the relationship is not exploitive, if the client requests it, if a clear written contract is established, and if such arrangements are an accepted practice among professionals in the community. (ACA, 1995, A.10.c.)
>
> Social workers should avoid accepting goods or services from clients as payment for professional services. Bartering arrangements, particularly involving services, create the potential for conflicts of interest, exploitation, and inappropriate boundaries in social workers' relationships with clients. Social workers should explore and may participate in bartering only in very limited circumstances where it can be demonstrated that such arrangements are an accepted practice among professionals in the local community, considered to be essential for the provision of service, negotiated without coercion and entered into at the client's initiative and with the client's informed consent. Social workers who accept goods or services from clients as payment for professional services assume the full burden of demonstrating that this arrangement will not be detrimental to the client or the professional relationship. (NASW, 1996, 1.13.b.)

Perhaps the safest course to follow as a general rule is to refrain from accepting goods or services in exchange for professional services because of the potential for conflicts, exploitation, and strains on the helping relationship. However, you will have to assess the real-life situations that confront you in your professional practice.

Case example.   For several months you have been seeing a client, Wayne, who has consistently paid for your services and who is currently making excellent progress in counseling. Wayne comes to a session very depressed because he lost his job as an auto mechanic at a large dealership. He can see no way of continuing to see you because of his other pressing financial commitments. Knowing that you had some car problems, he proposes that he do a complete engine overhaul as a way of making payment for some counseling sessions. He asks you if you would be willing to go along with this arrangement, because he really does not want to interrupt counseling at this point. On top of his other problems, he is now unemployed. Assuming that your car was in desperate need of major work, consider what you would do.

- Would you be inclined to enter into a bartering arrangement with Wayne? Why or why not?
- If so, what kind of understanding would you want to work out between you in advance? If not, would you terminate Wayne?
- Assume that you engaged in this exchange of services and that your car died on you on a busy freeway. How might this affect your work with Wayne, especially if the car problem was due to inferior work on his part?

- Assume that you told Wayne that you did not feel comfortable bartering and that he told you that he felt you were abandoning him in a time of dire need. How might you respond?

Dealing with Sexual Attractions

Some helpers feel guilty over an attraction toward a client, and they feel uncomfortable if they sense that a client is attracted to them. There is a tendency to treat sexual feelings as if they are something that shouldn't exist, which makes attractions difficult for helpers to recognize and accept. Pope, Sonne, and Holroyd (1993) maintain that the lack of research, theory, training, and opportunity to discuss sexual attractions has created a context that does not encourage helpers to explore such feelings when they occur. They add that the topic of sexual feelings in psychotherapy is surrounded by a taboo, which has created a sinister context for the helper's experience of sexual attraction. Typical reactions to sexual feelings in the helping relationship included: surprise, startle, and shock; guilt; anxiety about unresolved personal issues; fear of losing control; fear of being criticized; frustration at not being able to speak openly; frustration at not being able to make sexual contact; confusion about tasks; confusion about boundaries and roles; confusion about actions; anger at the client's sexuality; and fear over frustrating the client's demands.

In *Sexual Feelings in Psychotherapy: Explorations for Therapists and Therapists-in-Training*, Pope, Sonne, and Holroyd (1993) break the silence surrounding the taboo of acknowledging and dealing with sexual feelings in therapy. Their book is based on the following premises:

- Exploring helpers' sexual feelings and reactions should be a key aspect of training programs and continuing professional development.
- Sexual feelings must be clearly distinguished from sexual intimacies with clients.
- It is never permissible for helpers to exploit clients.
- Most helpers have experienced sexual attraction to a client, which often results in their feeling anxious, guilty, or confused.
- It is essential that helpers do not avoid recognizing and dealing with sexual attraction in the helping relationship.
- Helpers are best able to explore their feelings in a context with others that is safe, nonjudgmental, and supportive.
- Understanding sexual feelings is not a simple matter, which means that helpers need to be willing to engage in a personal, complex, and often unpredictable process of exploration.

We do not think that helpers should be distressed over experiencing sexual attractions to clients. Such attractions do not mean that they are guilty of therapeutic errors or that they are perverse. It is important, however, that helpers acknowledge their feelings and avoid acting obsessively or acting out by developing inappropriate sexual intimacies with their clients. There is a distinction between finding a client sexually attractive and being preoccupied with this attraction. It is critical for helpers to understand their behavior patterns when they become attracted to a client. Furthermore, helpers should become aware of warning signs so they can think and act in preventive ways. Gill-Wigal and Heaton (1996) identify some common reactions that may be indicative of exceeding appropriate therapeutic boundaries. Some of these helper behaviors serve as a caution:

- Wanting increased time with a particular client
- Feeling powerful when this particular client is present
- Experiencing increased pleasure with the client
- Enjoying discussion of sexual content
- Persistently engaging in sexual fantasies about the client
- Feeling sexually aroused when the client is present
- Wanting the client's approval
- Desiring physical contact with the client
- Feeling that you are the only one who can help this client
- Experiencing anxiety and guilt when thinking about the client
- Denying harm from turning a professional relationship into a sexual one

Part of learning how to deal effectively with attractions to clients involves recognizing your own feelings and taking steps to minimize the chances of an attraction interfering with the client's welfare. Gill-Wigal and Heaton (1996) recommend these strategies for managing an attraction to a client:

- Responsible management of attractions implies acknowledging that attractions must never be acted out, encouraged, or nurtured.
- Do not deny feelings of attraction, for responsible management is not possible if these feelings are disowned.
- Seek out a supervisor, a trusted colleague, or a therapist to discuss and come to a clearer understanding of your sexual attractions.
- Accept the responsibility of attending to your own therapeutic needs before your sexual feelings interfere with the progress of a client.
- Recognize that you have the responsibility for maintaining appropriate boundaries by setting clear limits.

Consider what you would do in each of the following case examples.

Case example. A single male colleague of yours tells you that he is having trouble with one of his female clients, whom he is very much attracted to. He finds himself willing to run overtime in the sessions, and if she were not a client, he would like to ask her out for a date. He is wondering if he should terminate the professional relationship and begin a personal one. He has shared with his client that he is sexually attracted to her, and she admits finding him attractive. Your colleague comes to you for your suggestions on how he should proceed. What do you think you would say to him? What do you think you would do if you found yourself in a similar situation?

Case example. In a counseling session, one of your clients discloses "finding you very sexually attractive." The client is uncomfortable making this admission and now wonders what you are thinking and feeling. If you heard this, how do you imagine it would affect you? What might you say in response to your client's concern?

Case example. One of your clients describes in great detail sexual feelings and fantasies. As you listen, you notice that you are getting uncomfortable and you begin to blush. The client notices that you are blushing and asks: "Did I say something that I shouldn't have?" How would you respond?

Implications for training programs. Stake and Oliver (1991) maintain that therapists should be prepared to respond ethically and therapeutically when they feel sexually attracted to their clients or when their clients express attraction for them. According to Pope, Keith-Spiegel, and Tabachnick (1986), a training program must acknowledge the need to prepare trainees to deal with sexual attractions in therapy. The taboo must be lifted so that therapy trainees can recognize and accept their sexual attractions as human responses. If this is not done, trainees are likely to think there is something very unprofessional about any sexual attractions they may experience.

Pope and his colleagues (1986) found clear evidence that attraction to clients is prevalent among both male and female therapists. Although most of the respondents (87%) reported having been sexually attracted to clients, the vast majority (82%) reported that they had never seriously considered actual sexual involvement with a client. Some of the reasons they gave for refraining from acting out their attractions to clients related to their professional values and their concern for the welfare of the client. Although acting on sexual feelings with clients appears to occur in relatively few cases, most practitioners reported feeling guilty, anxious, or confused about the attraction. However, 69% assumed that their feelings of sexual attraction may have some beneficial aspects in a professional relationship. Only 9% of the respondents believed that they had received adequate preparation in their graduate training to deal effectively with sexual attractions.

Pope and Vasquez (1991) stated that "to feel attraction to a client is not unethical; to acknowledge and address the attraction promptly, carefully, and adequately is an important ethical responsibility" (p. 107). They add that the practices of consulting with colleagues, obtaining supervision, and seeking our own therapy are useful ways to deal with sexual attractions. In a like manner, Bartell and Rubin (1990) have taken the position that education can play a crucial role in helping trainees be better prepared to recognize and monitor sexual attraction and to take the steps needed to avoid acting on such attractions. Bartell and Rubin advocate that injunctions against sexual relationships be well publicized as a way to eliminate dangerous liaisons in professional relationships.

Rodolfa, Kitzrow, Vohra, and Wilson (1990) have developed a training program that focuses on the personal, professional, ethical, and legal dimensions of sexual attractions in helping relationships. Their program helps interns examine the differences between being attracted to clients and acting out sexually with them. The authors acknowledged that most practitioners are bound to encounter sexual dilemmas during their careers and suggested that programs include formal training in learning how to deal with sexual attractions.

In light of the literature on the challenges of dealing with the reality of sexual attractions in the helping process, Herlihy and Corey (1997a) recommend that graduate programs in the counseling and human development fields place increased emphasis on the issue of sexual attraction. Helpers need to be assured that their feelings are natural and that with awareness they can learn to provide professional assistance to clients, even if they might experience sexual attraction at times. Herlihy and Corey stress the value of learning to monitor your own countertransference, consulting with colleagues, and being alert to the subtle ways that sexual attractions can cross the boundary into an inappropriate dual relationship. Ignoring this subject in programs conveys the message that this topic is unimportant, and it also interferes with the potential effectiveness of helpers.

Sexual Relationships with Current Clients

Research indicates that sexual misconduct is one of the major causes for malpractice actions against mental-health providers. Those who have studied the sexual relationships between helpers and clients generally report that such misconduct is more widespread than is commonly believed. Sonne and Pope (1991) report that clients who had been sexually involved with their therapists tended to exhibit reactions similar to those of survivors of incest and rape, including intense feelings of betrayal, confusion, and guilt. Pope and Vasquez (1991) have noted a fairly consistent decrease in the self-reported rate of sexual involvement with clients. They cautioned that this trend may reflect either a genuine decrease or increasingly less candid reporting.

In the last few years the greatest single category of complaints to the ethics committee of the APA involved sexual relationships. Judgments against therapists, dismissal of professors, revocation of licenses, and large damage awards are no longer unusual. The literature shows that sexual relationships with clients carry serious consequences in both ethical and legal terms.

As you read this, you may think that you would never become involved in sexual misconduct with any of your clients. The chances are that those practitioners who have engaged in sexual intimacies with clients made the same assumption. Realize that you are not immune to becoming sexually involved with those you help. Knowledge of the possibility of this involvement will at least allow you to be on the alert to your own needs and motivations and how they could get in the way of your work.

As a helper you are likely to receive respect and adulation and to be perceived as someone who can do no wrong. Clients may compare you with their significant others, and many times you will rank higher. Your clients are usually with you for a short time, and they are probably getting the best side of you. This unconditional admiration can become very seductive. You may learn to like their reactions to you too much. You can get in trouble as a helper if you cease to keep the feelings that your clients express to you in proper perspective.

As a beginning helper you are especially vulnerable to believing everything positive that your clients tell you about yourself. Thus, if clients tell you how sexually attractive you are, how understanding you are, and how different you are from anyone else they have met, it may be difficult to resist believing what they say. Without self-awareness and honesty, you may direct the sessions toward meeting your needs and may eventually become sexually indiscreet.

All of the professional organizations have some specific statement that condemns sexual intimacies in the client-therapist relationship. In addition to specifically prohibiting erotic contact, most codes of ethics warn against any activities on the helper's part that could lead to the risk of exploitation. If a client-helper relationship develops into a sexual one, most professional codes require termination of the relationship and a referral to another professional. The reasons that erotic contact is unethical center on the power that helpers have by virtue of their professional role. Because clients are talking about very personal aspects of their lives and making themselves highly vulnerable, it is easy to betray this trust by exploiting clients for your own personal motives. Erotic contact is also unethical because it fosters dependency and makes objectivity on the part of the helper impossible.

Perhaps the most important argument against sexual involvement with clients is that most clients report harm as a result. They typically become resentful and angry at having been sexually exploited and abandoned. They generally feel stuck with both unresolved problems and unresolved feelings relating to the traumatic experience.

Sexual Relationships with Former Clients

There is a trend for professional codes to specifically caution helpers against forming romantic relationships with former clients for at least two years after termination. This does not imply that such relationships with clients are ethical or professional after two years have elapsed. In fact, the codes of ACA (1995), NASW (1996), AAMFT (1991), and APA (1995) are quite specific about conditions pertaining to relationships with former clients. For example, it is not considered ethical to terminate with a client because of an attraction, wait the time period, and then begin a romantic relationship. Even after two years, it is incumbent upon helpers to examine their motivations, to continually consider what is best for the former client, and to be extremely careful to avoid any form of exploitation. In the exceptional circumstance of a sexual relationship with a former client after a two-year interval, the burden of demonstrating that there has been no exploitation clearly rests with the practitioner. The factors that must be considered include: the amount of time that has passed since termination of therapy; the nature and duration of therapy; the circumstances surrounding termination of the professional-client relationship; the client's personal history; the client's competence and mental status; the foreseeable likelihood of harm to the client or others; and any statements or actions of the helper suggesting a romantic relationship after terminating the professional relationship. The professional codes pertaining to sexual contact with former clients are explicit:

> Counselors do not engage in sexual intimacies with former clients within a minimum of 2 years after terminating the counseling relationship. Counselors who engage in such relationships after 2 years following termination have the

responsibility to examine and document thoroughly that such relations did not have an exploitative nature, based on factors such as duration of counseling, amount of time since counseling, circumstances of termination, client's personal history and mental status, adverse impact on the client, and actions by the counselor suggesting a plan to initiate a sexual relationship with the client after termination. (ACA, 1995, A.7.b.)

Social workers should not engage in sexual activities or sexual contact with former clients because of the potential for harm to the client. If social workers engage in conduct contrary to this prohibition or claim that an exception to this prohibition is warranted due to extraordinary circumstances, it is social workers—not their clients—who assume the full burden of demonstrating that the former client has not been exploited, coerced, or manipulated, intentionally or unintentionally. (NASW, 1996, 1.09.c.)

In discussing the ethics of sexual contact with former clients, Glosoff, Corey, and Herlihy (1996) point out that the topic is being extensively debated within the helping professions. Most agree that simply because a helping relationship is terminated, in and of itself, does not justify changing the professional relationship into a sexual one. The fact that the counseling relationship has been terminated does not present an adequate defense against charges of an ethical violation. Under the present ethics codes, if a helper considers getting romantically involved with a former client after two years have passed, a wise course to follow would be to consult with a colleague or seek a therapy session conjointly with the former client to explore mutual transferences and expectations. It is essential to remain aware of the potential harm that can result from sexual intimacies that occur after termination, of the aspects of the therapeutic process that continue after termination including residual transference, and of the continuing power differential (Herlihy & Corey, 1997a). If there are grounds to believe that treatment is ending to give the appearance of compliance with the ethical proscription against sexual intimacies between client and therapist, ethics committees will find that there has been a clear violation (Gottlieb, 1990).

From a legal perspective, several states prohibit sexual intimacies with former clients for one or two years after termination of therapy. Some professionals contend that the counselor-client relationship potentially continues for a long period of time, even after termination, which means that sexual relationships with former clients are unethical. This argument centers on the power imbalance in the helping relationship and the potential for exploitation, even after the professional relationship ends.

If you were a member of a committee with the task of revising ethical codes, what input would you have regarding the appropriateness of social, sexual, business, and professional relationships with former clients? Do you think that each of these relationships should be considered unethical under some or most circumstances? Can you think of exceptions? Can you think of situations where you might accept a social invitation from a former client? Would you see it as appropriate to engage in a business relationship with a former client? Can you think of any times when you might form professional relationships with former clients? In developing guidelines for your own practice, where would you begin in defining appropriate relationships with former clients?

Dual Relationships with Supervisors or Teachers

Those who teach or supervise students in the helping professions owe students and trainees the same kind of explanations they owe clients about the potential problems involved in dual relationships. The *Code of Ethics* of ACA (1995) deals directly and clearly with dual relationships in teaching and supervisory relationships. It is the responsibility of counselor educators and clinical supervisors to create and maintain appropriate relationship boundaries with students and trainees. Specifically, professionals in charge of educating and supervising students avoid engaging in sexual relationships with students or supervisees and avoid subjecting them to any form of sexual harassment. In addition, supervisors or counselor educators do not serve as counselors to students or supervisees over whom they have administrative, teaching, or evaluative roles—*unless* this is a brief role associated with a training experience. Although supervisors do have the responsibility to help trainees understand how their personal issues may interfere with working effectively with clients, it is not appropriate for supervisors to change the supervisory function to a therapy function.

We want to briefly discuss some ethical issues pertaining to sexual and romantic relationships between students and instructors, as well as between supervisors and supervisees. Not only are such relationships unethical, but they generally result in harm to students or supervisees. If a sexual relationship enters into a supervisory relationship, the entire process is confounded. The chances are that supervisees will not get the supervision they need if they are romantically involved with their supervisors (Herlihy & Corey, 1997a).

Sex in the supervisory relationship or in the professor-student relationship typically results in an abuse of power because of the role differences. The student is extremely vulnerable because of this difference in status. Faced with a faculty member who makes a sexual proposition, the student is likely to feel intimidated by the person with power. Students and interns recognize that their decision to reject a sexual proposition might well have a negative effect on their current performance. There is also the reality of poor modeling for students for their future relationships with their clients.

In a survey of the beliefs and behaviors of psychologists as educators, Tabachnick, Keith-Spiegel, and Pope (1991) identified several interesting findings:

- With respect to *educators who date their students,* 80% reported the *belief* that this behavior was never or only rarely ethical; 95% reported that they never or rarely engaged in this *behavior.*
- On the issue of *becoming sexually involved with students,* 91% reported the *belief* that such behavior was never or only rarely ethical; 99% reported that they had never or only rarely engaged in this *behavior.*
- On the issue of *being sexually attracted to a student,* 27% reported the *belief* that this behavior was never or only rarely ethical; 71% said that they had never or only rarely engaged in this *behavior.*

These researchers acknowledge that keeping clear boundaries appears to be a problem in academic settings. Their findings indicate that social and sexual relationships between faculty and students remain a problematic issue. It appears that sexual harassment is prevalent in academic settings (Hotelling, 1991; Riger, 1991).

As students, you have a right to expect a learning environment free from sexual harassment, both in the classroom and at your field placement. Ideally, you should not be expected to deal with situations involving unwanted sexual advances from those who function in teaching, supervisory, or consulting roles. Realistically, however, you need to know what to do in the event that you are faced with sexual harassment. Most agencies and institutions of higher education have specific policies regarding sexual harassment, as well as procedures to follow if you feel that you are subject to it.

Recognizing Unethical Behavior in Yourself

We encourage you to apply the general principles being discussed in this chapter to your own behavior rather than placing yourself in a judgmental position toward others. It is easier to see the shortcomings of others and to judge their behavior than to develop the attitude of honest self-examination. You can control your own professional behavior far more easily than you can that of your colleagues, so the proper focus is to look honestly at what you are doing. There is a tendency to think in terms of gross ethical violations while overlooking more subtle ways of being unethical. Consider for a moment some of the following behaviors, and ask yourself the degree to which you could picture yourself in each situation:

- A client calls you frequently and pleads that he is in great need of your direction. He is afraid to make decisions lest "I mess up my life even more than it is." Might you be flattered by being needed? Could you see yourself fostering his dependency out of your need to be needed?
- A client who is in private therapy with you is ambivalent about continuing counseling sessions. She wonders whether it is time to terminate and "try it alone." Things are rather tight financially for you right now, and several other clients have recently terminated. Would you be inclined to support her decision? Might you be inclined to encourage her to continue, partly out of financial motives?
- A client whom you find attractive tells you how accepting, kind, gentle, understanding, and strong you are. This client expresses a desire to hear more about your life. Might you take the focus off the client and engage in self-disclosure for your own needs? Could you see yourself getting carried away with personal conversations that are really not relevant to the therapeutic purpose of your relationship?

Unethical Behavior by Your Colleagues

Even though you do focus on being your own judge, there are times when you may encounter colleagues who are behaving in unethical and unprofessional ways. Professional codes of conduct generally state that in such cases the most prudent action is to approach the colleague and share your concerns directly in an attempt to rectify the situation. If this step fails, you are then expected to make use of procedures established by your professional organization, such as reporting the colleague.

Reflect for a few minutes on being in each of the following situations. Attempt to formulate what you would do in each case:

- A colleague frequently talks about his clients in inappropriate ways in places where others are able to hear him. The colleague says that joking about his clients is his way of "letting off steam" and preventing himself from taking life too seriously.
- A couple of female clients have told you that they were sexually seduced by another counselor at the agency where you work. In their counseling sessions with you, they are dealing with their anger over having been taken advantage of by this counselor.
- A colleague has several times initiated social contacts with her clients. She thinks that this practice is acceptable, because she sees her clients as consenting adults. Furthermore, she contends that time spent socializing with these clients gives her insights into issues with which she can productively work in the therapy sessions.
- You see that one of your colleagues is practicing beyond what you think is the scope of his competence and training. This person is unwilling to seek additional training and is also not receiving adequate supervision. He maintains that the best way to learn to work with unfamiliar problems that clients present is simply to "jump in and learn by doing."

Certainly, dealing with the unethical behavior of colleagues demands a measure of courage. If these people are in a position of power, you are obviously vulnerable. Even in the case of peers, confrontations may not be pleasant. The other person may react defensively and tell you to mind your own business.

ETHICAL AND LEGAL STANDARDS

Most professional organizations affirm that practitioners should be aware of the prevailing community standards and of the possible impact on their practice of deviation from these standards. Ethical and legal issues are frequently intertwined, which makes it imperative not only that practitioners follow the ethical codes of their profession but also that they know their state's laws and that they know their legal boundaries and responsibilities.

Ethical standards are different from legal standards. In the professional codes of ethics, standards of conduct usually describe the best practices of professionals. The aim is to ensure high quality of practice rather than to establish minimal standards of professional behavior. The codes of ethics are aspirational, which entails understanding the spirit behind the code and the principles on which it rests. Legal standards are minimal in nature and are enforced by the government. The government can order citizens to comply with legal standards and may punish those who refuse. Counselors must know and follow the law in their work with clients. In addition to acting in accordance with the laws and following the ethical codes of their profession, helpers agree to abide by the rules and regulations that have been established in their work setting. When helpers have problems relating to legal issues, they should seek legal advice. Colleagues and experts should be consulted for ethical issues (Remley, 1996).

Helpers who work with minors and certain involuntary populations are especially advised to learn the laws restricting their practices. Areas that may be governed by law include confidentiality, parental consent, informed consent, protection of client welfare, and civil rights of institutionalized persons. Because most helpers do not possess detailed legal knowledge, it is a good idea for helpers to obtain some legal advice about the procedures they use and their practices. Awareness of legal rights and responsibilities as they pertain to helping relationships protects not only the clients but also practitioners from needless lawsuits arising from negligence or ignorance.

MALPRACTICE IN THE HELPING PROFESSIONS

Malpractice is generally defined as the failure to render proper service, through ignorance or negligence, resulting in injury or loss to the client. Professional negligence consists of departing from the usual standard of practice or not exercising due care. For a malpractice suit to be filed against you, these three conditions must be present: (1) you must have a duty to the client, (2) you must have acted in a negligent or improper manner, and (3) there must be a causal relationship between that negligence and the damage claimed by the client.

Grounds for Malpractice Actions

The two areas that have probably received the greatest attention in the literature as grounds for malpractice are violations of confidentiality and sexual misconduct. (Both of these topics have been discussed in earlier sections of this chapter.) A review of articles dealing with frequent causes of malpractice actions against people in the helping professions shows the following as other key factors leading to a suit:

- Abandoning a client
- Failure to respect the client's integrity and privacy
- Improper death of a client
- Failure to supervise properly
- Failure to refer a client when the case warrants it
- Failure to protect others from a dangerous client
- Improper methods of collecting fees
- Misrepresenting one's professional training and skills
- Improper diagnosis and utilization of assessment techniques
- Breaching a contract with a client
- Failure to provide for informed consent
- Failure to have exercised reasonable care in cases of suicide

Other grounds for malpractice charges exist; this list simply describes actions that often lead to malpractice suits.

If you are a student, you may think that you have no worries about being sued for malpractice. Unfortunately, student practitioners are vulnerable to such action. At this time in your professional development you might well give serious consideration to ways in which you can lessen your chances of being sued for failing to practice in a professional manner. The reality of today is that even if you abide by the ethical codes of your profession and even if you practice within the boundaries of the law, you can still become embroiled in a malpractice action.

Case example.   One of your teenage clients might eventually commit suicide, regardless of how prudent your interventions have been. It is possible that the parents could fault you for not having known more and done more to prevent this final action. Although you do not have to prove that you are a superior or perfect being, you do have to demonstrate that you possess and exercise the knowledge and skill required for the services you offer. The questions that you might ask yourself are "Do I have to be able to predict a possible suicide? Assuming that I am able to spot a suicidal client, will I always know the best course of action to take?" You must be able to demonstrate that you acted in good faith, that you have been willing to seek supervision and consultation when needed, and that you have practiced within your competence. It is also essential that you can produce documentation to support your claims.

Ways to Prevent Malpractice Suits

We hope it is becoming clear that you would be wise to know your limitations in working with clients, to accept them, and to act only within the scope of your competence. Although making the best decision in every case is not always possible, we hope you will never hesitate to seek consultation, regardless of your professional experience. Consultation with colleagues often sheds light on a subject by providing a new and different perspective. Even if you are able to make wise decisions, it is validating to get support for your position from other professionals. If you are involved in litigation, it will be helpful to be able to demonstrate that your interventions were in accord with the standard of care exercised by other practitioners. If you employ exotic therapeutic techniques with little rationale behind them, you are likely to find yourself the loser in a civil action. Contending that you were following your instincts and doing what "felt right" is not likely to get you very far if you are asked to defend your therapeutic practices.

If you want a guarantee that you will not be sued for professional negligence, you probably should think about another career. Although there are no absolute protections in the mental-health professions, there are some practical ways to protect yourself from malpractice suits. In addition to the ways we have mentioned, here are some further guidelines:

- Make use of informed-consent procedures. Do not attempt to mystify the helping process. Professional honesty and openness with clients will go a long way in establishing genuine trust.

- Consider ways to define contracts with your clients that clearly structure the helping relationship. What are your clients coming to you for? How can you best help them obtain their goals?
- Because you can be sued for abandonment, take steps to provide coverage for emergencies when you are going away.
- Restrict your practice to client populations for which you are prepared by virtue of your education, training, and experience.
- Take steps to maintain your competence.
- At the outset of therapy, clearly define issues pertaining to fees.
- Carefully document a client's treatment plan.
- Become aware of local and state laws that limit your practice, as well as the policies of the agency you work for. Keep abreast of legal and ethical changes by becoming involved in professional organizations.
- Confidentiality must be maintained except in those cases where it is contraindicated. Be aware of the limits of confidentiality, and clearly communicate these to your clients. Attempt to obtain written consent whenever disclosure becomes necessary.
- Report any case of suspected child abuse as required by law.
- If you make a professional determination that a client is a danger to self or others, take the necessary steps to protect the client or others from harm.
- Do not barter services, except in cases where this is the cultural norm or where bartering is initiated by the client. Exchanging services is likely to lead to resentment on both your part and your client's.
- Avoid engaging in sexual relationships with either current or former clients or with supervisees or students.
- A dual relationship may occur whenever you interact with a client in more than one capacity. Be aware of your position of power, and avoid even the appearance of conflict of interest.
- Although you can be friendly and personal with clients, your relationships should be primarily professional.
- Treat your clients with respect by attending carefully to your language and your behavior. This practice generally leads to good relationships.
- Obtain written parental consent when working with minors. This is generally a good practice, even if not required by state law.
- Develop a diagnostic profile, and keep relevant notes on each client.
- Make it a practice to consult with colleagues or clinical supervisors whenever there is a potential ethical or legal concern. Find sources of ongoing supervision.
- Have a clear rationale for the techniques you use. Be able to intelligently and concisely discuss the theoretical underpinnings of your procedures.
- Have a clear standard of care that can be applied to your services, and communicate this standard to your clients.
- Don't promise clients anything that you can't deliver. Help them realize that their effort and commitment will be key factors in determining the outcomes of the helping process.
- If you work for an agency or institution, have a contract that specifies the employer's legal liability for your professional functioning.
- Abide by the policies of the institution that employs you. If you disagree with certain policies, first attempt to find out the reasons for them. Then

see if it is possible to work within the framework of institutional policies. Realize that you do not always have to agree with such policies to be able to work effectively.

- Adhere to billing regulations and paperwork requirements as prescribed.
- Make it a practice to assess the progress your clients are making, and teach them how to evaluate their progress toward their goals.
- Carry malpractice insurance. Students are not protected against malpractice suits.

These guidelines will lessen the chances of a malpractice suit, but we encourage you to continually assess your practices and keep up-to-date on legal, ethical, and community standards affecting your work setting and client populations. An excellent resource on malpractice issues is Austin, Moline, and Williams (1990).

A Word of Caution

Students sometimes burden themselves with the unrealistic expectation that they should have ready-made answers for the ethical issues we raise in this chapter. Quite the contrary is true. Indeed, seasoned professionals are aware that the complex nature of their work with people defies neat and absolute answers. They have an appreciation of the necessity for continuing learning, ongoing consultation and supervision, and for remaining humble.

Our intention has not been to overwhelm you but to stimulate you to develop habits of thinking and acting that will enhance your ability to base your practice on ethical and professional principles. Working in the helping professions is a risky as well as a rewarding venture. You are bound to make mistakes from time to time. Be willing to acknowledge those mistakes and learn from them. Make full use of supervision; you will not only learn from what may seem like mistakes but you will also minimize the chances of harming clients.

We hope you won't be frozen with anxiety over needing to be all-knowing at all times—or afraid to intervene for fear of becoming embroiled in a lawsuit. Perhaps the best way to prevent a malpractice action is by having a sincere interest in doing what is going to benefit your client. We encourage you to ask yourself throughout your professional career: "*What* am I doing, and *why* am I doing it?"

BY WAY OF REVIEW

- One of the trends in the helping professions is an increased interest in ethical and professional practice. This trend stems, at least in part, from a rise in malpractice actions against mental-health practitioners.
- Ethical decision making is a continuing process. Issues that you look at as a student can be examined from another perspective as you gain experience in your professional specialty.
- Ethical issues rarely have clear-cut answers. Ethical dilemmas, by their very nature, involve the application of professional judgment on your part. It is essential that you be familiar with the professional codes of ethics.

However, knowledge of ethical standards is not sufficient in solving ethical problems.

- Ultimately, you will have to make many difficult decisions as a practitioner. Responsible practice entails basing your actions on informed, sound, and responsible judgment. Be open to consulting with colleagues and supervisors throughout your professional career.
- Most of the professional codes explicitly state that it is unethical to practice outside the boundaries of your competence. It is important to learn what clients you can best work with and to understand when referral is appropriate.
- Either as an intern or on your job, you may be asked to take on clients or to provide therapeutic strategies that are beyond the scope of your training and experience. Learn to be assertive in staying within your limits.
- One way to increase your competence is by seeking supervision whenever it is called for and by remaining open throughout your professional career to learning new skills and techniques. Remember that continuing education is necessary to keep abreast of current developments in your field.
- Many clients have not even thought about their rights or responsibilities. As a helper you can do much to safeguard your clients by developing informed-consent procedures to help them make wise choices.
- Confidentiality is the cornerstone of the helping relationship. Although clients have a right to expect that what they talk about with you in the professional relationship will remain private, there are times when you will have to breach confidentiality. Clients have a right to know from the outset of the relationship the specific grounds for divulging confidences. It is essential that you know and follow the laws pertaining to confidentiality.
- Confidentiality takes on special meaning if you work with couples, families, or groups.
- At times you will have a professional and legal obligation to warn and to protect clients. It is essential that you know your duties in this area.
- It helps to keep your relationships with your clients on a professional, rather than a personal, basis. Mixing social relationships with professional relationships often works against the best interests of both the client and the helper.
- Your job is to teach clients how to help themselves and thus decrease their need to continue seeing you. Encouraging dependency in your clients is both unethical and untherapeutic.
- Sexual attractions are a normal part of helping relationships. It is important to learn how to recognize these attractions and how to deal with them in a therapeutic manner.
- Sexual misconduct is the leading cause of malpractice actions against mental-health providers. Sexual intimacies between helpers and clients are unethical for a number of reasons. One of the main ones is that they entail an abuse of power and trust.
- Sexual relationships between supervisors and supervisees or professors and students are unethical because of the harm that they typically do to the students or supervisees. Such relationships represent a clear misuse of power and also confound the supervisory or learning process.

- Although it is important to know how to deal with unethical behavior on the part of your colleagues, it is even more important to recognize your own potential unethical behaviors. These unethical acts are often subtle. Maintain a stance of honest self-exploration to ensure ethical behavior.
- Malpractice actions are on the increase. Not only are mental-health professionals being sued with increasing frequency but as a student you are also vulnerable. It is essential, therefore, that you understand what can lead to being sued and learn practical ways to lessen the chances of this happening.

WHAT WILL YOU DO NOW?

1. Find at least one person in the helping professions to whom you can talk about ethical issues in practice. Focus on the major ethical problem that this person has faced. How does this helper deal with this ethical concern?

2. Visit a community agency (such as a Child Protective Service) and ask about ethical and legal situations that are being reported. What are some key ethical concerns with which this agency has to cope? Are the staff members concerned about malpractice issues? How does the current malpractice crisis influence what they do in their agency?

3. Think about a particular ethical dilemma that you have experienced in one of your field placements. How did you deal with the situation? If you could replay the situation, would you do anything differently?

4. Look over the inventory of ethical issues at the beginning of this chapter and some of the case examples given throughout this chapter. Select what you consider to be the most pressing ethical issues you expect to face, and write about your concerns and ideas in your journal. If you are involved in fieldwork, keep journal entries about any potential ethical dilemmas, and bring your concerns to your supervision sessions or class meetings. You might write down specific ways you can increase your likelihood of becoming an ethical practitioner. What can you do now to move in this direction?

5. For the full bibliographic entry for each of the sources listed below, consult the References and Reading List at the back of the book.

For a useful handbook on the grounds for malpractice suits in the mental-health professions, see Austin, Moline, and Williams (1990). For a casebook geared to the ACA's code of ethics, see Herlihy and Corey (1996a). For a casebook geared to the APA's ethics code, see Canter, Bennett, Jones, and Nagy (1994). For a comprehensive handbook that deals with a wide range of topics in ethics, see Bersoff (1995). Consult Corey, Corey, and Callanan (1998) for a textbook dealing with ethical issues in the helping professions. Refer to the following journal articles in *The Counseling Psychologist* special volume on ethics: Meara, Schmidt, and Day (1996), Bersoff (1996), Ibrahim (1996), Kitchener (1996), and Vasquez (1996). For a treatment of many facets of the dual relationship controversy, see Herlihy and Corey (1997a) and Corey and Herlihy (1997).

Chapter 6

Values and the Helping Relationship

FOCUS QUESTIONS

1. Are you aware of your key values and of how they are likely to affect the way you work with clients?
2. Is it possible for you to interact with your clients without making value judgments? Do you think it is sometimes appropriate to make value judgments? If so, when?
3. Can you remain true to your own values and at the same time make allowances for the right of your clients to make their own choices, even if they differ from the ones you might make?
4. Do you have a need to push what you think is right on your friends and your family? If so, what are the implications for the way you are likely to function as a helper with your clients?
5. Are you able to make the distinction between exposing your values and imposing them?
6. Do you see it as your job to make decisions for clients, or is it your job to help your clients make their own decisions?
7. Are you able to give your clients the latitude to make their own decisions, even if you believe that they would be better served by following a different path?
8. How can you best determine whether a conflict between your values and those of a client dictates a referral to another professional?
9. When you become aware of difficulties in working with clients because of value differences, what is the appropriate course of action?
10. What basic values serve as the foundation for the helping process? Can you identify certain key values that are an essential part of effective helping? How would you communicate such values to your clients?

AIM OF THE CHAPTER

This chapter is designed to help you clarify your values and identify how they are likely to influence your work as a helper. Toward this end, we explore how values operate in the helping relationship and process. Our focus is on the critical distinction between making your values known to a client and indoctrinating him or her with a particular ethical code or philosophy of life. To assist you in clarifying your values and identifying ways in which they might interfere with effective helping, we describe practical situations about which you may find yourself perplexed.

Conflicts between clients and helpers often surface in situations involving sexual orientation, family values, sex-role behaviors, religious values, the issue of abortion, and sexual values. Value issues pertaining to multicultural populations are so important that we devote the next chapter to this subject.

THE ROLE OF VALUES IN HELPING

Although the professional literature reveals an interest in the role values play in the helping process, no consensus has been reached on which values are essential to helping or on how values should be used in the helping relationship (Bergin, 1991). Bergin compares the helping process to what occurs with effective parenting: After trust has been established in the relationship, helpers deal with values in a respectful way and offer guidance that allows for growth. Through the helping relationship, clients learn how to clarify and test their value choices, and they experiment with new behaviors and ideas until they become more mature and autonomous. As the person receiving help becomes stronger and more independent, the helper reduces external guidance. Helpers do not do for their clients what the clients are able to do for themselves.

Values are embedded in therapeutic theory and practice. What are some of the basic values that constitute the foundation of the helping process? A national survey of the mental-health values of practitioners (Jensen & Bergin, 1988) found a consensus that certain basic values are important for maintaining mentally healthy lifestyles and for guiding and evaluating the course of treatment. They include assuming responsibility for one's actions; developing effective strategies for coping with stress; developing the ability to give and receive affection; being sensitive to the feelings of others; practicing self-control; having a sense of purpose for living; being open, honest, and genuine; finding satisfaction in one's work; having a sense of identity and feelings of worth; being skilled in interpersonal relationships, sensitivity, and nurturance; being committed in marriage, family, and other relationships; having deepened self-awareness and motivation for growth; and practicing good habits of physical health. These values might be seen as universal ones on which helping relationships are based.

We suggest that you take the following self-inventory as a way of focusing your thinking on the role that your values will play in your work. As you read the following statements, decide the degree to which each most closely identifies your attitudes and beliefs about *your role as a helper*. Use this code: 3 = this statement is true for me; 2 = this statement is not true for me; 1 = I am undecided.

_____ 1. I see it as my job to challenge a client's philosophy of life.
_____ 2. I could work objectively and effectively with clients who had values that differed sharply from my own.
_____ 3. I see it as both possible and desirable for me to remain neutral with respect to values when working with clients.
_____ 4. Although I have a clear set of values for myself, I feel quite certain that I could avoid unduly influencing my clients to adopt my beliefs.

_____ 5. I think it is appropriate to express my views and expose my values, so long as I don't impose them on clients.

_____ 6. I might be inclined to subtly influence my clients to consider my values.

_____ 7. If I discovered sharp value conflicts between a client and myself, I would refer the person.

_____ 8. I have certain religious views that would influence the way I work.

_____ 9. I would not have any difficulty counseling a pregnant adolescent who wanted to explore abortion as one of her alternatives.

_____ 10. I have certain views pertaining to gender roles that might affect the way I counsel.

_____ 11. I would not have problems counseling a gay couple.

_____ 12. I see the clarification of values as the central task of the helping process.

_____ 13. My view of family life would influence the way I'd counsel a couple considering divorce.

_____ 14. I would have no trouble working with a woman (man) who wanted to leave her (his) children and live alone, if this is what my client decided.

_____ 15. I have generally been willing to challenge my values, and I think I have largely chosen them for myself.

_____ 16. I would have no trouble working in individual counseling with a married client who was having an affair, even if the client was not willing to disclose the relationship to his or her spouse.

_____ 17. I feel quite certain that my values will never interfere with my capacity to remain objective.

_____ 18. I think I will work best with clients who have values similar to mine.

_____ 19. I would be very willing to share my specific values on a given issue anytime a client asked me to do so.

_____ 20. I could work effectively with a person with AIDS who contracted the disease through IV drug use.

There are no "right" or "wrong" answers to these statements. The inventory is designed to help you think about how your values are likely to influence the way you carry out your functions as a helper. You might take some specific items that catch your attention and talk with a fellow student about your views. As you read the rest of the chapter, assume an active stance, and think about your position on the value issues we raise. A basic question is whether it is possible for helpers to keep their values out of their work.

EXPOSING VALUES VERSUS IMPOSING THEM

The clients with whom you work ultimately have the responsibility of choosing what values to adopt, what values to modify or discard, and what direction their lives will take. Through the helping process, clients can learn to examine values before making choices. You can play a significant role as a catalyst for this examination if you do not either conceal your values from your clients or try to impose your values on them.

Patterson (1989) makes several arguments against indoctrinating clients or attempting to inculcate a value system or a philosophy of life in them:

- Although people do share in some universally accepted values, each individual is unique. Therefore, each person's philosophy of life is unique.
- It is the individual's responsibility to develop this philosophy of life from many sources.
- It is unrealistic to expect that all counselors will have a fully developed and ideal philosophy of life ready to be impressed on clients.
- It is doubtful that the helping relationship is the appropriate place for instruction in ethics.
- Individuals typically do not adopt a system or code of ethics from one source at a particular time.

Patterson rightly emphasizes that because the values helpers hold cannot be kept out of their work, they should not refuse to discuss their core values. He believes that it is appropriate for them to make their values known when a client requests it, when they determine that it is necessary or desirable, or when they judge that the therapeutic relationship or process will be improved by it.

Bergin (1991) writes that the real challenge is to preserve client autonomy and simultaneously manage the inevitable value issues that emerge during treatment. He reminds us that it is unethical to trample on the values of clients and that it is a mistake to focus on a particular value issue when another issue may be at the heart of a client's problem. Bergin encourages helpers to develop a stance of openness about values with their clients.

Even if you think it is inappropriate to impose your values on clients, you may unintentionally influence them in subtle ways to embrace your values. The strategies you use provide your clients with clues to what you value. Your body messages give them indications of when you like or dislike what they are doing. Because your clients may feel a need to have your approval, they may respond to these clues by acting in ways that they imagine will meet with your favor instead of developing their own inner direction.

In addition to your own personal values, the helping professions have a set of core values. The NASW *Code of Ethics* (1996) cites these core values:

- *Service:* Social workers' primary goal is to help people in need and to address social problems.
- *Social justice:* Social workers challenge social injustice.
- *Dignity and worth of the person:* Social workers respect the inherent dignity and worth of the person.
- *Human relationships:* Social workers recognize the central importance of human relationships.
- *Integrity:* Social workers behave in a trustworthy manner.
- *Competence:* Social workers practice within their areas of competence and develop and enhance their professional expertise.

These core values serve as the foundation of social work's unique purpose and perspective.

The American Counseling Association recognizes the importance of being aware of your personal values: "Counselors are aware of their own values, attitudes, beliefs, and behaviors and how they apply in a diverse society, and avoid imposing their values on clients" (ACA, 1995, A.5.b.).

Guidelines such as these make it clear that helpers have personal values that influence their professional work. From an ethical perspective, it is imperative that helpers learn the difference between imposing and exposing values.

Our Perspective on Values in the Helping Relationship

In our view it is neither possible nor desirable for helpers to remain neutral or to keep their values separate from their professional relationships. Because values have a significant impact on the helping process, it is important to express them openly when it is appropriate. If you pay attention to your clients and why they are coming to see you, you will have clues to when that is.

There are certainly helpers who do not agree with our position about the role of values. On one extreme are those who see helping as very much a process of social influence. Some helpers, for example, have definite and absolute value systems, and they believe it is their proper function to influence their clients to adopt this view of the world. At the other extreme are helpers who are so concerned about unduly influencing their clients that they remain scrupulously neutral. Out of fear that their views might contaminate the client's decision, these helpers make it a practice not to expose their values. Or they err by assuming that the nonimposition of values means that they do not commit themselves to any set of values, when, in fact, some values are fundamental to the healing process.

Our position is that the helper's main task is to provide those who seek aid with the impetus needed to look at what they are doing, determine the degree to which what they are doing is consistent with their values, and consider whether their current behavior is getting them what they want. If clients conclude that their lives are not fulfilled, they can use the helping relationship to reexamine and modify their values or their actions, and they can explore a range of options that are open to them. Clients must ask themselves who and what they are, and they are the ones who will determine what they are willing to change.

Are Your Values Showing?

As a beginning helper, you may have a tendency to push your values. If you are strongly opposed to abortion, for example, you may not even consider that your client has a right to believe differently. On the basis of such convictions, you may subtly (or not so subtly) direct your client toward choices other than abortion. We see your job as helping your client clarify her values, struggling with what is best for her and for others in her situation, and assisting her in making the best choice. It is unfortunate that some well-intentioned helpers think that their job is to help people conform to acceptable absolute standards or to straighten out their clients.

Our own practice is to tell clients of some of our values that are likely to affect our work with them. To give you an idea of what we mean, we think that the examined life is better than the unexamined life. We operate on the assumption that people are not victims and that with awareness and hard work they can make substantial changes in their lives. Another bias we hold is that pain is frequently a useful source to explore. If clients identify painful experiences and are willing to express them, the chances are that they will be led to significant unfinished business, which is fertile material for exploration. One of the values that we promote is self-determination, or choosing for oneself and accepting the responsibility for these choices. Although some individuals would like others to choose for them, we assume that therapy is aimed at assisting people to find their own best decisions. These are but a few examples of the values that we are open about. Furthermore, if we have a difficult time with clients because it seems to us that they are behaving in ways that are inconsistent with their values, we confront them on this discrepancy.

VALUE CONFLICTS WITH CLIENTS

Exposing your values can be very useful. This is especially true in situations where you discover that you and your clients have sharp value differences. If you know that you would have a difficult time working objectively with someone because of such conflicts, ethical practice dictates that you not accept the person as a client. If you become aware of value conflicts once the relationship has been established, a referral might be in the best interests of your client. You could discuss the possible difficulties you or your client might have if the professional relationship were not terminated. If your client subscribed to strongly fundamentalist religious values and had a certain vision of how she should live her life as a good person, for example, you might have trouble accepting her attitudes and choices if you did not embrace her values. You might find that you wanted to continually challenge her values and liberalize her thinking.

As another example, assume that you are seeing a gay man who wants to talk about his relationship with his lover and the difficulties they have in communicating with each other. As you are working with him, you become aware that it is difficult for you to accept his sexual orientation. You find yourself challenging him about this, and you are not concentrating on what he says he wants to work on. Instead, you are focused on his sexual orientation, which is totally unacceptable to you, for it goes against what you think is morally right. These reactions are so much in the foreground that you and your client recognize that you are not helping him. In such cases the ethical course of action is to refer the client to a professional who is able to work with him more objectively than you can because of your value system. In making such referrals, it is essential that you avoid giving clients the impression that there is something wrong with them. Instead, it is best to put the focus on yourself and how your values are likely to make it difficult to maintain your objectivity and work effectively with them. In short, if you feel a need to refer a client, the problem may reside more in you than in a particular client.

Tjeltveit (1986) suggests that referrals are appropriate when moral, religious, or political values are centrally involved in a client's presenting problems and when any of the following situations exist on the helper's part: the boundaries of competence have been reached, there is extreme discomfort with a client's values, the helper is unable to maintain objectivity, or the helper has grave concerns about imposing values on a client. In such cases, it is appropriate to refer a client to a professional who does not have these limitations or who shares the client's values. Merely having a conflict of values does not necessarily imply a referral, for it is possible to work through a conflict successfully. We hope that you will not be too quick to refer when there are conflicting value systems but that you will challenge yourself to determine what it is about a client that prompts you to want to make the referral.

There may be times when referral resources are not available, due to budgetary considerations or limited services in your area. This reality makes it imperative that you do your best to see that your values do not obstruct your ability to work with certain clients. Getting supervision or consulting with a colleague might shed some light on your reasons for thinking that you could not work with a certain client. What is essential is that you respect your clients' right to hold a set of values different from yours. Even if you do not endorse their values, you may still be able to work effectively with them if you are able to refrain from pushing your values onto them.

In the remainder of this chapter, we consider some value-laden issues that you are likely to encounter in your work with a range of client populations. Some of these areas include concerns of gay and lesbian individuals, family issues, values pertaining to sex-role identity, religious and spiritual values, abortion, and sexuality.

Gay and Lesbian Issues

The question of how values affect the outcomes of the helping process is often manifest when working with gay or lesbian clients. Many helpers have blind spots, biases, and misconceptions about gay and lesbian issues. Fassinger (1991b) emphasizes the importance of mental-health professionals' accepting the responsibility for developing the attitudes, knowledge, and skills necessary to work effectively with gay men and lesbians. She adds that "all practitioners should take time often in the therapy hour to process their interaction with their clients in order to ensure mutual comfort levels, to check the effectiveness of their interventions, and to uncover any blind spots that may be impeding the therapeutic alliance" (p. 172).

If you hope to work effectively with gay and lesbian clients, it is absolutely essential that you begin by challenging your own assumptions about homosexuality, that you be aware of your own biases, that you challenge any myths and misconceptions that you might hold, and that you be open to understanding how your values are likely to affect your work. Put yourself in the following situation and consider how your values are likely to influence the way in which you would work with Art.

The situation.   You are doing an intake interview with a gay man, age 33. Art tells you that he is coming to counseling because he often feels lonely and isolated. He has difficulty in intimate relationships, with men or women. His concern is that once people get to know him, they will not accept him and somehow won't like him. During the interview you find out that he has a lot of pain over his father, with whom he has very little contact. He would like a closer relationship with his father, yet his gayness stands in the way. His father has let him know that he feels guilty that Art "turned out that way." He just cannot understand why Art is not "normal" and why he can't find a woman and get married like his brother. Art mainly wants to work on his relationship with his father, and he also wants to overcome his fears of rejection by others with whom he'd like a close relationship. He tells you that he has accepted his gayness and would like those he cares about to accept him as he is.

Your stance.   What are your initial reactions to Art's situation? Considering your own values, do you expect that you would have any trouble establishing a therapeutic relationship with him? In light of the fact that he lets you know that he does not want to change his sexual orientation, would you be able to respect this decision? As you think about how you would proceed with Art, reflect on your own attitudes toward gay men. Think especially whether you might be inclined to push any of your values, regardless of your stance. For example, if you have personal difficulty in accepting homosexuality on moral or other grounds, might you encourage Art to give up his ways and become heterosexual? You might focus on a number of issues in your counseling sessions with Art, some of which are his fear of rejection, pain with his father, desire for his father to be different, difficulty in getting close to both men and women, sexual preference, and values. With the information you have, which of these areas are you likely to emphasize? Are there other areas you might want to explore with Art?

Discussion.   A survey of psychologists designed to identify major themes of both biased and sensitive therapeutic practice with lesbians and gay men found evidence of both beneficial and harmful practices (Garnets, Hancock, Cochran, Goodchilds, & Peplau, 1991). The authors write that most practitioners will eventually find themselves working with gay males and lesbian clients, which necessitates an awareness of how their values and potential biases can emerge in subtle ways and can influence the outcomes of the therapeutic relationship. Below are some themes that illustrate biased, inadequate, or inappropriate practices:

- Therapists might automatically attribute a client's problems to his or her sexual orientation.
- Therapists sometimes operate on the assumption that a client is heterosexual and might discount a client's self-identification as gay or lesbian.
- Some therapists focus on sexual orientation as the core issue in therapy when it is not relevant.
- Therapists can underestimate the possible consequences of a gay client's disclosure of homosexuality to others.
- Therapists are sometimes insensitive to the nature and diversity of lesbian and gay male relationships and inappropriately use a heterosexual perspective.
- Therapists might express beliefs that trivialize or demean a gay or lesbian orientation.

- Therapists might be insensitive to the effects of prejudice and discrimination on lesbians and gay male parents and their children.

The researchers also identified themes illustrating exemplary practice. Some examples of these sensitive practices follow:

- Therapists understand that homosexuality, by itself, is not a form of psychopathology or developmental arrest, and they recognize that gays and lesbians can live fulfilling lives.
- Therapists understand that societal prejudice and discrimination are often experienced by gay clients and use this knowledge to help their clients overcome their negative views about themselves.
- Therapists recognize that their own sexual orientation, attitudes, and misinformation can hamper therapeutic efforts; recognizing their limitations, they seek consultation and suggest referrals when appropriate.
- Therapists respect their clients' autonomy in that they do not try to change their clients' sexual orientation without evidence that this is the appropriate course of action and that this change is desired by the clients.
- Therapists assist clients with the development of a positive gay male or lesbian identity.
- Therapists understand that the family of origin of lesbians and gay men may need education and support.
- Therapists are familiar with the needs and treatment issues of gay clients; they use relevant mental-health, educational, and gay and lesbian resources in the community.

Gay and lesbian political issues tend to evoke much negative reaction, as you are aware from the news media. If you have a conservative value system, this could easily present a challenge for you if you work with gay or lesbian clients. Although you may tell yourself and others that you accept the right of others to live their lives as they see fit, you may have trouble when you are in an actual encounter with a client. There could be a gap between what you can intellectually accept and what you can emotionally accept. If you have negative emotional or intellectual reactions to gay men or lesbians, there is a danger that you could try to impose your own values if you accepted such clients.

If you find that your values are such that you'd have difficulty counseling gays and lesbians, we think it is essential that you know and accept your limitations and make an appropriate referral. You will be doing both yourself and your potential clients a service in the long run.

As a way of clarifying some of your values pertaining to homosexuality, take the following inventory, using this code: 3 = I agree, in most respects, with this statement; 2 = I am undecided in my opinion about this statement; 1 = I disagree, in most respects, with this statement.

_____ 1. Gay and lesbian clients are best served by gay and lesbian counselors.

_____ 2. A counselor who is homosexual is likely to push his or her values on a heterosexual client.

_____ 3. I would have trouble working with either a gay male couple or a lesbian couple who wanted to adopt children, even if they were fit parents.

_____ 4. Homosexuality is a form of mental illness.

____ 5. A lesbian or a gay man can be as well adjusted (or poorly adjusted) as a heterosexual person.

____ 6. Homosexuality is immoral.

____ 7. I would have no difficulty being objective in counseling gay men and lesbians.

____ 8. I have adequate information about referral sources in the local gay community.

____ 9. I feel a need for specialized training and knowledge before I can effectively counsel gay men or lesbians.

____ 10. I expect that I would have no difficulty conducting family therapy if the father were gay.

After you finish the inventory, look over your responses for any patterns. Compare some of your responses with a survey that assessed psychological practitioners' attitudes, knowledge, concerns, and strategies in counseling lesbians and gay men (Graham, Rawlings, Halpern, & Hermes, 1984). With respect to attitudes, the survey revealed that:

- Eighty-eight percent of the therapists agreed with the position that homosexuality is not a form of mental illness.
- Seventy-seven percent felt that a homosexual person could be as well adjusted as a heterosexual person.
- Seventy-four percent felt that lesbians and gays should be allowed to adopt children if they are fit parents.

With respect to knowledge about same-sex relationships, the results were:

- Despite seemingly positive attitudes toward homosexuals as a group, the therapists demonstrated only scant knowledge about homosexuality, even though information was available in the scientific literature.
- Therapists' major concerns were about their lack of "objectivity," their lack of information about referrals to local lesbian and gay helpers, and the inadequacy of training in counseling these clients. They specifically stated a need for such training.

Family Issues

A situation involving a restless mother. Veronika has lived a repressed life. She got married at 17, had four children by the age of 22, and is now going back to college at 32. She is a good student—excited, eager to learn, and discovering all that she missed. She finds that she is attracted to a younger peer group and to professors. She is now experiencing her second adolescence, and she is getting a lot of affirmation that she did not have before. At home she has been taken for granted, and the members of her family are mostly interested in what she can do for them. At school she is special and is respected for her intellect.

Ultimately, Veronika becomes involved in an affair with a younger man. She is close to a decision to leave her husband and her four children, ages 10 to 15. She comes to see you at the university counseling center. Veronika is in turmoil over what to do, and she wants to find some way to deal with her guilt and ambivalence.

Your stance.   For a moment, consider your own value system. If Veronika were asking for your advice, what would you be inclined to say? What are your thoughts about her leaving her husband? her four children? Would you encourage her to "do her own thing"? If Veronika gave this matter considerable thought and then told you that, as painful as it would be for her own growth and well-being, she needed to leave her family, what would be your stance? Would you be inclined to encourage her to bring her entire family in for some counseling sessions? What values do you think you might push, if any? If she told you that she was leaning toward staying married and at home, even though she would be resentful, what interventions might you make? If you had been left yourself, either as a child or by a spouse, how might this trauma affect you in working with Veronika?

A situation involving a family in crisis.   A wife, husband, and three adolescent children come to your office. The family was referred by the youngest boy's child-welfare and attendance officer. The boy is acting out by stealing and is viewed as the problem person in the family.

The husband is in your office reluctantly. He appears angry and resistant, and he lets you know that he doesn't believe in this "therapy stuff." He makes excuses for the boy and says he doesn't see that there is much of a problem, either in the marriage or in the family.

The wife tells you that she and her husband fight a lot, that there is much tension in the home, and that the children are suffering. She is fearful and says that she is afraid of what might happen to her family. She has no way of supporting herself and her three children and is willing to work on the relationship.

Your stance.   If you were sitting with this family, would you feel some hope because at least they were all in your office? Would the fact that the father had come to the session, though reluctantly, be an indication that he might be willing to work out the difficulties? Or would you feel hopeless with this family? If so, would you counsel the couple to get a divorce? In light of the fact that the children appear to be negatively affected by the couple's problems, would you suggest a separation or divorce? Consider your own values on family stability, on working hard to make a marriage work, on separating when problems arise, and on divorcing and getting on with a new life. Some counselors are likely to say: "Well, you don't seem to be making it with each other. Your kids are being hurt by your bickering, and neither of you seems very happy in your relationship. I wonder why you would want to stay together and continue hurting each other?" Another counselor with a different bias might say: "You know, it's your decision either to stay together or to separate. I very much hope that the two of you can decide whether you're willing to work at making a go of your marriage. I hope you don't quit too soon, without exploring all the options and the consequences of your decision."

In light of your values pertaining to the family, what might you say, and what values might you express? Would you expose your own values to this family, even if the members did not ask you? If they asked you what you thought of their situation and what you thought they should do, what would you say?

A situation involving an affair.   A couple enters your office for marital counseling. The husband has confessed to his wife that he is having an affair, and the incident has precipitated the most recent crisis in their relationship. Although the wife is highly distraught, she wants to stay married. She realizes that their marriage needs work and that there is boredom between the two of them, yet she thinks it is worth it to work on their problems. They have children, and the family is well respected and liked in the community.

The husband wants to leave and live with his newfound lover, yet he is struggling with conflicting feelings and is not sure what to do. He is very confused, for he still loves his wife and children. He is aware that he is going through a midlife crisis, and each day he comes up with a different decision. His wife is in a great deal of pain and feels desperate. She has been totally dependent on him, with no means of support.

Your stance.   What are your values pertaining to affairs in a marriage? Do you think that an affair is a sign of betrayal? a troubled marriage? certain problems with the family? growth and change? a midlife crisis? personal conflicts within the person having the affair? something that just happens and can't be helped? What would you want to say to the wife? to the husband? Given your value system, would you counsel them to divorce? to have a trial separation? to work hard on saving the marriage?

In thinking about the direction you might pursue with this family, consider if you have ever been in this situation yourself in your own family. If so, how do you think this experience would affect the way you worked with the couple? If the husband said he was confused, desperately wanted an answer, and was hoping that you would point him in some direction, would you be inclined to tell him what you thought he should do? Or would you tell him that this was his struggle and he would have to find his own answer? Would you be inclined to tell the couple your values? Or would you keep them to yourself so as not to unduly influence them?

Sex-Role Identity

The situation.   Frank and Judy describe themselves as a "traditional couple." They are in marriage counseling with you to work on the strains in their relationship that arise from rearing their two adolescent sons. The couple talk a lot about their sons. Both Judy and Frank work full time outside the home. Besides working as an elementary school principal, Judy has another full-time job as mother and homemaker. Frank says he is not about to do any "women's work" around the house. Judy has never really given much thought to the fact that she has a dual career. Neither Judy nor Frank shows a great deal of interest in critically examining the cultural stereotypes that they have incorporated. Each of them has a definite vision of what women and men "should be." Rather than talking about their relationship or the inequalities of the distribution of tasks at home, they focus the attention on troubles with their sons. Judy wants advice on how to deal with their problems.

Your stance.   If you become aware of the tension between this couple over rigid sex roles, will you call it to their attention in your counseling with them? Do you see it as your job to challenge Frank on his traditional views? Do you see it as your job to encourage Judy to want more equality in their relationship? If you were counseling this couple, what do you think you might say to each of them? How would your values influence the direction in which you might go? Would you encourage the couple to focus more on their relationship and less on the behavior of their sons? What bearing would your own sex-role conditioning and your own views have on what you did?

Discussion.   If you will be working with couples and families, it is essential that you appreciate the fact that sex-role stereotypes serve a purpose and, therefore, are not easily modified. You need to examine your own beliefs about appropriate family roles and responsibilities, child-rearing practices, multiple roles for women, and traditional and nontraditional family arrangements. You should be able to present your views on issues such as stereotyped sex roles and the distribution of responsibilities between parents and children.

Margolin (1982) has given recommendations on how to be a nonsexist family therapist and how to use the therapeutic process to confront negative expectations and stereotyped roles in the family. One of her suggestions is that helpers examine their own behavior and attitudes that would imply sex-differentiated roles and status. For example, helpers can show their bias in subtle ways by looking at the husband when talking about making decisions and looking at the wife when talking about home matters and rearing children. Margolin also contends that practitioners are especially vulnerable to the following biases: (1) assuming that remaining married would be the best choice for a woman, (2) demonstrating less interest in a woman's career than in a man's career, (3) encouraging couples to accept the belief that child rearing is solely the responsibility of the mother, (4) showing a different reaction to a wife's affair than to a husband's, and (5) giving more importance to satisfying the husband's needs than to satisfying the wife's needs. Margolin raises two critical questions for those who work with couples and families:

- How does the counselor respond when members of the family seem to agree that they want to work toward goals that (from the counselor's vantage point) are sexist in nature?
- To what extent does the counselor accept the family's definition of sex-role identities rather than trying to challenge and eventually change these attitudes?

Religious and Spiritual Values

Contrary to the myth that psychologists have little interest in spiritual matters, Elkins (1994) suggests that the majority of clinicians are now paying more attention to the spiritual dimensions of the human being. Many clients are hungry for therapeutic experiences that offer them help with the spiritual and existential issues of life. Elkins calls for a "soulful psychology" and concludes that psychotherapy ought to be considered a journey of the soul in search of its own healing.

Miranti and Burke (1995) state that helpers must be prepared to deal with spiritual issues that lie at the very core and essence of the client's being. For many clients who are in crisis, the spiritual domain offers them solace and comfort and is a major sustaining power that keeps them going when all else seems to fail. According to Miranti and Burke, the guilt, anger, and sadness that clients experience often result from a misinterpretation of the spiritual and religious realm, which can lead to depression and a sense of worthlessness. It is essential that helpers be open and nonjudgmental to their clients who may be going through some life transition, for their spiritual beliefs can be a major source of strength as they make crucial life decisions. Miranti and Burke remind us: "For counselors, the challenge is not whether the issue of spirituality should be addressed, but how it can best be addressed by well-prepared and sensitive professionals" (1995, p. 3).

The situation.   Your client has a strong fundamentalist background. Peter has definite ideas about right and wrong, sin, guilt, and damnation, and he has accepted the teachings of his church without question. When he encountered difficulties and problems in the past, he was able to pray and find comfort in his relationship with his God. Lately, however, he has been suffering from chronic depression, an inability to sleep, extreme feelings of guilt, and an overwhelming sense of doom that God is going to punish him for his transgressions. He consulted his physician and asked for medication to help him sleep better. The physician suggested that he seek psychological counseling. At first Peter resisted this idea, for he strongly felt that he should find comfort in his religion. With the continuation of his bouts of depression and sleeplessness, he hesitantly came to you for advice.

He requests that you open the session with a prayer so that he can get into a proper spiritual frame of mind. He also quotes you a verse from the Bible that has special meaning to him. He tells you about his doubts about seeing you for counseling, and he is concerned that you will not accept his religious convictions, which he sees as being at the center of his life. He inquires about your religious beliefs.

Your stance.   Would you have any trouble counseling Peter? He is struggling with trusting you and with seeing the value in counseling. What are your reactions to some of his specific views, especially those pertaining to his fear of punishment? Do you have reactions to his strong fundamentalist beliefs? If you have definite disagreements with his beliefs, could you be accepting of him? Would you challenge him to think for himself and do what he thinks is right? Would you encourage him to question his religion?

Assume that you have a religious orientation, yet you believe in a God of love whereas Peter believes in a God of fear. You let him know that you have differences in the way the two of you perceive religion. Yet you also say that you want to explore with him how well his religious beliefs are serving him in his life and also examine possible connections between some of his beliefs and how they are contributing to his symptoms. With these assumptions, do you think you could be helpful to Peter? Would you accept him as a client?

Now assume that you don't share any of Peter's religious values, that you are intolerant of fundamentalist beliefs, and that you see such beliefs as doing far more harm than good for people. Given these values, would you accept a client like Peter? Would you be able to work with him objectively, or would you try to find ways to sway him to give up his view of the world?

Discussion. In a national survey of counselor values, Kelly (1995a) reports that almost 64% of the respondents believed in a personal God, while another 25% believed in a transcendent or spiritual dimension to reality. Approximately 70% expressed some degree of affiliation with organized religion, with almost 45% indicating that they regularly participate in religious services. Counselors who identified themselves as religious tended to view religion as a guide to life rather than valuing its social benefits or the comfort it brings to individuals. Counselors affirmed spirituality more extensively than they acknowledged affiliation with an organized religion.

In a national survey of counselor education programs, Kelly (1994) found that religious and spiritual issues are being dealt with as a course component in fewer than 25% of the programs. What may be more surprising is his finding that only about half the counselor educators who participated in the study believe that religious/spiritual issues are either "very important" or "important" in the education and training of counselors. Clearly, if counselors are to meet the challenge of addressing the role of spirituality in counseling, they not only need training in this area in both their coursework and their fieldwork experiences but they also need inspiration and leadership from their teachers.

The situation. Fran is a student intern who feels deeply committed to spirituality and also claims that her religious faith guides her in finding meaning in life. While she does not want to impose her values on her clients, she does feel it is essential to at least make a general assessment of the client's spiritual/religious beliefs and experiences during the intake session. One of her clients, Donald, tells Fran that he is depressed most of the time and feels a sense of emptiness. He wonders what is the meaning of his life. In Fran's assessment of Donald, she finds that he grew up without any kind of spiritual or religious guidance in his home, and he states that he is agnostic. He never has explored either religion or spirituality, for these ideas seem too abstract to help with the practical problems of everyday living. Fran becomes aware that she is strongly inclined to suggest to Donald that he open up to spiritual ways of thinking, especially because of his stated problem with finding meaning in his life. She brings her struggle to her supervisor.

Your stance. It is very likely that you will experience conflicts in values with your clients in the spiritual realm. If you hold a definite system of religious values, you may have a tendency to want your clients to adopt these values. Without blatantly pushing your values, you might subtly persuade clients to your religious beliefs or lead them in a direction you hope they will take. Conversely, if you do not place a high priority on spirituality and do not view religion as a salient force in your life, you may not be open to assessing your client's religious and spiritual beliefs. Whatever your personal beliefs are concerning spirituality and religion, we hope that you exercise caution when talking to your clients about spirituality. Consider Fran's situation as you reflect on how your values might influence your approach with clients. If you had a client who held radically different views on spirituality/religion than you did, would this present a problem for you? If you sought consultation from your supervisor, what key issues would you most want to explore and clarify? Could you maintain your objectivity? When would you consider suggesting a referral because of conflicts between you and your client with respect to spiritual/religious beliefs and values?

Discussion.   Faiver and O'Brien (1993) have devised a form to assess the religious beliefs of clients that they use to glean relevant information on the client's belief system for diagnostic, treatment, and referral purposes. Kelly (1995b) contends that a first step is to include the spiritual and religious dimensions as a regular part of the intake procedure and the early phase of the counseling process. Actually including items pertaining to general information about the client's spirituality and religion serves the purpose of: (a) obtaining a preliminary indication of the relevance of spirituality and religion for each client, (b) gathering information that the helper might refer to at a later point in the helping process, and (c) indicating to the client that it is acceptable to talk about religious and spiritual concerns.

There are many paths toward fulfilling spiritual needs, and it is not the helper's task to prescribe any particular pathway. However, we think that it is the helper's responsibility to be aware that spirituality is a significant force for many of their clients. It is especially important for a practitioner to pursue spiritual concerns if the client initiates them. Clinicians inquire about their clients' general physical health and their attitudes and practices about their physical health. In a like manner, it is in the realm of duty for helpers to inquire about their clients' values, beliefs, and the sources from which they have attempted to find meaning in life. As part of the assessment process, it is good practice to ask about a client's spiritual and religious beliefs and values. If clients indicate that they are concerned about any of their beliefs or practices, this is a useful focal point for exploration. The key here is that the practitioner remain finely tuned to the client's story and to the purpose for which he or she sought professional assistance.

An increasing number of students are expressing interest in the relationship between religion and counseling. Many of them wonder whether the goals of religion and those of counseling are compatible. Some of them are attracted to the field of counseling because they see it as a vehicle for teaching people about the value of religion as a way to find meaning in life. Some students are concerned that their religion will not be respected by other students and professors in the counseling field. Thus, they feel that they must hide their values. Others wonder about their ability to work objectively with people who don't embrace a religion.

Quackenbos, Privette, and Klentz (1986) and Bergin (1991) take the position that religion is a pervasive force in our society and yet is excluded from counseling practices. They support an integration of religious values with counseling and suggest that the clergy need rigorous training in counseling and that secular counselors also need preparation for dealing with religious issues. Bergin (1991) offers recommendations for including education in values and religious issues in the training of mental-health practitioners so that the vast population of religious clients can be better served. He argues that there is a spiritual dimension of human experience that can contribute to improving both psychological and social conditions. He cites a growing professional literature that provides evidence of the usefulness of spiritual dimensions in enhancing change.

Peck (1978), a psychiatrist and author of *The Road Less Traveled,* writes that psychotherapists tend to pay too little attention to the ways in which their clients view the world. He encourages counselors to be specifically aware of the view of the world held by their clients. From his perspective, this world view is always an essential part of clients' problems, and a correction of it is necessary if they are to get better. Peck advises psychotherapists whom he supervises to become aware of their clients' religion, even if they maintain that they do not have a religion. In this broader frame of reference, a religion is a basic part of how individuals view the world and, consequently, how they decide to act.

In clarifying your values pertaining to religion and counseling, consider these questions: Does an exploration of religion belong in formal helping relationships? Is the helping process complete without a spiritual dimension? If a client's religious needs arise in the therapeutic relationship, is it appropriate to deal with them? Are helpers pushing their values on their clients when they decide what topics can and cannot be discussed in counseling? Do you have to hold the same religious beliefs to work effectively with clients who have religious struggles?

Abortion

The situation.   Connie, a 19-year-old college student, has not seriously considered using a diaphragm or condoms, because she likes the idea of being a "spontaneous person." She doesn't want to use birth-control pills, because she is afraid she will gain weight. She has had an abortion, which was difficult for her. Now she is pregnant again.

Connie is wondering whether she wants to have another abortion. A part of her wants that, and another part of her wants to have the child. She is thinking about telling her parents, especially since she is wondering what it would be like to have her child and live at home with them. She is also considering the option of having her child and giving it up for adoption. She is unable to sleep, feels guilty for having gotten herself into this situation again, and is very undecided. Although she has talked to her friends and solicited their advice, she has gotten many contradictory recommendations. Connie lets you know that she is not at all sure that she did the "right thing" by having the abortion a year ago. She asks you for advice on what to do.

Your stance.   With the information you have, what are some things you'd say to Connie? You could pursue any number of options with her, including the following:

- You could encourage her to tell her parents and let them advise her what to do.
- You might explore her guilt with her to find out the meaning of it.

- You might suggest that she follow her inclination to have the child, especially as she felt unsure about the abortion a year ago.
- You could persuade her to have another abortion, especially because she is uncertain about what to do.
- You could encourage her to have her child and give it up for adoption.
- You might refer her to another agency or practitioner because of your values on abortion, either for or against.

Think about your values pertaining to abortion. Are you clearly opposed to it on moral and religious grounds? If so, would you tell her so? Would you attempt to dissuade her from having an abortion and suggest other options? Would you attempt to keep your values out of the session? If your values are that women have the right to decide whether they will have a child, would you try to persuade her to accept your view? Would the fact that she had had a prior abortion make any difference to you? If you sensed that she was using abortion as a method of birth control, would this make a difference in how you proceeded?

Sometimes we hear students say that they would refer a pregnant client who was considering an abortion to another professional because of their values. They would not like to sway the woman, and they fear that they could not remain objective. Does this apply to you? What would you do if a client of yours happened to get pregnant while she was in treatment with you? Would you refer her at this point? If so, might she feel that you were abandoning her?

Sexuality

Situation involving sex in a nursing home.   You are working in a nursing home. You discover that several of the unmarried elderly residents have sexual relationships. At a staff meeting several other workers begin to complain that supervision is not tight enough and that such "goings on" should not be permitted. What input would you want to have in this staff meeting? What are your thoughts about unmarried elderly people engaging in sex? Would you be inclined to promote this practice? Would you agree that more careful supervision was needed to prevent it? How would your own values affect your recommendations?

Situation involving a sex-education program.   You are working in a facility for adolescents and are doing a good deal of individual and group counseling. You discover that many young teenagers are sexually active and that a number of them have gotten pregnant. Abortion is common. Many of these girls keep their babies, whether or not they get married. The agency director asks you to design a comprehensive education program for preventing unwanted pregnancy.

In thinking about the kind of program you would suggest, consider these questions: What are your values with respect to teenagers' being sexually active? What are your attitudes about providing detailed birth-control information to children and adolescents? How would your own values influence the design of your program?

Assessing your sexual values.   Consider your values with respect to sexuality, as well as where you acquired them. How comfortable do you feel in discussing sexual issues with clients? Are you aware of any barriers that could prevent you from working with clients on sexual issues? How would your experiences in sexual relationships (or the lack of them) influence your work with clients in this area? Would you promote your sexual values? For example, if a teenage client was promiscuous and this behavior was in large part a form of rebellion against her parents, would you be inclined to challenge her behavior? Or if a teenage client took no birth-control precautions yet was sexually active with many partners, would you urge him or her to use birth control? Or would you encourage abstinence? Or would you recommend that he or she be more selective in choosing sexual partners?

Although you may say that you are open-minded and that you can accept sexual attitudes and values that differ from your own, we think you could be tempted to try to change clients who you believed were involved in self-defeating practices. It would be good to assess your attitudes toward casual sex, premarital sex, sex with many partners, group sex, teenage sexuality, and extra-marital sex. What are your attitudes toward monogamy? What do you consider to be the physical and psychological hazards of sex with more than one partner? How would your views on this issue influence the direction you'd take with clients in exploring sexual concerns?

When you've made this assessment, ask yourself whether you would be able to work objectively with a person who had sexual values sharply divergent from yours. If you have very conservative views about sexual behavior, for example, will you be able to accept the liberal views of some of your clients? If you think their moral values are contributing to the difficulties they are experiencing in their lives, will you be inclined to persuade them to adopt your conservative values?

From another perspective, if you see yourself as having liberal sexual attitudes, how do you think you'd react to a person with traditional values? Assume your unmarried client says that he'd like to have more sexual experiences but that his religious upbringing has instilled in him the belief that premarital sex is a sin. Whenever he has come close to having sexual experiences, he has been burdened with guilt. He would like to learn to enjoy sex without feeling guilty, yet he does not want to throw his values away. He is in conflict and wants your advice. What do you think you'd say to him if your values were liberal? Would you be inclined to challenge his moral upbringing? Would you encourage him to discard his values, which seem to be bringing him grief and anxiety? Could you be supportive of his choices if they were in conflict with your values?

BY WAY OF REVIEW

- Ethical practice dictates that helpers seriously consider the impact of their values on their clients and the conflicts that might arise if values are sharply different.

- Ultimately, it is the responsibility of clients to choose in which direction they will go, what values they will adopt, and what values they will modify or discard.
- It is neither possible nor desirable for helpers to remain neutral or to keep their values separate from their professional relationships.
- It is not the helper's role to indoctrinate clients or to push them to adopt the value system of the helper.
- At times, it can be useful for helpers to expose their values to their clients, yet it is counterproductive to impose these values on them.
- Simply because you do not embrace a client's values does not mean that you cannot effectively work with the person. The key is that you be objective and respect your client's right to autonomy.
- There are numerous areas in which your values can potentially conflict with the values of your clients. You may have to refer some clients because of such differences.

WHAT WILL YOU DO NOW?

1. Write down some of your central values pertaining to the helping process. Under what circumstances might you want to share and perhaps explore your values and beliefs with your clients? Can you think of situations in which it might be counterproductive for you to do so?

2. Consider a personal value that could get in the way of your being objective in working with a client. Take a value that you hold strongly, and challenge it. Do this by going to a source who holds values opposite to your own. If you are strongly convinced that abortion is immoral, for instance, consider going to an abortion clinic and talking with someone there. If you are uncomfortable with homosexuality because of your own values, go to a gay organization on campus or in your community and talk with people there. If you think you may have difficulty with religious values of clients, find out more about a group that holds religious views different from yours.

3. Spend some time reflecting on the role you expect your values to play as you work with a range of clients. How might your values work for you? against you? Reflect also on the source of your values. Have you internalized your own value system? Are you clear where you stand on the issues raised in this chapter? In your journal, write some of your thoughts about the ACA'S (1995) ethical guideline that pertains to the role of the helper's personal values: "Counselors are aware of their own values, attitudes, beliefs, and behaviors and how these apply in a diverse society, and avoid imposing their values on clients."

4. For the full bibliographic entry for each of the sources listed below, consult the References and Reading List at the back of the book.

For books dealing with the role of spiritual values in the helping process, see Burke and Miranti (1995), Kelly (1995b), and Peck (1978). For an examination of religious and spiritual values consult Grimm (1994), Mattson (1994), Faiver and O'Brien (1993), and Kelly (1994).

Chapter 7

CULTURAL DIVERSITY IN THE HELPING PROFESSIONS

FOCUS QUESTIONS
AIM OF THE CHAPTER
SELF-ASSESSMENT: CULTURAL DIVERSITY AND GENDER EQUITY
A MULTICULTURAL PERSPECTIVE ON HELPING
OVERCOMING CULTURAL TUNNEL VISION
EFFECTIVE MULTICULTURAL HELPERS
BY WAY OF REVIEW
WHAT WILL YOU DO NOW?

FOCUS QUESTIONS

1. How much thought have you given to your own cultural background and the assumptions that you have developed? To what degree are you open to expanding your vision of reality?
2. How prepared are you to work with client populations that differ from you significantly in a number of dimensions (age, gender, culture, ethnicity, sexual orientation, socioeconomic status, and educational background)? What life experiences can you draw from to bridge any gap of differences between you and your clients?
3. What ethical issues are involved in failing to take cultural factors into account in the helping relationship?
4. What problems and pitfalls are associated with a multicultural perspective?
5. What values do you hold that could make it difficult for you to work with clients who have a different worldview or a different cultural background? For example, if you value self-determination and this is not a central value in your client's culture, could this pose problems?
6. What might you do if a client who sought your help wondered if you would be able to help him or her despite cultural or lifestyle differences?
7. In your college program, how much attention is given to developing awareness of your cultural assumptions, knowledge about diverse cultural groups, and skills for working in a pluralistic society?
8. What can you do to increase your ability to make contact with clients who are different from you? How can you move toward becoming a culturally skilled helper?

AIM OF THE CHAPTER

In most places where you might work, it will be necessary for you to relate effectively to a wide variety of clients. At this point in your development as a helper, it is essential that you be open to considering how to establish contact with clients who differ from you in age, gender, ethnicity, race, culture, socioeconomic status, sexual orientation, lifestyle, life circumstances, or basic values.

You don't need to be the same as your client or to have experienced the same life circumstances to form a therapeutic alliance. But it is necessary that you have a range of experiences on which you can call as a basis for understanding the human condition. Universal human themes link people in spite of their differences. What is crucial is your openness to learn from the lessons that life has presented to you, your respect for contrasting perspectives, your interest in understanding the diverse worldviews of the clients you will meet, and your capacity for breaking out of the narrow partitions that filter reality. If you have grown up in a monocultural world, it is not impossible for you to understand people with a different worldview, but it will demand a good deal of challenging and changing of your attitudes and views.

In the previous chapter we focused on the influence that your values have on the interventions you make as a helper. This theme continues as we examine the basic role that cultural values play in every helping relationship. Both you and the person seeking your help bring attitudes, behaviors, and life perspectives into the relationship. If these values are clashing, there is little chance for a helping relationship to form. To function effectively as a helper, you need to remain aware of clients' cultural attributes and to realize how cultural values operate in the helping process. You need to know about specific cultural differences and realize how certain cultural values affect your work. It is crucial that all helpers seriously consider these issues, regardless of their racial, ethnic, and cultural background. To achieve these ends, we will explore several themes:

- Recognizing cultural encapsulation and beginning to adopt a multicultural perspective
- Contrasting the underlying values of Western and Eastern approaches to helping
- Recognizing biases, prejudices, and racism
- Challenging stereotypical assumptions
- Identifying the characteristics of culturally skilled helpers

This chapter is not designed to teach you all you need to understand about diversity. Our intention is to offer a perspective on learning how to appreciate and work with diversity in the helping relationship. We stress coming to an understanding of the ways in which your own cultural background has contributed to who and what you are and honestly examining your basic views about diversity. If you have not given much thought to how your cultural frame of reference will affect your work as a professional helper, this chapter could initiate a process of reflection about the intricate manifestations of culture in all human endeavors. You will probably take a course in cultural diversity, which is likely to cover gender concerns, ageism, racism, multicultural issues, physical disabilities, and issues pertaining to sexual orientation. We would hope that you don't view such a course as merely a "requirement" to get through but as a challenging and awakening experience that can broaden your vision of the world. A good course in cultural diversity is a necessity in helping you formulate alternative perspectives and in giving you tools for working with all client populations.

SELF-ASSESSMENT: CULTURAL DIVERSITY AND GENDER EQUITY

Before delving into the issues related to a multicultural and diversity perspective on the helping process, we think it makes sense to identify your present attitudes and beliefs about cultural diversity and gender equity issues. We hope you'll take and score the social-attitude survey on pages 178 and 179. This survey, called the Quick Discrimination Index, is designed to assess sensitivity, awareness, and receptivity to cultural diversity and gender equity. Because this is a self-assessment inventory, it is essential that you respond to each item as honestly as possible. This inventory is designed to assess subtle racial and gender bias. You can use this inventory to become more aware of your attitudes and beliefs pertaining to these issues.

A MULTICULTURAL PERSPECTIVE ON HELPING

Multicultural counseling refers to practices that integrate culture-specific awareness, knowledge, and skills in the helping process. The United States is a pluralistic or multicultural society that includes individuals from different ethnic, racial, and cultural backgrounds (Arredondo, Toporek, Brown, Jones, Locke, Sanchez, & Stadler, 1996). When you become a helper, you will encounter many individuals from cultures different from your own. In many instances, your first step toward helping these clients will be coming to an understanding of their cultural values.

Culture can be defined narrowly or broadly. Lee and Richardson (1991a) contend that the term *culture* should be limited to categories of race or ethnicity and focus on the mental-health issues and developmental needs of those racial and ethnic groups in the United States that do not have European roots. Pedersen (1994) looks at culture from a broader perspective, defining cultural groups by *ethnographic* variables (nationality, ethnicity, language, and religion), *demographic* variables (age, gender, and place of residence), *status* variables (educational and socioeconomic background), and formal and informal *affiliations.* According to Pedersen, the multicultural perspective provides a conceptual framework that both recognizes the complex diversity of a pluralistic society and suggests bridges of shared concern that link all people, regardless of their differences. This perspective looks both at the unique dimensions of a person and at how this person shares common themes with those who are different.

Arredondo and her colleagues (1996) make a distinction between multiculturalism and diversity. Multiculturalism puts the focus on ethnicity, race, and culture. In the context of training helpers, the term *multicultural* refers to five major cultural groups in the United States and its territories: African/Black, Asian, Caucasian/European, Hispanic/Latino, and Native American. *Diversity* refers to other individual differences and characteristics by which persons may self-define. This includes but is not limited to an individual's age, gender, sexual orientation, religion or spiritual identification, physical ability/disability, social and economic class background, and residential location.

Ethical Dimensions in Multicultural Practice

Becoming an ethical and effective helper in a multicultural society is a continuing process, not a destination that we reach once and for all. Sue (1996) suggests that ethical and effective multicultural counseling evolves from three primary

(text continues on page 180)

Quick Discrimination Index*

Directions: Remember there are no right or wrong answers. Please circle the appropriate number to the right.

		Strongly Disagree	Disagree	Not Sure	Agree	Strongly Agree
1.	I do think it is more appropriate for the mother of a newborn baby, rather than the father, to stay home with the baby (not work) during the first year.	1	2	3	4	5
2.	It is as easy for women to succeed in business as it is for men.	1	2	3	4	5
3.	I really think affirmative-action programs on college campuses constitute reverse discrimination.	1	2	3	4	5
4.	I feel I could develop an intimate relationship with someone from a different race.	1	2	3	4	5
5.	All Americans should learn to speak two languages.	1	2	3	4	5
6.	It upsets (or angers) me that a woman has never been president of the United States.	1	2	3	4	5
7.	Generally speaking, men work harder than women.	1	2	3	4	5
8.	My friendship network is very racially mixed.	1	2	3	4	5
9.	I am against affirmative-action programs in business.	1	2	3	4	5
10.	Generally, men seem less concerned with building relationships than women.	1	2	3	4	5
11.	I would feel OK about my son or daughter dating someone from a different race.	1	2	3	4	5
12.	It upsets (or angers) me that a racial minority person has never been president of the United States.	1	2	3	4	5
13.	In the past few years, too much attention has been directed toward multicultural or minority issues in education.	1	2	3	4	5
14.	I think feminist perspectives should be an integral part of the higher education curriculum.	1	2	3	4	5
15.	Most of my close friends are from my own racial group.	1	2	3	4	5
16.	I feel somewhat more secure that a man rather than a woman is currently president of the United States.	1	2	3	4	5

*The Quick Discrimination Index (QDI) is copyrighted by Joseph G. Ponterotto, Ph.D. No further reproduction or Xeroxing of this instrument is permitted without the written permission of Dr. Ponterotto. If you are interested in using this instrument for any purpose, write to Joseph G. Ponterotto, Ph.D. (at the Division of Psychological and Educational Services, Fordham University at Lincoln Center, Room 1008, 113 West 60th Street, New York, NY 10023-7478) and request the "User Permission Form," the QDI itself, and the latest reliability and validity information.

	Strongly Disagree	Disagree	Not Sure	Agree	Strongly Agree
17. I think that it is (or would be) important for my children to attend schools that are racially mixed.	1	2	3	4	5
18. In the past few years too much attention has been directed toward multicultural or minority issues in business.	1	2	3	4	5
19. Overall, I think racial minorities in America complain too much about racial discrimination.	1	2	3	4	5
20. I feel (or would feel) very comfortable having a woman as my primary physician.	1	2	3	4	5
21. I think the president of the United States should make a concerted effort to appoint more women and racial minorities to the country's Supreme Court.	1	2	3	4	5
22. I think white people's racism toward racial-minority groups still constitutes a major problem in America.	1	2	3	4	5
23. I think the school system, from elementary school through college, should encourage minority and immigrant children to learn and fully adopt traditional American values.	1	2	3	4	5
24. If I were to adopt a child, I would be happy to adopt a child of any race.	1	2	3	4	5
25. I think there is as much female physical violence toward men as there is male physical violence toward women.	1	2	3	4	5
26. I think the school system, from elementary school through college, should promote values representative of diverse cultures.	1	2	3	4	5
27. I believe that reading the autobiography of Malcolm X would be of value.	1	2	3	4	5
28. I would enjoy living in a neighborhood consisting of a racially diverse population (Asian, blacks, Latinos, whites).	1	2	3	4	5
29. I think it is better if people marry within their own race.	1	2	3	4	5
30. Women make too big a deal out of sexual-harassment issues in the workplace.	1	2	3	4	5

The total score measures overall sensitivity, awareness, and receptivity to cultural diversity and gender equality. Of the 30 items on the QDI, 15 are worded and scored in a positive direction (high scores indicate high sensitivity to multicultural/gender issues), and 15 are worded and scored in a negative direction (where low scores are indicative of high sensitivity). Naturally, when tallying the total score response, these latter 15 items need to be *reverse-scored*. Reverse scoring simply means that if a respondent circles a "1" he or she should get five points, a "2" four points, a "3" three points, a "4" two points, and a "5" one point.

The following QDI items need to be *reverse-scored*: 1, 2, 3, 7, 9, 10, 13, 15, 16, 18, 19, 23, 25, 29, 30.

Score range = 30 to 150, with high scores indicating more awareness, sensitivity, and receptivity to racial diversity and gender equality.

practices. First, helpers must be aware of their own assumptions, biases, and values about human behavior, and of their own worldview as well. Second, helpers need to become increasingly aware of the cultural values, biases, and assumptions of diverse groups in our society, understanding the worldview of culturally different clients in nonjudgmental ways. Third, with this knowledge helpers will begin to develop culturally appropriate, relevant, and sensitive strategies for intervening with individuals and with systems.

Recognizing diversity in our society and embracing a cross-cultural approach in the helping relationship are fundamental tenets of professional codes of ethics. Respecting diversity implies a commitment to acquiring the knowledge, skills, and personal awareness that are essential to working effectively with diverse client populations. The reality of working in a pluralistic society is that helpers are required to learn a variety of perspectives to meet the unique needs of clients. ACA's (1995) code states: "Counselors will actively attempt to understand the diverse cultural backgrounds of the clients with whom they work. This includes, but is not limited to, learning how the counselor's own cultural/racial identity impacts her or his values and beliefs about the counseling process."

The *Ethical Standards of the National Organization for Human Service Education* (1995) contain at least six principles aimed at the human-service professional's responsibility to the community and society, with a specific emphasis on ethics and human diversity. These specific standards state that human-service profesionals:

- Advocate for the rights of all members of society, particularly those who are members of minorities and groups at which discriminatory practices have been directed
- Provide services without discrimination or preference based on age, ethnicity, culture, race, disability, gender, religion, sexual orientation, or socioeconomic status
- Are knowledgeable about the cultures and communities within which they practice
- Are aware of their own cultural backgrounds, beliefs, and values, recognizing the potential for impact on their relationships with others
- Are aware of sociopolitical issues that differently affect clients from diverse backgrounds
- Seek the education and supervision necessary to ensure their effectiveness in working with culturally diverse client populations

Herlihy and Corey (1996a) emphasize that working in a pluralistic society entails a willingness on the part of helpers to apply ethical codes from a perspective that recognizes and respects diversity.

The Need for a Multicultural Emphasis

The helping professions have yet to fully address the special issues involved in working with people of various cultures. Many of the clients you will work with will bring with them specific values, beliefs, and actions conditioned by their race, ethnicity, gender, religion, historical experiences with the dominant culture, socioeconomic status, political views, lifestyle, and geographic region. D.W. Sue

(1996) reminds us that the complexion of the United States is rapidly changing. He cites United States Census figures indicating that sometime between the years 2030 and 2050 racial and ethnic minorities will become the majority population. Sue contends that the values, assumptions, beliefs, and practices of monocultural society are structured to serve only one narrow segment of the population. He also maintains that educational systems and traditional counseling approaches have often done harm to minority individuals:

> Rather than educate or heal, rather than offer enlightenment and freedom, and rather than allow for equal access and opportunities, historical and current practices have restricted, stereotyped, damaged, and oppressed the culturally different in our society. (Sue, 1996, p. 195)

From Sue's (1992) perspective, the mental-health professions are confronted with making a choice at the crossroads. The road more traveled is that of monoculturalism and ethnocentrism. This is the road that has served many well and offers comfort and security. The road that is less traveled is multiculturalism, which recognizes and values diversity. This path provides a picture of our society as a cultural mosaic rather than a melting pot. The path of multiculturalism offers a basis for helpers to develop new structures, policies, and practices that are responsive to all groups in society.

It is important for human-service professionals to embrace a broad multicultural perspective. Pedersen (1991b) clearly states the link between culture and behavior:

- Our perceptions of the world are culturally learned and culturally mediated.
- People from different cultural backgrounds perceive their world differently.
- Counseling requires an accurate and profound understanding of the world of each client.

Pedersen (1994) maintains that human-service workers have two choices—to ignore the influence of culture or to attend to it. Whatever choice is made, culture will continue to influence the behavior of both the client and the helper.

Adopting a multicultural perspective allows us to think about diversity without polarizing issues into "right" or "wrong" (Pedersen, 1991b). For many of the questions we can raise, there is no right or wrong answer. When two people argue from culturally different assumptions, they can disagree without one being right and the other being wrong. Depending on the cultural perspective from which a problem is considered, there can be several appropriate solutions. In some cases, a similar problem may have very different solutions depending on one's culture.

A multicultural perspective takes into consideration all of the complex dimensions of our pluralistic society. Such a perspective respects the needs and strengths of diverse client populations, and it recognizes the experiences of these clients. However, don't get into the trap of perceiving individuals as simply belonging to a group. Remember that the differences between individuals within the same group are often greater than the differences between groups. Pedersen (1994) indicates that individuals who share the same ethnic and cultural background are likely to have sharp differences. Not all Native Americans have the same experience, nor do all blacks, all Asians, all women, all old people, or all people with disabilities. Helpers must be prepared to deal with the complex differences among individuals from every cultural group. Sue, Arredondo, and McDavis (1992) point out that although all of us are racial, ethnic, and cultural beings belonging to a particular group, we are not innately endowed with the competencies and skills necessary to be culturally skilled helpers.

We hope that you will not view the tapestry of culture that is woven into the fabric of all helping relationships as a barrier to break through but that you will approach cultural diversity as something positive. As Pedersen (1994) reminds us, multiculturalism can make your job as a helper easier and more fun; it can also increase rather than decrease the quality of your life. You can adopt a perspective that cultural differences are positive attributes that add richness to relationships.

Some Trends in the Multicultural Emphasis

There is a growing awareness of and sensitivity to ethnic and cultural issues in the helping professions. A variety of multicultural concerns have received increased attention over the last decade. These recent developments can be summarized as follows:

1. Multiculturalism has now become the "fourth force in counseling" (Pedersen, 1991b, 1994; D'Andrea & Daniels, 1991).
2. Given the major demographic changes taking place in our society, the impact of multiculturalism in the 1990s will be as widespread as the influence of the client-centered movement was in the 1950s and 1960s (D'Andrea & Daniels, 1991).
3. Embracing multiculturalism is not an easy path, yet it is becoming the only viable option in our pluralistic society. Increasingly, working with minority populations will become the norm rather than the exception (Sue, 1992, 1996).
4. There is a concern about adapting techniques and interventions to culturally varied clients.
5. There is recognition that the helper's self-awareness is as important as cultural awareness in multicultural helping situations.
6. There is a trend toward developing multicultural competencies and standards and infusing this perspective throughout training programs (Sue, Arredondo, & McDavis, 1992; Arredondo et al., 1996).
7. Guidelines have been established for delivery of services to ethnic, linguistic, and culturally diverse populations (APA, 1993) and for integration of diversity perspectives in codes of ethics (ACA, 1995).
8. There is an increased call for accepting the challenge of multiculturalism in assessment, treatment, and research and in making a commitment to moving out of cultural encapsulation (Ivey, 1992; Sue, 1992; Sue, Ivey, & Pedersen, 1996).
9. There are implications for practice in the value orientations and differing basic assumptions underlying Eastern and Western therapeutic systems.

OVERCOMING CULTURAL TUNNEL VISION

Our work with students in a human-services training program has shown us that many of them have cultural "tunnel vision." They have limited cultural experiences, and in some cases they see it as their role to transmit their values to their clients. We find that many students are unaware of the difficulty of dealing with clients who have a cultural background different from their own. Some students have made inappropriate generalizations about a particular group of clients. For example, helpers often assert that minorities are unresponsive to psychological intervention because of a lack of motivation to change or a "resistance" to seeking professional help.

Regardless of your cultural heritage, it is essential that you honestly examine your own expectations, attitudes, and assumptions about working with various cultural and ethnic groups. In a sense, all helping relationships are multicultural to some extent. Both those providing help and those receiving help bring to their relationship attitudes, values, and behaviors that can vary widely. One mistake is to deny the importance of these cultural variables; another mistake is to overemphasize such cultural differences to the extent that helpers lose their spontaneity and thus fail to be present for their clients. You need to understand and accept clients who have a different set of assumptions about life, and you need to be alert to the likelihood of imposing your own worldview. In working with clients with different cultural experiences, it is important that you resist making value judgments for them.

Cormier and Hackney (1993) note that values and lifestyles of clients from other cultures may well differ from the predominant values of the culture. Encapsulation is a potential trap that all helpers must be wary of falling into. It results in believing that one way of thinking is correct and refusing to entertain alternative positions. If you accept the idea that certain cultural values are necessarily supreme, you become limited by refusing to consider alternatives.

If you possess cultural tunnel vision, you are likely to misinterpret many patterns of behavior displayed by clients who are culturally different from you. Unless you understand the values of other cultures, you are likely to misunderstand these clients. Because of this lack of understanding, you may label certain client behavior as resistant, you may make an inaccurate diagnosis of a particular behavior as maladaptive, and you may impose your own value system on the client. For example, many Hispanic women might resist changing what you view as dependency on their husband. If you work with Hispanic women, you need to appreciate that they are likely to live by the value of remaining with their husband, even if he is unfaithful. Hispanic tradition tells these women that no matter what, it is not appropriate to leave one's husband. If you are unaware of this traditional value, you could make the mistake of pushing such women to take an action that will violate their belief system.

Avila and Avila (1988) caution helpers that certain basic values are a part of the Mexican-American heritage and should not be challenged, attacked, or degraded. If helpers are not aware of these core characteristics that are deeply ingrained in the character of many Mexican Americans, they may irrevocably alienate some clients. Avila and Avila see the notion of acculturation as an insult, for it implies that one set of principles, values, and actions is right, whereas another is wrong. If helpers push clients toward acculturation, they may give them the message "Leave your heritage behind, and allow me to show you a better way." Many members of minority groups want to be included in mainstream society without sacrificing those qualities that make them different. On a similar note, Sage (1991) comments that for Native Americans adopting the values and behaviors of another culture means alienating themselves from their own culture. According to Sage, the paradox is that even if American Indians do adopt values of the dominant culture, they rarely find acceptance, understanding, or success in the non-Indian culture.

These examples illustrate how important it is that helpers respect the cultural heritage of their clients and that they avoid encouraging clients to "give up" this culture so that they can "make it" in the dominant culture. Certainly, clients need to consider the consequences of not accepting certain values of the society in which they live, but they should not be pressured to accept wholesale a set of values that may be alien to them. Although clients who inhabit more than one culture are likely to struggle in finding ways to integrate what is best for them from both cultures, the synthesis is bound to be richer with possibilities.

Helpers from all cultural groups need to honestly examine their expectations and attitudes about the helping process. Realize that there is no sanctuary from cultural bias. We tend to carry our bias around with us, yet we often do not recognize this fact. Most of us are culture-bound and encapsulated to some extent, and it takes a concerted effort and vigilance to monitor our biases and value systems so that they do not interfere with establishing and maintaining successful helping relationships.

Western and Eastern Values

Most of the theories and practices of the helping process that you have learned are grounded in Western assumptions. But many of the clients with whom you will work have a cultural heritage associated with Eastern values. In short, some of the interventions you have learned will be of questionable relevance if you do not modify your techniques. Indeed, as Cormier and Hackney (1993) observe, the skills and strategies of most models of professional helping are derived from counseling approaches developed by and for white, middle-class, Western clients and therefore may not be applicable to clients from different racial, ethnic, and cultural backgrounds. The Western model of helping has major limitations when it is applied to minority groups such as Asian Americans, Hispanics, Native Americans, and blacks. Seeking psychological professional help is not typical for many of these groups. In most non-Western cultures, in fact, informal groups of friends and relatives provide a supportive network. Informal helping consists of the spontaneous outreach of caring people to others in need (Brammer, 1985).

A comparison of Western and Eastern systems shows some striking differences in value orientations. Saeki and Borow (1985) and Ho (1985) discuss some of these contrasts. Western culture places prime value on choice, the uniqueness of the individual, self-assertion, and the strengthening of the ego. By contrast, the Eastern view stresses interdependence, downplays individuality, and emphasizes losing oneself in the totality of the cosmos. From the Western perspective, the primary values are the primacy of the individual, youth, independence, nonconformity, competition, conflict, and freedom. The guiding principles for action are found in the fulfillment of individual needs and individual responsibility. From the Eastern perspective, the primary values are the primacy of relationships, maturity, compliance, conformity, cooperation, harmony, and security. The guiding principles for action are found in the achievement of collective goals and collective responsibility.

Behavioral orientations are also different. The Western view encourages expression of feelings and striving for self-actualization, whereas the Eastern view encourages control of feelings and striving for collective actualization. There are also differences in therapeutic practices between these systems. Western approaches emphasize outcomes such as improving the environment, changing one's coping behavior, learning to manage stress, and changing objective reality in other ways to improve one's way of life. Eastern approaches emphasize acceptance of one's environment and inner enlightenment.

Some time ago we presented a series of workshops in Hong Kong for human-service professionals. It gave us the opportunity to rethink the challenges of applying Western approaches to working with non-Western clients. Almost all the participants in these workshops were Chinese, but some of them had obtained their graduate training in social work or counseling in the United States. These professionals were challenged with retaining the values that were basic to their Chinese heritage while integrating a counseling viewpoint.

In talking with these practitioners, we learned that their focus is on the individual in the context of the social system. In their interventions they pay more attention to the family than to the individual's interests. They are learning how to balance a stress on personal growth with what is in the best interest of the family and society. They are able to respect the values of their clients, who are also mostly Chinese, yet at the same time they are able to challenge their clients to think of some ways to change. Many of the helping professionals in Hong Kong told us that they had to demonstrate patience and understanding with their clients. They saw it as essential to form a trusting relationship before engaging in confrontation. Although this necessity applies to counseling in general, it seems especially important for non-Western clients.

Case example. A student is seeing you because he continues to get "B" and "C" grades, which is a source of embarrassment to his family. He is in great difficulty because he feels that he is letting his family down and actually bringing shame to them by what he considers his "academic failure." If you were working with this student, how would you help him deal with his feelings of guilt and failure and at the same time be cognizant of his cultural values? Would you challenge your client? Would you try to change his reactions to his family? Would you help him become more self-accepting? Would you tend to focus on the issue of what constitutes academic success, or would your focus be on what constitutes "bringing shame to the family"?

Challenging Your Cultural Assumptions

Culturally learned basic assumptions deeply influence the ways in which we perceive and think about reality and how we act. A willingness to examine such assumptions opens doors to seeing others from their vantage point rather than from a preconceived perspective. Helpers often make cultural assumptions that they are unaware of. We give a few examples of assumptions that could interfere with effective helping in multicultural situations. By reflecting on them, you can begin to see ways to challenge your assumptions as you work with any client.

Assumptions about time.   If your clients are primarily concerned with making it through on a day-to-day basis, they are not likely to take well to a 50-minute-hour appointment that is made weeks in advance. They are expecting to get expert help and advice now on what they can do to better cope with their problems (Cormier & Hackney, 1993).

Kottler (1993) writes of being surprised when he was a visiting professor at a university in Peru that his students were not as compulsive about arriving on time as he was. When he was ready to begin class at 9 A.M., he found himself standing before an empty room. He would be interrupted every few minutes by students casually strolling into class. Kottler's students taught him to appreciate whatever was happening at the moment. He learned that in Latin cultures there is a great respect for the present but less concern for the future. Many people in these cultures are not ruled by the clock and simply will not be rushed. This trait does not mean, however, that they are uncooperative or resistant to authority. Rather, it means that time will wait; and, if not, who cares?

Assumptions about self-disclosure.   Self-disclosure is highly valued in traditional counseling. Most helpers assume that no effective helping can occur unless clients reveal themselves. This assumption ignores the fact that self-disclosure is foreign to the values of some cultural groups. For example, some European ethnic groups stress that problems should be kept "in the family." According to D. W. Sue and D. Sue (1985), those Asian Americans who are described as the "most repressed of all clients" may well be holding true to their cultural background. For economically and educationally disadvantaged clients, "talk therapies" based on self-disclosure may be incompatible with their cultural values (D. W. Sue, 1992). The helper might serve some of these clients better by focusing more on active intervention in the system (which we explore in greater detail in Chapter 8). A different perspective on this issue is given by Patterson (1985), who contends that the inability to self-disclose is something to be overcome, not accepted. For him, unless clients are willing to verbalize and communicate their thoughts, feelings, attitudes, and perceptions, there is no basis for empathic understanding by the helper.

We generally agree with Patterson that unless clients challenge the obstacles to some level of disclosure, they will be unable to participate in the helping relationship. However, you can recognize and appreciate that some of your clients will struggle in letting you know the nature of their problems. This struggle in itself is a useful focus for exploration. Rather than expecting such clients to disclose freely, you can demonstrate respect for their values and at the same time ask them what they want from you. With your support and encouragement, they can sort through their values and conditioning pertaining to self-disclosure and decide the degree to which they want to change. You can also realize that there are other forms of helping that place less stress on verbal disclosure. These can include music therapy, occupational and recreational therapy, and other forms of activity therapy. Helpers can also assume an advocacy role for the client in the system, can help clients build on their natural sources of support, or can teach them to use the resources within the community. As you will see in Chapter 8, a number of community-based interventions may be more appropriate for some clients than traditional approaches to helping.

Assumptions about family values.   D. Sue and D. W. Sue (1991) have written about some traditional Chinese family values. Filial piety is a significant value in Chinese-American families. They emphasize obedience to parents and respect and honor for them. They value self-determination and independence less than family bonds and unity. Family communication patterns are based on cultural tradition and emphasize appropriate roles and status. Academic achievement is prized. Helpers who fail to understand and appreciate these values are likely to err by pushing Chinese-American clients to change in directions that are not consistent with their values.

In one of his multicultural workshops, Pedersen related that many Asian students with whom he worked reflected values from their family when they were confronted with a problem. They first tended to reflect inward for some answer. If they did not find an answer within themselves, they tended to go to someone in the family. If neither of these routes worked, they were likely to seek a teacher, a friend, or someone with wisdom for guidance. If all of these avenues did not result in a satisfactory solution, they might consult a professional helper.

Assumptions about nonverbal behavior.   Clients can disclose themselves in many nonverbal ways, and thus it is a mistake to rely solely on what they talk about. Mainstream Americans often feel uncomfortable with silence and tend to fill in quiet gaps with words. In some cultures, in contrast, silence indicates a sign of respect and politeness. You could misinterpret a quiet client's behavior if you did not realize that she might be waiting for you to ask her questions. There are no universal meanings of nonverbal behaviors. Thus, it is essential that you acquire sensitivity to cultural differences to reduce the probability of miscommunication, misdiagnosis, and misinterpretation of behavior (Wolfgang, 1985).

You may have been systematically trained in attending and responding skills, which include keeping an open posture, maintaining good eye contact, and leaning toward your client (Egan, 1994). Clients from some ethnic groups, however, may have trouble responding positively to or understanding the intent of your body language. You have probably been taught that good eye contact is a sign of presence and that the lack of such contact is evasive. Yet Devore (1985) cautions that Asians and Native Americans may view direct eye contact as a lack of respect. In some cultures lack of eye contact may even be a sign of respect and good manners. Attneave (1985) writes that Native Americans consider a direct gaze as indicative of aggressiveness; in cross-gender encounters it usually means sexual aggressiveness. Thus, you can make a mistake if you prematurely label clients as "resistant" or "pathological" if they avoid eye contact and do not respond to your invitation of attending behavior.

Assumptions about trusting relationships. Many Americans of European background tend to form quick relationships and to talk easily about their personal life. This characteristic is often reflected in their helping style. Thus, the helper expects that the client will approach their relationship in an open and trusting manner. Doing this is very difficult for some clients, however, especially given that they are expected to talk about themselves in personal ways to a stranger. Among many cultures it takes a long time to develop meaningful relationships. What is more, you will have to *earn* the trust of these clients before they will confide in you.

Assumptions about self-actualization. Helping professionals commonly assume that it is important for the individual to become a fully functioning person. But some clients are more concerned about how their problems or changes are likely to affect others in their life. You will recall that in the Eastern orientation one of the guiding principles is achievement of collective goals. Likewise, Native Americans judge their worth primarily in relation to how their behavior contributes to the harmonious functioning of their tribe. Native Americans have a value system that is fundamentally different from that of the dominant culture, determining their self-worth in reference to the betterment of the tribe rather than their own gain (Anderson & Ellis, 1988).

Assumptions about directness. Although the Western orientation prizes directness, some cultures see it as a sign of rudeness and as something to be avoided. If you are not aware of this cultural difference, you could make the mistake of interpreting a lack of directness as a sign of being unassertive rather than as a sign of respect. Some Latin-American cultures value finding indirect ways of communicating.

Assumptions about assertiveness. If you are operating from a Western orientation, you will assume that your clients are better off if they can behave in assertive ways, such as telling people what they think, feel, and want. Some training programs teach participants coping skills that involve taking an active stance toward life.

As is true of directness, being assertive is not always viewed as appropriate behavior. Native-American clients are likely to be seen by some helpers as shy, unassertive, passive, and highly sensitive to the opinions of their peers (Anderson & Ellis, 1988). Thus, you could offend certain clients by automatically assuming that they would be better off if they became more assertive. Assume that you are working with a woman who seems very unassertive to you. She rarely asks for what she wants, she allows others to decide her priorities, and she almost never denies a request or demand from anyone in her family. If you worked hard at helping her become an assertive woman, it could very well create conflicts within her family system. If she changed her role, she might no longer fit in her culture. Therefore, it is crucial that both you and your client consider the consequences of making too many such changes.

Given all of these assumptions, we hope you see the importance of challenging some of the views about clients that you take for granted. One way to respect your clients is to ask them to tell you about themselves and listen to their underlying values. We are not suggesting that you merely listen in an accepting way, for you can still challenge clients who are culturally different from you. For example, the client who expresses little emotion can be asked if that is a problem for her or if it is something she might consider changing. You can ask another client if he sees any problem with not being assertive or direct. Perhaps he may change certain aspects of his cultural conditioning yet retain other aspects that he deems important. Asking your clients what they want from you is a way of decreasing the chances that you will impose your cultural values on them.

Go back over the basic cultural assumptions that influence helping practices, and check where you stand with regard to them. What forces have shaped your basic assumptions? Are you open to considering the relevance of such assumptions in working with a variety of clients?

Challenging Your Stereotypical Beliefs

Although you may think you are without bias, stereotypical beliefs could well affect your practice. Stereotyping involves assuming that the behavior of an individual will reflect or be typical of that of most members of his or her cultural group. This assumption leads to statements such as these: "Asian-American clients are emotionally repressed." "Black clients are suspicious by nature and will not trust professional helpers." "White people are arrogant." "Native Americans have very low motivation." Some of the authors we quoted in the last section come perilously close to such generalizations.

Helpers who view themselves as being without any stereotypes, biases, and prejudices are underestimating the impact of their socialization. Such helpers can be even more dangerous than those who are more open about their biases and prejudices. According to Pedersen (1994), this form of racism emerges unintentionally from well-meaning and caring professionals who are no more nor less culturally biased than segments of the general public. He believes that unintentional racists must be challenged either to become intentional racists or to modify their attitudes and behaviors. The key to changing the unintentional racist lies in examining basic underlying assumptions, such as those we described earlier.

Besides cultural stereotypes, there are stereotypes associated with other special populations, such as people with disabilities, the elderly, and the homeless. Statements that lump together individuals within a group reflect a myth of uniformity. Helpers need to realize that there are variations within cultural groups and that such differences may be at least as important as those among different groups.

Although cultural differences both among and within groups are obvious, we think that it is important not to go to the extreme of focusing exclusively on the differences that can separate us. In working with mental-health professionals in foreign countries, we have become even more convinced that there are some basic similarities among the peoples of the world. Universal experiences can bind people together. Although personal circumstances differ, most people experience the pain of making decisions and attempting to live with integrity in their world. It is essential to be respectful of the real cultural differences that exist, and it is equally critical that we not forget the common denominators of all people.

EFFECTIVE MULTICULTURAL HELPERS

Increasingly, helpers will come into contact with culturally diverse client populations who may not share their worldview of what constitutes normality and abnormality. Because the helping professions continue to emphasize a monocultural approach to training and practice, many helpers are ill prepared to deal effectively with cultural diversity (Sue, Arredondo, & McDavis, 1992).

Training programs need to reflect the fact that no one style of helping, nor a single school or theory, will be appropriate for all populations and situations. Instead, helpers must be able to adapt their interventions to meet not just the developmental needs of clients but also their cultural dimensions. Training programs grounded primarily in a single theoretical school may be doing a disservice to trainees (Sue, 1992).

According to Sue (1996), helpers need to recognize that culture is central to everything they do. Both clients and helpers are carriers of their cultures. Training programs should foster flexibility in applying skills in working with culturally diverse populations. Sue (1992) advocates teaching ways of using intervention strategies that consider not only individual characteristics but cultural factors as well:

> We can no longer afford to treat multiculturalism as an ancillary, rather than an integral, part of counseling. If we truly believe that multiculturalism is intrinsic and crucial for our nation, then monoculturalism and ethnocentrism should be seen as forms of maladjustment in a pluralistic society. (p. 14)

Developing Multicultural Competencies and Standards

Working with culturally diverse client populations requires that helpers possess the awareness, knowledge, and skills to effectively deal with the concerns of the people with whom they work. Although it is unrealistic to expect that you will have an in-depth knowledge of all cultural backgrounds, it is feasible for you to have a comprehensive grasp of general principles for working successfully amid cultural diversity. If you are open to the values inherent in a diversity perspective, you will find ways to avoid getting trapped in provincialism, and you will be able to challenge the degree to which you may be culturally encapsulated (see Wrenn, 1985). This would be a good time to take an inventory of your current level of awareness, knowledge, and skills. Reflect on the following questions:

- Are you familiar with how your own culture has a present influence on the way you think, feel, and act? What steps could you take to broaden your base of understanding, both of your own culture and of other cultures?

- Are you able to identify your basic assumptions, especially as they apply to diversity in culture, ethnicity, race, gender, class, religion, and lifestyle? To what degree are you clear about how your assumptions are likely to affect your practice as a helper?
- How open are you to being flexible in applying the techniques you use with clients?
- How prepared are you to understand and work with clients of different cultural backgrounds?
- To what degree are you now able to accurately compare your own cultural perspective with that of a person from another culture?
- Is your academic program preparing you to gain the awareness, knowledge, and skills you'll need to work with diverse client populations?
- What kinds of life experiences have you had that will better enable you to understand and counsel people who have a different worldview?
- Can you identify any areas of cultural bias that could inhibit your ability to work effectively with people who are different from you? If so, what steps might you take to challenge your biases?

Sue, Arredondo, and McDavis (1992) developed a conceptual framework for multicultural counseling competencies and standards in three areas: beliefs and attitudes, knowledge, and skill. Arredondo and her colleagues (1996) developed a revised set of multicultural competency standards that clarify and define these three domains. These competencies take the profession further along in the process of institutionalizing counselor training and practices to be multicultural at the core. A brief version of the multicultural competencies and standards identified by Sue and his colleagues (1992) and by Arredondo and her colleagues (1996) follows. You can use this checklist to identify areas of competence you now possess as well as areas in which you need to acquire skills.

Beliefs and Attitudes of Culturally Skilled Helpers

Put a check mark in the box before each of the beliefs and attitudes in this section that you think you already hold or each area of awareness that you already possess.

With respect to beliefs and attitudes, culturally skilled helpers . . .

- ☐ recognize and understand their own stereotypes and preconceived notions that they may hold toward other racial and ethnic minority groups.
- ☐ do not allow their personal biases, values, or problems to interfere with their ability to work with clients who are culturally different from them.
- ☐ believe that cultural self-awareness and sensitivity to one's own cultural heritage are essential for any form of helping.
- ☐ are aware of their negative and positive emotional reactions toward other racial and ethnic groups that may prove detrimental to establishing collaborative helping relationships.
- ☐ are aware of how their own cultural background and experiences have influenced attitudes, values, and biases about what constitutes psychologically healthy individuals.
- ☐ have moved from being culturally unaware to knowing their cultural heritage.

☐ are able to recognize the limits of their multicultural competence and expertise.

☐ seek to examine and understand the world from the vantage point of their clients.

☐ respect clients' religious and spiritual beliefs and values.

☐ recognize their sources of discomfort with differences that exist between themselves and others in terms of race, ethnicity, culture, and beliefs.

☐ welcome diverse value orientations and diverse assumptions about human behavior and, thus, have a basis for sharing the worldview of their clients as opposed to being culturally encapsulated.

☐ rather than maintaining that their cultural heritage is superior, are able to accept and value cultural diversity.

☐ are able to identify and understand the central cultural constructs of their clients and to avoid applying their own cultural constructs inappropriately to people with whom they work.

☐ respect indigenous helping practices and respect help-giving networks within the community.

☐ monitor their functioning through consultation, supervision, and further training or education.

☐ realize that traditional concepts and helping strategies may not be appropriate for all clients or for all problems.

Knowledge of Culturally Skilled Helpers

Put a check mark in the box before each type of knowledge in this section that you think you already possess.

With respect to knowledge areas, culturally skilled helpers . . .

☐ possess knowledge about their own racial and cultural heritage and how it affects them personally and in their work.

☐ possess knowledge and understanding about how oppression, racism, discrimination, and stereotyping affect them personally and professionally.

☐ acknowledge their own racist attitudes, beliefs, and feelings.

☐ do not impose their values and expectations on their clients from differing cultural backgrounds and avoid stereotyping clients.

☐ understand the worldview of their clients and attempt to learn about their clients' cultural backgrounds.

☐ understand the basic values underlying the helping process and know how these values may clash with the cultural values of various minority groups.

☐ are aware of the institutional barriers that prevent minorities from utilizing the mental-health services available in their communities.

☐ have knowledge of the potential bias in assessment instruments and use procedures and interpret findings keeping in mind the cultural and linguistic characteristics of clients.

☐ possess specific knowledge and information about the particular individuals with whom they are working.

☐ are aware of the values, life experiences, cultural heritage, and historical background of their culturally different clients.

☐ possess knowledge about their social impact on others.

☐ are knowledgeable about communication style differences and how their style may clash with or foster the helping process with persons from different cultural groups.

☐ are knowledgeable about the community characteristics and the resources in the community as well as those in the family.

☐ have knowledge about sociopolitical influences that impinge upon the lives of ethnic and racial minorities, including immigration issues, poverty, racism, stereotyping, and powerlessness.

☐ view diversity in a positive light, which allows them to meet and resolve the challenges that arise in their work with a wide range of client populations.

☐ know how to help clients make use of indigenous support systems. In areas where they are lacking in knowledge, they seek resources to assist them.

Skills and Intervention Strategies of Culturally Skilled Helpers
Put a check mark in the box before each of the skill areas in this section that you think you already possess.

With respect to specific skills, culturally skilled helpers . . .
☐ take responsibility for educating their clients to the way the helping process works, including matters such as goals, expectations, legal rights, and the helper's orientation.

☐ familiarize themselves with relevant research and the latest findings regarding mental health and mental disorders that affect diverse client populations.

☐ are willing to seek out educational, consultative, and training experiences to enhance their ability to work with culturally diverse client populations.

☐ are open to seeking consultation with traditional healers or religious and spiritual leaders to better serve culturally different clients, when appropriate.

☐ use methods and strategies and define goals consistent with the life experiences and cultural values of their clients. They also modify and adapt their interventions to accommodate cultural differences.

☐ are not limited to only one approach in helping but recognize that helping strategies may be culture bound.

☐ are able to send and receive both verbal and nonverbal messages accurately and appropriately.

☐ are able to exercise institutional intervention skills on behalf of their clients.

☐ become actively involved with minority individuals outside of the office (community events, celebrations, and neighborhood groups) to the extent possible.

☐ are committed to understanding themselves as racial and cultural beings and are actively seeking a nonracist identity.

☐ actively pursue and engage in professional and personal growth activities to address their limitations.

☐ consult regularly with other professionals regarding issues of culture to determine whether or where referral may be necessary.

Recognizing Your Own Limitations

As a culturally skilled helper, you are able to recognize the limits of your multicultural competency and expertise. When necessary, you will refer clients to more qualified individuals or resources. Furthermore, it is not realistic to expect that you will know everything about the cultural background of people with whom you will work. There is much to be said for letting your clients teach you about relevant aspects of their culture. Ask clients to provide you with the information you will need to work effectively with them. In working with culturally diverse individuals, it helps to assess the degree of acculturation and identity development that has taken place. This is especially true for individuals who have had the experience of living in another culture. They often have allegiance to their own home culture but find certain characteristics of their new culture attractive. They may experience conflicts when integrating the values from the two cultures in which they live. These core struggles can be productively explored in the context of a collaborative helping relationship.

As a way of getting the most from your training, we encourage you to accept your limitations and to be patient with yourself as you expand your vision of how your culture continues to influence the person you are today. It is not helpful to overwhelm yourself with all that you do not know or to feel guilty over your limitations or parochial views. You will not become a more effective and culturally skilled helper by expecting to be completely knowledgeable about the cultural backgrounds of all your clients, by thinking that you should have a complete repertoire of skills, or by demanding perfection. Instead, recognize and appreciate your efforts toward becoming a more effective person and professional. The first step is to become more comfortable in accepting diversity as a value and in taking actions to increase your ability to work with a range of clients. You can also recognize when referral is in the best interest of your client.

Multicultural Training

To enable helpers to utilize a multicultural perspective in their work, we support specialized training through formal courses and supervised field experiences with diverse client populations. We believe that a self-exploratory class should be required for helpers so that they can better identify their cultural and ethnic blind spots. In addition to enabling students to learn about cultures other than their own, such a course could offer opportunities for trainees to learn more about their own race, ethnicity, and culture. In addition, a good program should include at least one course dealing exclusively with multicultural issues and minority groups.

It is essential that a multicultural perspective be integrated throughout the curriculum. For example, a fieldwork or internship seminar can introduce ways that helping strategies can be adapted to the special needs of diverse client populations and show how some techniques may be quite inappropriate for culturally different clients. The integration of multiculturalism and gender awareness can certainly be a thread running through relevant formal courses. In addition, there could be at least one required field placement or internship in which trainees have multicultural experiences. Ideally, the supervisor at this agency will be well-versed in the cultural variables of that particular setting and also be skilled in cross-cultural understanding. Further, trainees should have access to both individual and group supervision on campus from a faculty member.

Supervised experience, along with opportunities for trainees to discuss what they are learning, is the core of a good program. We encourage you to select supervised field placements and internships that will challenge you to work on gender issues, cultural concerns, developmental issues, and lifestyle differences. You will not learn to become an effective multicultural counselor by working exclusively with clients with whom you are comfortable and who are "like you." Lee (1991) maintains that although courses and workshops are valuable sources of learning about cultural diversity, more can be learned by going out into the community and interacting with diverse groups of people who face a myriad of problems. Through well-selected internship experiences, you will not only expand your own consciousness but increase your knowledge of diverse groups. This will provide a basis for acquiring intervention skills.

The basic components of an effective multicultural training program have been identified by Loesch (1988) and Pedersen (1994). These components include: awareness, knowledge, skill development, and experiential interaction, all of which are integrated in actual practice (Ibrahim, 1991; Loesch, 1988; Pedersen, 1994). As you have seen, awareness of personal attitudes and of attitudes toward diverse client populations is integral to becoming an effective helper. From a knowledge perspective, helpers need to understand what makes a diverse population special. They need to know what is acceptable behavior within the diverse population and how this behavior differs from that of other groups. Skill development is a necessary but not sufficient component of learning to work with diverse populations. The skills themselves are not unique, but the ways in which these kills are applied to particular clients should be the focus of training.

Effective training will pay sufficient attention to each of these domains. If any of them are neglected, helpers are at a disadvantage. Training in multiculturalism often bogs down because of the tendency to focus on one area, while dealing insufficiently with the other domains. According to Pedersen (1994), multicultural training programs often fail in the following three ways:

- If there is an overemphasis on awareness, trainees may not know what to do with this awareness in terms of increasing their knowledge or learning appropriate action.
- If knowledge objectives are overemphasized, or if the knowledge dimension is presented as an exclusive focus, students may be overwhelmed with the accumulation of information yet not be able to apply this knowledge to particular situations.
- Teaching that overemphasizes skill without providing appropriate awareness and knowledge about a culture can leave trainees uncertain that they are making changes for the better.

In his multicultural training workshops, Pedersen often states that the temptation is to focus too quickly on teaching skills without sufficient emphasis on promoting awareness of trainees' underlying assumptions. We fully agree with Pedersen's position that effective multicultural development is a continuous learning process based on the integration of awareness, knowledge, and skills. The awareness stage focuses on assumptions of similarities and differences of behavior, attitudes, and values. The knowledge stage enhances information about culturally learned assumptions. The skills stage provides helpers with the tools to work within the framework of awareness of cultural differences and to apply accurate knowledge to bring about change.

Arredondo and her colleagues (1996) offer a number of suggestions that we think are well worth considering as a way to gain and maintain competence when working from a multicultural perspective.

- Read materials regarding identity development. Not only is it a good idea to read about your own cultural and ethnic identity development but it is important to read about others' identity development processes.
- Attend annual conferences and workshops that deal with multicultural concerns.
- Read newspapers and other periodicals targeting specific populations different from your own.
- Engage a mentor from your own culture who you see as working toward becoming a culturally competent counselor and who is making the kind of strides that you'd like to be making.
- Engage a mentor or two from cultures different from your own who are willing to provide you with honest feedback regarding your attitudes, beliefs, and behavior.
- Enroll in an ethnic studies course at a community college or university that focuses on cultures different from your own.
- Spend time in communities different from your own (such as shopping in grocery stores, attending churches, and walking in marches).
- Take part in activities and celebrations within communities different from your own.
- Accept that it is your responsibility to learn about other cultures and the implications for counseling, and do not expect or rely on individuals from those cultures to teach you.
- Learn another language relevant to clients as a way of beginning to understand the significance of that language in the transmission of culture.
- Seek out and engage in consultation with professionals from cultures relevant to the clients with whom you work.
- Spend some time in a civil service office, and observe the service orientation toward people of color. Contrast that with the service orientation toward white individuals. Also observe any differences in service orientation that may be based on class issues.
- Actively communicate to your organization the need for multicultural training.

Training programs have come a long way in the past decade, but they still have some way to go if they are to meet the challenges of equipping helpers to acquire the knowledge and develop the skills required to meet the needs of diverse clients. As a student, you can begin to meet this challenge by taking some small, yet significant, steps toward recognizing and examining the impact of your own cultural background and learning about cultures different from your own.

Deciding to act upon even a few of the suggestions listed here is one way to move in the direction of becoming a culturally skilled helper.

BY WAY OF REVIEW

- Multiculturalism can be considered as the fourth force in the helping professions. This perspective recognizes and values diversity in helping relationships and calls on helpers to develop strategies that are culturally appropriate.
- A multicultural perspective on the helping process takes into consideration specific values, beliefs, and actions related to race, ethnicity, gender, religion, socioeconomic status, lifestyle, political views, and geographic region.
- To function effectively with clients of various cultures, you need to know and respect specific cultural differences and realize how cultural values operate in the helping process.
- Be aware of any tendencies toward cultural tunnel vision. If you have limited cultural experiences, you may have difficulties relating to clients who have a different view of the world. You are likely to misinterpret many patterns of behavior displayed by such clients.
- It is important to pay attention to ways in which you can express unintentional racism through your attitudes and behaviors. One way to change this form of racism is by making your assumptions explicit.
- There are some striking differences in value orientations between the Western and the Eastern systems. These differences have important implications for the process of helping.
- In working with people from other cultures, avoid stereotyping, and challenge your assumptions about the use of time, self-disclosure, nonverbal behavior, trusting relationships, self-actualization, directness, and assertiveness.
- Effective multicultural helpers have been identified in terms of the specific knowledge, beliefs and attitudes, and skills they possess.
- Helpers who view differences as positive attributes will be most likely to meet and resolve the challenges that arise in multicultural helping situations.
- Rather than thinking of cultural differences as barriers to effective helping relationships, learn to welcome diversity as something positive. Recognize that consciously dealing with cultural variables in helping can make your job easier, not more difficult.

WHAT WILL YOU DO NOW?

1. If your program does not require a course on cultural diversity, consider taking such a course as an elective. You might also ask if you can sit in on some class sessions in various courses that deal with special populations. For example,

in one university these are a few of the courses offered: The Black Family, The Chicano Family, American Indian Women, The African Experience, The Chicano and Contemporary Issues, Afro-American Music Appreciation, The White Ethnic in America, Women and American Society, The Chicano Child, and Barrio Studies.

2. On your campus you will probably find a number of student organizations for particular cultural groups. Approach some members of one of these organizations for information about the group. See if you can attend one of their functions to get a better perspective on their culture.

3. There are a number of ways to challenge yourself to broaden your cultural horizons. Decide if you are willing to take any of the following steps, or others that you might think of, as a way to introduce yourself to other patterns:

- Go to an ethnic restaurant and order a meal that is different from your usual meals.
- Go to a play or a movie that depicts ethnic or cultural themes.
- Go to a restaurant, social event, church service, concert, play, or movie with a person from a cultural background that is different from yours. Ask this person to teach you about salient aspects of his or her culture.

4. If your grandparents originally came from another country, interview them about their experiences growing up in their culture. If they are bicultural, ask them about any experiences with combining both cultures. What have been their experiences in assimilation? Do they retain their original cultural identity? What do they most value in both cultures? Do what you can to discover the ways in which your cultural roots have some influence on your thinking and behavior today. In Chapter 10 you will be introduced to the importance of discovering how your family of origin continues to influence you. This exercise can help you develop a richer appreciation of your cultural heritage.

5. Take a few minutes to look at the results of the self-assessment inventory (QDI) pertaining to awareness and receptivity to cultural diversity and equity that is found in the early part of this chapter. After reading this chapter, are you more aware of your attitudes and beliefs pertaining to cultural diversity? In your journal, write about strengths that you see in yourself that will assist you in becoming a culturally competent helper. Write also about any of your beliefs, values, and assumptions that could inhibit your ability to make good contact with individuals who are culturally different from you. Then review the checklist of knowledge, skills, and awareness competencies that appeared later in this chapter and determine your current level of proficiency in these competencies. List some steps you can take to either acquire or refine your knowledge and skills.

6. For the full bibliographic entry for each of the sources listed below, consult the References and Reading List at the back of the book.

For a state-of-the-art book on multicultural perspectives on supervision and training, practice, and research and on models of racial and ethnic identity development, see Ponterotto, Casas, Suzuki, and Alexander (1995). For a good overview of counseling strategies and issues for various ethnic and racial groups, consult Atkinson, Morten, and Sue (1993). Pedersen (1994) deals extensively with the topic of developing multicultural awareness, knowledge, and skills. An in-depth treatment of multicultural counselor preparation is contained in Wehrly

(1995). For an excellent treatment of unintentional racism in counseling, see Ridley (1995). Sue, Ivey, and Pedersen (1996) deal in a comprehensive manner with multicultural counseling from the perspectives of theory, practice, and research. Sue and Sue (1990) have written a comprehensive text on helping diverse client populations. Lee and Richardson (1991a) deal with the implications of cultural diversity for education, training, and research.

Chapter 8

WORKING IN THE COMMUNITY

FOCUS QUESTIONS

1. What role would you like to play in your community? To what degree do you think you should focus on the needs of the community as well as on those of individuals?

2. Some helpers direct their efforts to helping clients understand factors within themselves that contribute to their problems. Other helpers focus on the environmental forces that need to be changed that are resulting in an individual's problems. Which perspective do you favor? What are the advantages or disadvantages of an integrated approach that combines both individual and environmental factors? How might your perspective influence the manner in which you work in a community setting?

3. Community workers devote some of their attention to educating the community about pressing social problems and about making use of the human services within the community. In what area might you be interested in developing an educational program?

4. Outreach work is a basic community intervention. If you were working in a community agency at this time, what target group would you particularly want to reach? Would you go into the community to provide services for a client population that might not seek out your services?

5. Are target populations only those in need, or does your definition include groups that have potential for contributing resources to a common effort? For example, how could a parent-teacher association be a target group?

6. What assumptions or beliefs do you hold about people's ability and willingness to walk into an agency and seek assistance? What can get in their way? Does the way you see services being provided reflect your understanding or differ from it?

7. Sue, Ivey, and Pedersen (1996) contend that the values, assumptions, beliefs, and practices of our monocultural society are structured to serve only one narrow segment of the community and that delivery of psychological services tends to be ethnocentric and inherently biased against racial/ethnic minorities and women. If this charge is valid, what challenges will you face as a community worker? What might you do to

We are indebted to Mark Homan of Pima County Community College in Tucson, Arizona, for his detailed review of this chapter and his collaboration with us in updating the material in the third edition.

include more appropriate interventions for more diverse client populations in the community?

8. What are some creative uses of paraprofessional peer helpers for community projects? What ideas do you have for training, supervising, and supporting paraprofessionals?

9. AIDS is becoming an increasing problem in all our communities. What kind of education or action program is needed for a community? What role would you want to play in this endeavor?

10. What are some myths and stereotypes pertaining to people with disabilities? How have you been involved with these individuals? How do you generally feel in their presence? What assumptions are you likely to hold in working with people with disabilities, and how might your assumptions affect the manner in which you work?

11. Have you been involved with older people? How do you generally feel in their presence? How do they generally respond to you? What personal characteristics could enable you to work effectively with the elderly?

12. What are some myths and stereotypes pertaining to the elderly? Can you think of some ways to educate people in the community about the needs of the elderly? about correcting their negative perceptions of the elderly?

13. Crisis intervention is a short-term helping strategy that has particular relevance for dealing with many of the problems individuals in a community face. Are you interested in learning more about crisis intervention? What has been your experience with it in your own community? How could crisis intervention methods result in community change or strengthen a community?

AIM OF THE CHAPTER

Many people argue that professional helpers can foster real and lasting changes only if they have an impact on the total milieu of people's lives. The aspirations and difficulties of clients intertwine with those of many other people and, ultimately, with those of the community at large. Herr (1991) advocates an active role for mental-health professionals in social planning and in politics.

Individuals are part of a community system and are best viewed in relation to others, family, and culture. The systems perspective views the community as a functioning unit, and as an entity unto itself that is made up of more than the sum of its members. The community provides the context for understanding how individuals behave in relationship to each other. Actions by individuals will influence others in the community.

In this chapter we focus on some special responsibilities as a helper in the community. Practitioners who view the community as a "client" will have many roles to play in helping it to improve. Although some of the issues we present pertain mainly to practitioners employed by a community agency, it is essential that helpers, even if they do not work in an agency setting, avoid working in isolation. You can benefit by knowing how to work with community resources. Regardless of your work setting, you will want answers to questions such as the following: How are the human-services needs in your community met? What are the special needs of low-income people? What are some pressing economic needs in addition to mental-health concerns? Can you think of ways to work with a community's efforts in establishing recreational facilities? Where can people go for the social and psychological services they need? If people ask you what resources are available to assist them, can you direct them? What are some of the forces within your community that contribute to the problems individuals and groups are experiencing? What are some of the prevailing attitudes of people in your community about the range of human services? How might you build on these attitudes if they are positive? What can you do to change these attitudes if they are negative? What role would you like to play as a helper in improving your community? What gets in the way of community improvement?

We begin by looking at the community approach, which emphasizes understanding clients by examining their social setting. Whereas the traditional approach to understanding and treating human problems focuses on resolution of internal conflicts as a pathway to individual change, the community approach focuses on ways of changing the environmental factors causing individual problems. This approach stresses social change rather than merely helping people adapt to their circumstances. The community approach also includes meeting unmet community needs, helping the community identify and develop its resources, and employing other measures that ultimately strengthen the community itself. This perspective is based on the premise that the community rather than the individual is the most appropriate focus of attention.

THE COMMUNITY APPROACH

The helping process does not take place in a vacuum isolated from the larger sociopolitical influences of society. Many human-services specialists see a need for new approaches to augment individual counseling. Some call for developing intervention strategies that deal with the societal factors that adversely affect the lives of many members of minority groups (Sue, 1996; Sue, Arredondo, & McDavis, 1992). It is becoming increasingly clear that the values, assumptions, beliefs, and practices of our society are structured to serve only one narrow segment of the population and that the delivery of mental-health services is often ethnocentric and inherently biased against racial/ethnic minorities and women (Sue, Ivey, & Pedersen, 1996).

Helpers have a responsibility to understand that social and political forces affect both their personal and professional lives. Herr (1991) clearly presents a case for developing broader strategies that do not ignore these factors. The changing nature of client populations, pressing social problems, and the impact of advanced technology present a challenge to human-services practitioners to develop problem-solving strategies and techniques with a multidisciplinary perspective. Herr's comments echo the traditional social work perspective of working with the "person in the environment." Rather than focusing on individual dynamics or environmental factors, a process that considers both aspects is often most beneficial to clients.

Professionals who serve in the community need to work harder to change society so it better fits the needs of individuals rather than encouraging people to adapt themselves to some dysfunctional aspects of society. Many of the problems people face are the result of being disenfranchised as individuals or as members of a community or group from systems that hold valued resources for them. The challenge for community workers is to work toward greater degrees of enfranchisement. Culturally skilled community workers particularly understand how the sociopolitical influences impinge on the experiences of racial and ethnic minority groups. For example, immigration issues, racism, stereotyping, poverty, and powerlessness can all severely damage individuals (Arredondo et al., 1996; Sue, Arredondo, & McDavis, 1992).

The traditional approach tends to treat dysfunctions as belonging to the individual, and the helper teaches the individual to adjust to the "realities" of living in a society. In contrast, the community approach assesses these dysfunctions in the context of a larger system; individuals are taught ways of empowering themselves so that they can begin to change some of the inequities in society (Lewis & Lewis, 1989).

Multiple Roles of Community Workers

Increasingly it has become clear that helpers need to move beyond a problem or deficits approach and begin working with communities, building on the strengths and resources in the community. By creating opportunities for community members to develop skills and abilities that contribute to the vitality of their community, community workers help to develop the community, not merely attend to some of its problems. This elevates the quality of life in the community and expands the members' capacity to confront current and future challenges.

Training programs must focus on proactive approaches that include prevention and early intervention strategies for at-risk groups in the community (Hanson, Skager, & Mitchell, 1991). Workers can provide valuable assistance by organizing members of the community and helping them develop their power and set their own agenda on a range of issues, some small or narrowly drawn, and some quite substantial. This approach is possible for agency-based workers and provides for much more active roles for community members and workers alike.

Working with the community usually means working with a specific group or in a situation in which competing or collaborating groups are dealing with an issue or set of issues in a community. These groups usually have a strong identity or a potential for one and can be readily organized for action. In fact, the work of community change is really the work of small groups. That is, within the community group with whom you are working there will be a smaller group of people who take an active part in change efforts. Most of the work of this group will be done in a small group context. In Chapter 9 on group work, we will describe how important it is for human-services workers to capitalize on the value of using group approaches. In working as a change agent within the community, small group skills are essential.

The helping professions must recognize that many problems reside outside the person—such as prejudice and discrimination—and not within the person. Helpers must assume nontraditional roles if they hope to make an impact on social systems. These roles may include advocate, educator, consultant, change agent, facilitator of indigenous support or healing systems, and adviser (Atkinson, Thompson, & Grant, 1993). Although these nontraditional roles are often the most effective interventions from a multicultural perspective, most training programs do not provide education and training in these roles.

According to Mark Homan (1994), if you want to assume an active role in mobilizing the resources within a community, it is useful to have certain knowledge and skills. To maximize your efforts in a community, you need to:

- Know the community's needs, resources, decision-making methods, frames of reference, leadership, and information networks
- Achieve credibility and standing within the community
- Promote meaningful involvement of members of the community being served in community change efforts
- Develop leadership among members of the community
- Develop and build on the strengths or capabilities of members of the community
- Know your target, your issue, your troops, and your resources
- Identify the stakeholders, those who are potential allies and opponents
- Develop investors in the change effort
- Establish and maintain a personal network, especially involving people who may be in a position to assist client groups
- Apply an understanding of systems theory to problems
- Understand the transferability of skills used in working with individual clients to working with the community
- Understand planning and its relationship to action
- Acknowledge that power is used to maintain or change conditions within the community
- Learn that power *with* is at least as important as power *over*
- Make sure that the power and resources you have are greater than the issue you are handling
- Assist the community to declare its needs in a way that allows people to act on them
- Keep people who are involved in the change effort connected to one another
- Link people who want to know with people who do know
- Hold the target accountable and keep the pressure on

- Make sure that your strategies and tactics fit the situation
- Understand that people must *feel* something before they will *do* something
- Use the "cycle of empowerment": involvement, communication, decisions, action
- Listen as assertively as you speak
- Assume responsibility for instigating change
- Avoid setting arbitrary limits on yourself
- Believe in your own capabilities
- Understand that things may well be more important to you who have made the initial decision to get things done than to anyone else involved in the change effort
- Commit yourself to learning—about yourself, your community, your issue, your strategies and tactics
- Remember that it's not only "they" who need to change but "we" who must change what we are doing
- Accept the reality of certain problems or conditions without letting these barriers stop productive efforts
- Confront ethical issues in the delivery of services
- Believe in the rights of members of the community to lead full and satisfying lives

In his book *Promoting Community Change: Making It Happen in the Real World,* Homan (1994) promotes five guidelines for effective helpers: (1) adopt a success attitude, (2) enter into a situation well prepared and with a clear picture of the outcomes you intend to achieve from change projects, (3) follow through with your commitments, (4) acknowledge that you have heard and understood the message of others, and (5) remember to express your appreciation by saying "thank you."

Some uncertainty is natural when you are trying to decide how you can make a difference in your community. Remember, you already have many of the skills you will need to analyze situations and build relationships. It is also important to recognize that idealism can be a valuable asset. Like any other asset, it is strengthened when put into practice. Once you have chosen a community project to become involved with, evaluate your readiness to succeed by answering these questions on Homan's (1994, p. 324) checklist for action:

- From whom do you want to get a response?
- What response do you want to get?
- What action or series of actions has the best chance of producing that response?
- Are the members of your organization able and willing to take these actions?
- How do the actions you decide to take lead to the needed development of your organization?
- How do your actions produce immediate gains in a way that helps achieve your long-term goals?
- Is everything you are doing related to the outcomes you want to produce?
- How will you assess the effectiveness of your chosen approach and refine the next steps you should take?
- What are you doing to keep this interesting?

Take a moment to reflect on what you have already read about the community approach. Think about your educational background, level of professional training, and work experiences. If you plan to go into the human-services field, you are likely to spend some time working in a community agency setting, and you will be working with many different groups within the community. If you were working in such a setting at this time, how prepared are you, both personally and academically, to assume a broader view of helping that encompasses being an agent for change within the community? How can you learn what you will need to know to assume the role of a helper in the community? What specific skills do you need to acquire? What fears would you need to challenge to work effectively in the community? How might you translate your idealism into a practical set of strategies to bring about constructive change within the community?

Facets of the Community Approach to Helping

Lewis and Lewis (1989) define *community counseling* as "a multifaceted approach combining direct and indirect services to help community members live more effectively and to prevent the problems most frequently faced by those who use the services" (p. 10). They describe the activities that make up a comprehensive community counseling program as having the following four distinct facets:

1. *Direct client services* focus on *outreach activities* to a population that might be at risk for developing mental-health problems or that tends to underuse psychological services in the community. For example, older adults are the most underrepresented group among those receiving outpatient mental-health services, yet they are overrepresented in inpatient mental-health populations. More than 60% of public mental hospitals are occupied by people over the age of 65. Efforts such as early intervention and community programs could well prevent or postpone many of these hospitalizations of the elderly (Myers, 1990). It is clear that outreach activities are critically needed to help older people deal with the life transitions they face. Outreach programs find ways to bring services to populations in need of them.

2. *Direct community services* in the form of *preventive education* are geared to the population at large. Examples of these programs include life-planning workshops, AIDS-prevention workshops, the creative use of leisure, and training in interpersonal skills. Because the emphasis is on prevention, these programs help people develop a wider range of competencies.

3. *Indirect client services* involve *client advocacy*, or intervening actively for an individual or group. Those who work in the community aim to empower disenfranchised groups that have become split off from the mainstream community, such as the unemployed, the homeless, people with handicaps, racial and ethnic minorities, elderly people, and people with AIDS. Advocacy doesn't empower people, even though it is a key step toward empowerment. An advocate represents the interests of a group rather than working with a group so that it can effectively promote its own interests. Actively engaging a group with the intention of assisting it to develop its own power is a necessary facet of community work. There will be increased opportunities for the mental-health worker to play a

major role in advocacy for individuals at risk. Helping professionals need to advocate social policies that lead to effective day-care programs, interventions to deal with child abuse or spouse abuse, strategies for early identification and treatment, parent education, and formal programs to develop self-esteem and coping skills (Herr, 1991).

4. *Indirect community services* are attempts to change the social environment for the purpose of meeting the needs of the population as a whole and are carried out by influencing social policy. Community intervention deals with the victims of poverty, sexism, ageism, and racism, who typically feel powerless. The emphasis is on *influencing policymakers* and bringing about positive changes within the community.

The Outreach Approach

As mental-health professionals have become more aware of the need to provide services to a wider population, effective outreach strategies have received increased attention. These strategies are particularly useful for reaching ethnic minorities because of the traditional mistrust of primarily white mental-health professionals who have often mislabeled minorities and excluded them from services. Many people of color perceive counseling as a process that the dominant society employs to forcibly control their lives and well-being (Lee & Richardson, 1991b). As you saw in Chapter 7, if practitioners hope to reach and effectively deal with a cultural group different from their own, they must acquire a broad understanding of culturally diverse client populations. It is essential that helpers use intervention techniques that are consistent with the life experiences and cultural values of culturally diverse groups in the community if they hope to succeed in their outreach efforts (Sue, Arredondo, & McDavis, 1992).

The community psychology model, with its emphasis on creating responsive social systems, is perhaps best suited for people of color. White and Parham (1990) write that this kind of outreach model differs from the traditional model used in the helping professions in the sense that the community worker does not wait for people to come in for help. Instead, the worker reaches out to the community with a coordinated package of preventive mental-health services aimed at improving the psychological health of people throughout the life cycle.

White and Parham (1990) view the community as the client and the community worker as a social engineer who orchestrates a variety of functions involving various levels of the social system that impinge on the psychological well-being of minority groups. It is essential that the community perspective be reflected in the design and delivery of psychological services. White and Parham (1990) state:

> Too often in the past, service models have been developed to do things for Black folks rather than with them. Ideally, a community mental health center in the Black community is a cooperative effort with mental health professionals and community people as equal partners, with community representation at every level of policy making and service delivery. (p. 122)

The "Right of Passage" program (cited in Marino, 1996) is an excellent example of an outreach effort that is exposing a community to counseling and developing a community program for preventing potential problems with young people. Ron Coley and Thomas Parham are both very active in developing the "Right of Passage" program, which is part of the "Passport to the Future" program organized by the 100 Black Men of Orange County. The Right of Passage program includes counseling for a group of African-American young men, ages 14 and up, on a variety of issues. The students in this program meet every other week until they are 18, and the program includes discussion of these pertinent issues:

- Self-awareness
- History of African-American culture
- Relationships with family, women, and other men
- Skill development, including conflict resolution and career development
- Leadership skills such as economic empowerment
- Community service

Parham (cited in Marino, 1996) hopes that the program demonstrates how counseling can become more relevant to the reality of these young men. Parham sees this program as an example of how counselors can design interventions that address specific needs within a community.

There is a growing need to provide programs for populations such as school dropouts, alcohol and drug abusers of all ages, the homeless, victims and perpetrators of child and elderly abuse, suicidal individuals, victims of violent crimes, persons with AIDS, and adolescent mothers. Traditional mental-health concepts and techniques are often inappropriate with such at-risk groups. One of the future challenges for the mental-health practitioner will be to work with institutions (schools, churches, and employers) to offer outreach services for these groups (Hanson, Skager, & Mitchell, 1991; Herr, 1991).

The outreach approach includes developmental and educational efforts, such as skills training, stress management training, education of the community about mental health and the benefits of counseling, and consultation in a variety of settings. These efforts must be made in a way that makes sense to the community, not just the practitioner. If people in the community do not utilize services, it is appropriate to question the value of the services or the appropriateness of the way these services are delivered. Community workers must be willing to learn *from* and *with* the community when organizing services.

You do not have to be all things to potential clients in the community. If you work in a community agency, you will most likely be part of a team working with individual clients. The case management approach involves a number of helping professionals, each with a different specialty. Managed care systems also utilize a team approach, so you need to learn how to build collaborative relationships with the members of a professional team at your agency. Once a need is identified within a community, a group of workers has more power to reach client groups than does a single worker functioning in isolation.

Ask yourself what kind of outreach work you might be inclined to do in your own community. If you have a field placement or a job in a community agency, what ideas do you have for outreach projects? Can you seek out mental-health professionals in your community, or faculty members at your college, who have the expertise to provide you with direction in meeting critical needs of certain client groups? How might you and some fellow students combine your talents and efforts to develop a program for reaching a neglected segment of your community? What agencies and resources within your community could you use in developing an outreach project? Your program does not have to involve a grand design; even a small change can help individuals who are not likely to ask for the assistance they need.

Educating the Community

Educating the community includes educating the professionals regarding the existence and dimensions of problems as well as some steps for dealing with them; educating the broad community about the same things and, in addition, about the costs to the community of maintaining the problem; and educating the potential consumers about the availability of services as well as their right to demand that they be delivered with quality.

Some community workers stay within the agency and do very little to inform the community about existing services and how to utilize them. It is hardly surprising that many people who need psychological help never get it if no one has set up an effective program to educate the public and deal with people's difficulties in getting services. Practitioners must take responsibility for educating their clients about aspects of the helping process such as goals, expectations, and rights and responsibilities.

There are many reasons why people do not make use of available resources: they may not be aware of their existence, they may not be able to afford these services, they may have misconceptions about the nature and purpose of counseling, they may be reluctant to recognize their problems, they may harbor the attitude that they should be able to take charge of their lives on their own, they may believe that professional helpers are attempting to control their lives, they may perceive that these services are not intended for them because they view such services as culturally insensitive, or they may believe that they are not worthy to receive services.

One goal of the community approach is to educate the public and attempt to change the attitudes of the community toward mental-health programs. Perhaps the most important task in this area is to demystify the notion of mental illness. Many people still cling to misconceptions and archaic notions of mental illness. Professionals face a real challenge in combating these faulty notions. Helpers also need to be able to present the array of services they offer to the community in terms that the target groups can understand. Many people still consider seeking any form of professional psychological treatment as something only for those who are seriously mentally ill. Others see professional helpers as having answers for every problem a client brings to the agency. And others hold the belief that professional help is only for the weak or for those who simply cannot solve their own problems. Unless professionals actively work on presenting helping services in a way that is understandable to the community at large, many people who could benefit from professional help may not seek it out. Later in this chapter we go into detail on the role of helping professionals in educating the community about the problems pertaining to AIDS. The ideas we discuss about this topic can easily be applied to any critical need within your community. Educating the community can awaken people to what is available to empower various groups.

Client Advocacy

It is our view that an increasing number of people are unable to cope with the demands of their environment and are receptive to the idea of professional assistance. As more people overcome the stigma attached to seeking psychological help, the demand for community services increases. Helpers need to assume an advocacy role for disenfranchised clients whose backgrounds make it difficult for them to utilize professional assistance. They need to challenge long-standing traditions and preconceived notions that stand in the way of optimal mental health and development.

This challenge might take the form of social and political activism to help client groups learn how to overcome barriers and empower themselves (Lee & Richardson, 1991b). For example, today's older people were raised in a time when mental-health services were available only to people with severe impairments, and thus they often attach a negative stigma to receiving such services (Myers, 1990). The elderly are more difficult to reach, for they may not be so likely to seek a counselor when they are facing problems. They may be more resistant and skeptical about the effectiveness of counseling than are other populations, and it may take special efforts and more time to establish trust. A coordinated effort is needed to remove the stigma that older people have often associated with counseling and to stimulate community mental-health practitioners in designing appropriate programs for the elderly (Weikel, 1990).

Another example of an advocacy role that helpers might assume involves the civil rights of gay and lesbian clients. Dworkin and Gutierrez (1992) challenge mental-health professionals to inform lawmakers and government administrators who determine public policy about the reality of the gay, lesbian, and bisexual population so that decisions will not be based on fears, misconceptions, and stereotypes. Dworkin and Gutierrez present some steps that helpers can take as agents of social change within the community and as advocates for the rights of gay, lesbian, and bisexual people:

- Helpers can demonstrate a spirit of activism by becoming involved with special-interest groups of professional organizations that are designed to examine gay, lesbian, and bisexual issues.
- Practitioners can become activists on the local, state, and national levels. For example, school counselors can work with school boards to bring about in-service education and training pertaining to the needs of gay and lesbian youths.
- Mental-health professionals can assist in the struggle for recognition of gay and lesbian couples and families by supporting bills that provide equality for them. They can also lend support to the removal of bias based on sexual orientation in the evaluation of gay and lesbian parents during custody cases.
- Helpers can play a crucial role in advocating fairness in housing and employment, regardless of sexual orientation. An example might be assist-

ing in the national movement to change the discriminatory policies of the military against gay and lesbian people.

Besides the elderly population and the gay and lesbian population, there are other groups where helpers can exert their influence in changing discriminatory policies. The same principles that were described with these populations can be applied to many other special client populations who could benefit from activism on the part of the mental-health professions.

We also believe that it is essential for helpers to demonstrate a willingness to deal with the client's economic survival needs from the outset. Too often practitioners ignore the fact that before people can be motivated toward growth and actualization, these basic needs must be met. Mental-health services can no longer be tailor-made for the upper middle class. People who are unable to afford the services of professionals in private practice are equally entitled to high-quality treatment programs. Consequently, the community approach is needed to serve people of all ages and backgrounds and with all types and degrees of problems.

Influencing Policymakers

The need for community-based programs is compounded by such problems of our contemporary society as poverty, the plight of the homeless, crime, AIDS, absent parents, divorce, domestic violence, child abuse, unemployment, tension and stress, alienation, addictions to drugs and alcohol, delinquency, and neglect of the elderly. One role that community helpers can assume is shaping social policy and working with legislators who make policy. Helpers need to work within the sociopolitical arena to instigate change. For instance, research into the prevention of AIDS has come about largely through lobbying efforts and political pressure.

It is critical that professional training programs prepare helpers to become competent advocates for at-risk individuals and groups and that they teach students the skills they will need to influence policymaking. If helpers are to be competent in these areas, they will need planning and consultation skills, and they will need to study organizational systems and community resources. They will also need to know (1) what affects policy at the state, local, or national level, (2) what laws or regulations can be applied to gain services for at-risk individuals, and (3) what processes are involved in bringing programs and services to at-risk clients (Hanson et al., 1991).

Community workers can easily feel overwhelmed, especially when there are constraints on funding. A problem facing helpers in community agencies is that they are often underfunded and understaffed. Without adequate funding, creative programs can only remain on the drawing board, and agencies often resort to crisis work and treat problems rather than preventing problems. Because helpers are frequently overworked and have many conflicting demands on their time, it may be difficult for them to do much work in the areas of education, influencing policymakers, outreach, and advocacy. However, helpers must find a way to legitimize the use of time for these activities, because these tasks will not be accomplished if they are considered to be an afterthought.

The Role of the Paraprofessional

There are not enough mental-health professionals to meet the demand for psychological assistance. Faced with this reality, many people in the mental-health field have concluded that nonprofessionals should be given the training and supervision they need to provide some psychological services. There has therefore been a trend toward the use of paraprofessionals in counseling and related fields. Service agencies have discovered that paraprofessionals can indeed provide many direct services as effectively as full professionals, for much lower salaries. Schools and colleges are finding that training peer counselors is an effective strategy for reaching certain individuals who might otherwise go unserved. The paraprofessional movement emerged partially in response to the exclusive practices of the counseling profession, which made mental-health services available only to those who could afford to pay. Moreover, the profession was unwilling to recognize or attempt to remedy the environmental stressors facing their clients. It should be added that professionals are not always supportive of the use of paraprofessionals.

However, a large part of the success of community mental-health programs will depend on these nontraditional workers' receiving training, support, and supervision from professionals. It is essential for both professionals and paraprofessionals to acquire understanding of culturally diverse populations and learn multicultural competencies, as we discussed in Chapter 7. The trend toward the increased use of paraprofessionals means that professionals will have to assume new and expanding roles. They can be expected to spend less time providing direct services to clients, so that they will have time for indirect services such as teaching and consulting with community workers, volunteers, and paraprofessionals. Rather than devoting the bulk of their time to doing case work, interviewing, and counseling, they may need to spend that time offering in-service workshops for paraprofessionals and volunteer workers. Utilizing paraprofessionals can benefit the community. It can benefit paraprofessionals, for they will receive training and supervision. It can also benefit professional practitioners, for it gives them opportunities to develop new roles in carrying out community programs.

An example of the creative use of paraprofessionals is the role of professionals in providing training, supervision, and support for workers with the elderly. Stone and Waters (1991) describe how peer counselors can work with older people in group counseling. The Continuum Center, a community outreach unit of Oakland University in Rochester, Michigan, offers a variety of peer-group counseling programs for older adults. Existing peer counselors recommend those group participants who demonstrate a caring attitude and an ability to listen to the other members in the group. The candidates for new peer-counselor positions attend an orientation and selection process. Those who are selected receive training in the basic helping skills of active listening, effective questioning, and group facilitation. As a part of their training they lead small groups that are videotaped and critiqued. At times, a professional person will sit in the group and provide modeling and feedback. There are frequent in-service meetings at which peer counselors have opportunities to discuss what is going on in their groups.

For the duration of the program, there is supervision, feedback, and support from the professional staff member.

Stone and Waters report that the peer-group counseling program has been quite successful. They point out that such counselors have both advantages and limitations. One of these advantages is that peer counselors are often perceived more as friends and role models than as therapists, which tends to make them less threatening than professionals. One of the limitations is that the skills of peer counselors are not as well developed as those of professionals. Thus, these paraprofessionals need to be aware when problems are beyond their level of competence and to know when and how to refer. This limitation underscores the need for professional supervision as the cornerstone of an effective paraprofessional program. Stone and Waters believe that although peer-counselor programs entail a good deal of training and supervision, they are worth the time and effort because they are effective. This outreach program at the Continuum Center can serve as a model for how paraprofessional peer counselors could be used in community agencies to deliver a wide variety of services to a range of client populations. There are many creative possibilities for professionals and paraprofessionals in working collaboratively to meet the mental-health needs of the community.

AIDS: EDUCATING THE COMMUNITY

Because the AIDS crisis shows no signs of easing, education to stop the spread of the disease is becoming a priority in many of the helping professions. We encourage you to think about your role and responsibility in dealing with the issues surrounding this crisis.

AIDS already affects a wide population with diverse demographics and will continue to be a major health problem in communities. It was not until this disease put a large segment of the population at risk that there was much responsiveness. Along with Earvin ("Magic") Johnson's disclosure of his positive HIV test in November 1991 came the realization that even athletic heroes are vulnerable. He may well be a catalyst who will eventually provoke communities into action.

As a helper you will inevitably come in contact with people who have tested positive as carriers of the virus, people who have AIDS, people who have had sexual contact with those who have tested HIV-positive, people who are the "worried well," and people who are close to AIDS patients. You simply cannot afford to be unaware of the many issues that have emerged from the AIDS epidemic. You need to keep yourself updated with the recent findings as they affect clinical practice. You might be expected to offer direct services to clients with the disease or to provide indirect services in the community geared to education and prevention. You will not be able to educate those with whom you come in contact unless you are educated about the problem yourself. This principle of educating yourself about basic issues can be applied to a range of problems, such as poverty, substance abuse, homelessness, domestic violence, racism, sexism, ageism, and unemployment. Although it is not realistic to expect that you will have in-depth knowledge of the range of problems confronting a community, you can have a general knowledge of these problems and familiarize yourself with resources to direct people with specific needs. In working in a community you will probably be a part of a team of human-services professionals. Each member of the team will have different areas of expertise, and through interprofessional collaboration the combined strengths of practitioners can bring a diverse range of resources to a problem such as preventing AIDS.

We have decided to give prominence to this disease because of the ignorance and fear surrounding the AIDS crisis, both within the community and among members of the helping professions. Remember that there are conflicting reports and evidence about this disease. The changing nature of information about AIDS and misinformation about the ways in which the disease is spread result in apprehension and frustration among helping professionals. Our intent is not to provide you with all the relevant facts about AIDS but, rather, to encourage you to explore your own attitudes, values, and fears about working with people with AIDS-related concerns.*

The Helper's Role
and Responsibility in the AIDS Crisis

Resistance within the helper. The AIDS crisis has created anxiety among many medical personnel and mental-health professionals. This fear brings such helpers into a real conflict. Although they have dedicated their lives to helping those in need, they may have a variety of reasons to justify their unwillingness to help people afflicted with the AIDS virus or AIDS-related problems. Never before have mental-health professionals had concern that they would be infected with a fatal disease that their clients were carrying. Thus, these helpers often resist close contact with those who have been infected.

Overcoming your resistance through education. Mental-health providers may say "I don't know anything about this disease, and I'm not competent to deal with people who are affected by the problem." If you find yourself identifying with this statement and feeling somewhat overwhelmed, it is not necessary to remain this way. You can get the basic information you need about this disease by reading current literature. You can also attend a workshop on AIDS or contact one or more of the many clinics all over the country and use it as a resource for learning what you need to know.

In addition to this basic information about AIDS, it is imperative that you have skills in crisis intervention. Hoffman (1991a) maintains that offering services to individuals who are infected with the human immunodeficiency virus (HIV) will challenge helpers to rethink typical therapy goals and instead develop a framework for utilizing strategies such as reducing stress, helping victims cope, promoting healthful behaviors, and promoting active change. She points out that helpers need to address a range of common issues with these clients, such as sexuality and sexual practices, drug practices, anticipatory grief, declining abilities in daily functioning, spirituality, death, and loss. Perhaps the major challenge

*We want to express our appreciation to Jerome Wright, of Savannah State University in Savannah, Georgia, for his thoughtful reading of this section on AIDS and his constructive suggestions for refining this discussion.

is helping AIDS clients come to terms with loss: "At its simplest, AIDS is about loss. It is about loss of one's health, vitality, sensuality, and career—and most profoundly, the letting go of the future as one had envisioned it" (Hoffman, 1991a, p. 468).

People who come to you because they believe or know that they are carriers of HIV are typically highly anxious. Both those who have tested positive and those who have contracted AIDS are typically in need of short-term help. On learning of their infection, they not uncommonly experience a gamut of emotional reactions, from shock and anger to fear and anxiety, grief over the loss of their previous sexual freedom, and uncertainty over the future. Indeed, some may feel that they have been given a death sentence. They will surely need to find a system to support them through the troubled times that lie ahead. Not only can you be of support by listening to them and helping them deal with their immediate feelings, but you can assist them in finding a broader network. This may take the form of a support group at the agency where you work or a support system among friends and family members.

Some topics frequently shared and explored in an AIDS support group are the grief and loss process, assertiveness training, family issues, spirituality, medication and other health care concerns, nutrition and exercise, learning ways of being sexually safer, coping with homophobia and discrimination, and coping with depression. A group experience teaches people that they are not alone in their plight. For a description of how an AIDS support group can be initiated and maintained in the community, see Steven Lanzet's "One Counselor's Story: Starting an HIV/AIDS Support Group," in M. Corey and G. Corey (1997).

Lanzet began AIDS support groups in his community by consulting with other health care professionals in the community. He worked with a nurse epidemiologist at the local health department who was administering HIV tests. To find out what help was available in his community, he called the National HIV and AIDS Hotline at 800-342-AIDS. He then looked for a suitable location to hold the group meetings and eventually decided to use the YMCA. He found the Gay Community Center to be a helpful resource in spreading the word about the group he was forming. Lanzet suggests that in a large community it is possible to create various groups to meet the specific needs of categories of people such as those who are HIV-positive with symptoms, those with terminal-stage AIDS, those who have been newly diagnosed, and family and friends. Perhaps the key to success in a project like Lanzet's is to realize that relevant people and organizations within a community need to be contacted for their support. An individual practitioner who works in isolation will not have the rich range of resources that is available in many communities. It is the mobilization of these resources that can provide the team effort needed to launch and successfully implement any program in the community.

Special Needs of Clients with the AIDS Virus

The stigma of AIDS.   In addition to clients who have manifested the more severe symptoms of AIDS, you will see clients who have discovered that they have the virus within them. They live with the anxiety of wondering whether they will come down with this incurable disease. Most of them also struggle with the stigma attached to AIDS. They live in fear not only of developing a life-threatening disease but also of being discovered and thus being rejected by society in general and by friends and loved ones.

The stigma is attached to the fact that most of those in the United States who have contracted AIDS are either sexually active gay or bisexual men or present or past abusers of intravenous drugs. For some, the stigma may be worse than the diagnosis itself. Indeed, this stigma may be the filter through which society has viewed the AIDS crisis (Hoffman, 1991a). Yet it is a mistake to identify the problem of AIDS with any particular group. AIDS has been called an "equal-opportunity disease," for it affects a wide segment of society. It is a myth that AIDS is a disease that is restricted to the gay male population.

Among the mainstream population, there is still a general negative reaction toward lesbians, gay men, and bisexuals. Educational programs must be directed at challenging and changing stereotypes, misconceptions, and negative attitudes toward certain populations. Typically, people who develop AIDS are afflicted with a double-edged stigma, one due to their lifestyle and the other due to the disease, which is often seen as the result of their homosexual activities or drug behavior. People afflicted with AIDS often stigmatize themselves and perpetuate beliefs such as "I feel guilty and ashamed," "I feel that God is punishing me," "I am a horrible person, and therefore I deserve to suffer," and "I am to blame for getting this disease."

AIDS patients' anger.   In addition to feeling different and stigmatized, those with AIDS typically have a great deal of anger. They often feel left alone and without support. This feeling is frequently grounded in reality. In some cases family members actually "disown the outcast." Patients often feel a sense of disillusionment, for after getting better for a time, they become sicker. They also feel isolated. For some, this isolation is expressed through their feeling of utter rejection by others: "I'm gay, and now I've got AIDS. No one wants anything to do with me." "I'm a drug user, and I engage in criminal and deviant behavior." It is hard for them to see any meaning in their plight, and thus they often slip into depression. Consequently, they develop anger at having a life-threatening condition. They express this anger by asking over and over: "What did I do to deserve this? Why me?" This anger is sometimes directed at God for letting it happen, and then they may feel guilty for having reacted this way. Anger is also directed toward others, especially those who are likely to have given them the virus. Anger is aimed at health professionals as well. Patients are angry because their lives have been unalterably changed.

If you expect to provide help to HIV-positive clients, patients with AIDS, and their loved ones, it is critical that you confront any biases and misconceptions you may have. One study revealed that the psychologists and social workers who were sampled consistently held negative and biased views toward HIV-positive people and those with AIDS (Crawford, Humfleet, Ribordy, Ho, & Vickers, 1991). Many professionals in this study expressed the view that people with AIDS were more responsible for their illness, less deserving of compassion, and more dangerous to society than people who had leukemia. The respondents consistently indicated that they did not want to provide service to clients with AIDS. If helpers have negative views toward people with the virus, the chances are slim that they will be able to work effectively with this population.

How You Are Affected as a Helper

If you are involved in providing help and support for people who have developed AIDS, many of these clients will be dying, which will certainly have an impact on you. Reflect on the following questions:

- Your clients may well displace some of their anger onto you. How do you think you will handle such anger?
- Your clients will probably be affected by relationship issues and shifts in roles. How will they adapt to these changes? How might you be affected by their struggles to adapt?
- How do you prepare yourself as a helper to respond to questions such as "Why did this happen to me?"
- How might the hopelessness that your clients feel affect you? Could their despair lead you to feel that your work with them was futile?
- As your clients bring up unfinished business with key people in their lives, how might it affect you?
- What specific values and biases might you hold that could make it difficult for you to be objective in working with people who have AIDS? Are you open to examining and changing these attitudes?
- Your clients are likely to bring up the issue of meaning in their lives now that they are afflicted with a disease that prevents them from doing many of the things that gave them meaning. How might their crisis in discovering meaning have an impact on you? Many times these clients will say: "I simply can't see any point in living anymore. I can't do anything. All I have to look forward to is suffering." What would you have to offer them?
- If clients bring up their fears of dying or what lies beyond death, do you see yourself as able to assist them in giving expression to their fears? Will their fears trigger your own fears?
- How do you think losing relatively young AIDS patients is likely to affect you?
- In working with clients who are at risk for contracting AIDS, you cannot avoid talking about sexually explicit topics. Do you feel able to discuss such topics?
- Gray and House (1991) maintain that sexually active clients must make responsible decisions, change familiar patterns, and learn new sexual behaviors. They add that it is unrealistic to expect clients to do this without the active assistance of professionals. Do you see yourself being able to fulfill this role? If not, how will you deal with clients who want to explore their sexual behavior?
- If you do a good deal of work with AIDS patients and their family members, what concerns do you have about burnout? What are some ways in which you could prevent it? Do you see yourself as willing to ask for sup-

port from others as you work with this difficult population? Do you have a support group?

- Assume that you were working with people who had tested HIV-positive or had AIDS and were confronted with the question "How can you possibly understand what I am going through; you haven't walked in my shoes?" How would you respond?

The Helper's Role in Educating the Community

Regardless of what type of helper you happen to be, one of your most important functions is to dispel myths and misconceptions about AIDS and to help the community acquire realistic knowledge and attitudes. As we have mentioned, to be able to carry out this function effectively, you need to differentiate between fact and fiction about this disease. Information about some aspects of AIDS seems to be changing daily, so facts we provide here might be outdated by the time this book is published. Therefore, as we have stressed, it is imperative that you keep up with the latest research in this field.

Education of various target groups is the key in preventing sharp rises in the number of AIDS victims. According to Hoffman (1991a), prevention of the disease must be given priority in working with all clients. For her, education is the best way to avert the devastation of HIV infection; prevention is the best means of ending this epidemic. To educate various segments of the community, you will need to know your community and be aware of the values, mores, and cultural backgrounds of the various groups you serve. In attempting to change the habits of racial, cultural, and religious groups, you are likely to run up against considerable resistance unless you are able to "speak their language." Furthermore, in educating members of the community, it is important to realize that AIDS patients can easily become the scapegoats of people's projections of their unconscious fears and hatred. People who are highly intolerant of those who are different from them often engage in denial and seek a target for their resentments. Any educational program must be directed toward minimizing denial and homophobia.

Because information is changing rapidly, it is difficult for people who are at risk to trust what they hear from the medical profession. They may be defensive about further education because they don't believe what is presented to them. They may also remain in a state of denial because they do not want to change their sexual lifestyle. These difficulties will challenge you to find a meaningful way to provide education. A few key elements of the educational effort are listed below:

- As a helper, explore your own attitudes, and eliminate those beliefs that make it difficult for you to make contact with those who need your help.
- Take steps to understand AIDS yourself. Learn updated information on both the medical and the psychological aspects of the disease.
- Emphasize prevention. A comprehensive sex-education program, for all age groups, is essential if AIDS is to be prevented.
- Rather than thinking in terms of "safe sex," consider practices that are "unsafe," "relatively save," and "safer." If people are going to be sexually

active, they will not be safe, and they need to recognize the risks of infection. Whether or not they are infected with the virus, clients should be informed and encouraged to adopt safer sex practices to reduce risks.

- Seek training in crisis intervention in the issues facing HIV-positive individuals and people with AIDS.
- Community efforts need to be made to care for people with AIDS. Part of your job as a helper could be to mobilize people in the community to become active and to serve in various capacities as volunteers.
- In developing educational programs, keep in mind the special needs of minority groups. Certainly, many minorities are not responsive to education as it is typically presented. Alternatives to the usual means of education might include training ministers to work with their congregations, using a spokesperson or a role model to whom young people can relate, creating videos with educational goals, and using AIDS victims as resource people to teach others about the disease.

Advances in medical technology, birth control, and artificial reproduction methods allow for an increased range of sexual choices. At the same time, AIDS and other sexually transmitted diseases make the consequences of sexual choices more serious than at any time before. Human-services professionals have an ethical responsibility to help their clients identify and explore any sexual issues that are relevant to their lifestyle or to refer clients to helpers who are prepared to address sexual concerns. Helpers will not be able to carry out this responsibility if they are lacking in knowledge about human sexuality. If helpers are uncomfortable dealing with sexual matters with their clients, the helping relationship may be sabotaged.

Case Example of AIDS Education

You are working in a community mental-health agency, and the director asks you and several of your colleagues to design a comprehensive education program to promote awareness of AIDS in the community. The director tells you that her goal is to do everything possible to prevent people from contracting AIDS and that she would like members of the community to develop a realistic understanding of the issues involved in this major health problem. She wants people to have detailed information about AIDS and would like to see them discuss the issue at community meetings in the center. Once you and your colleagues have written up a proposal, she wants your group to make a presentation to the board members of the agency, who represent a range from very conservative to very liberal.

Your group works diligently and comes up with a comprehensive program. Your proposal calls for focusing on the schools from elementary to community college. Your group is suggesting workshops and short courses to be conducted by community workers and health care providers. Although your program involves a frank and comprehensive discussion of all major issues pertaining to AIDS, it also calls for dealing with the topic in a manner that is sensitive to the community and that is appropriate for the target groups. The key features of your proposed workshops include the following: information on the state of the disease, identification of who is at risk, psychosocial dimensions of the disease, attitudes toward those who have contracted AIDS, ethical and legal issues, medical facts and concerns, prevention of AIDS, and implications for the future. You intend to have AIDS patients talk to classes at the schools, along with physicians and other professionals with knowledge about this disease. Your program will also focus on teaching specific methods of "safer sex" and encouraging these practices.

After your group finishes presenting its findings to the board of directors, several members loudly and passionately protest on the grounds that your group is promoting immorality and interfering with their rights as parents. They don't want the schools encouraging their children to practice "safer sex" when in their home they are teaching them how to live morally decent lives. They attempt to convince you that AIDS is a natural consequence of rampant immorality that has been spreading through the country.

On the basis of your values, what arguments might you give these board members? How would you answer their opposition? Would you be willing to omit the more controversial aspects of your program? Would you be willing to make room in your program for advocates of abstaining from sexual relationships outside of marriage? Would you be willing to give equal time to representatives who opposed your point of view? Your values will certainly enter into the picture as you develop your views toward your responsibilities in dealing with the AIDS crisis.

UNDERSTANDING TWO SPECIAL POPULATIONS

In this section we deal with assumptions and attitudes pertaining to two special populations, people with disabilities and the elderly. People with disabilities have to face prejudice, hostility, lack of understanding, and discrimination on the basis of their physical, emotional, or mental handicap. Nondisabled individuals frequently view this group through the same distorted spectacles with which they see others who differ from them. The clarity of a helper's vision can be impaired by myths, misconceptions, prejudices, and stereotypes about people with disabilities. We also include a treatment of the needs of the elderly because they are often a neglected client population and because many human-services programs are being developed to provide help to the elderly. Our discussion focuses on the importance of the helper's attitudes as a key factor in successfully intervening in the lives of people with disabilities and with older people. Some guidelines are given for better serving the diverse range of individuals in these groups in the community.

Assumptions about People with Disabilities

Vacc and Clifford (1988) maintain that physically disabled people do not want to be labeled in a general way as handicapped but tend to view themselves as individuals who have a disability. Some paraplegics are concerned that others may view them as being paralyzed from the neck up as well as from the waist down. Nonhandicapped individuals often try to hide their feelings of awkwardness in the presence of a person with a disability through exaggerated attention and kindness. Vacc and Clifford emphasize the importance of helpers' being willing to examine their own attitudes when they are working with clients who have any kind of disability. Helpers need to avoid categorizing individuals as all being the same, even though they have some common concerns due to their disability.

As with any special population with which you work, it is essential that you identify your assumptions pertaining to people with disabilities. For example, you could assume that certain careers might be out of reach for a client with a disability. But to make this assumption without checking it out with your client is tantamount to limiting his or her options. This would be a good time for you to reflect on any stereotypes that you may have toward this group and to challenge your assumptions. A few examples of myths and misconceptions associated with this special population are:

- If you are physically disabled, you are also mentally and emotionally disabled.
- People with disabilities do not have the same feelings as the nondisabled.
- Individuals with a disability have a limited capacity to be normal.
- They are totally dependent on others.
- They are disabled as people, and their goals should be modest.

I (Marianne) gave a talk to people with disabilities at a residential facility. The kinds of questions they raised were not any different from those of other groups that I have addressed, and many of the residents emphasized that they were no different from people without disabilities. Later, I asked a staff member at this institution to ask a few residents this question: "What would you like to tell helpers in training about yourself to assist them in better dealing with special populations?" Three different residents gave these responses:

- "I would like them to know that I want to be treated as a normal person even though I am in a wheelchair. Look at the person, not at the wheelchair. Don't be afraid of us."
- "I'm a very good person. I'm a very smart person. I have a disability, but I also have intelligence."
- "I can think and feel just like a normal person."

The staff member said a great deal in very few words in a letter to me about her perceptions of the people she helps:

They have lived in institutions for most of their adult lives. They say they are no different from people without disabilities, but I think that they have enormous hearts. The people I have known have no prejudice and are very loving and giving. They also have a greater appreciation for the very simple things in life that most of us take for granted each day. They are unique individuals and I feel fortunate to have worked with them.

Special Needs of the Elderly

The way you approach aging has a great deal to do with how you will treat older people. Rather than focusing on old age as being exclusively a time of loss, you can see it as a time of both positive and negative transformations. Be open to what older people can teach you, even if you are in the role of helping them. Elderly people have a vast wealth of life experiences and coping skills, which they are likely to share with you if they sense that you have a genuine interest in them. They can draw on their experiences as they are deciding on ways to respond to the circumstances of later life. In working with the elderly, avoid making assumptions, and instead listen carefully to learn about their coping resources (Myers, 1990).

Working with the elderly demands an awareness of the particular life issues they face. Some themes that are more prevalent with the elderly than with other age groups include loneliness and social isolation, loss of friends, loss of bodily and mental functions, feelings of rejection, the struggle to find meaning in life, feelings of uselessness and despair, fears of death and dying, and regrets about past events.

During the period known as "maturity" (ages 50–65) and "old age" (65 years to death), the core transitional theme is the resolution of a sense of "generativity" versus stagnation. Erikson's concept of generativity suggests an interest going beyond caring for one's own offspring to include a concern with the next generation. This is a time for both consolidation of experience and resources and a reorientation toward one's later years. Slaikeu (1990) outlines a range of possible developmental crises associated with this phase of life, some of which are health problems, retirement, conflicts with adult children, divorce, death of a spouse, conflicts with parents, financial difficulties, neglect by adult children, and the death of friends.

Challenging myths and stereotypes about the elderly.   If you are working with the elderly, one of your first tasks is to debunk some of the myths and negative perceptions about the elderly that you may have incorporated, either consciously or unconsciously. If you accept the many misconceptions about older people, there is little chance that your behavior with them will be helpful. Not only do you need to explore your own beliefs about the elderly, but it would be well to think of ways in which you could educate the community about the aging process. It is also important in your work with the elderly to find ways of helping them question any self-limiting beliefs they may have accepted from their society. Some stereotypes associated with older people that need to be challenged are:

- All elderly people eventually become senile.
- Old people are nonproductive and cannot contribute to society.
- Most older people are depressed.
- Growing old always entails having a host of serious physical and emotional problems.
- Older people are set in their ways, are stuck in rigid patterns of thinking and behaving, and are not open to change.

- When people grow old, they are no longer capable of learning.
- Old people are no longer beautiful.
- Most elderly people are lonely.
- Old people are no longer interested in sex.

These are some negative perceptions and stereotypes of older people that are common in our society. The basic myth that the elderly are resistant to change, combined with many helpers' lack of experience with this age group and unfamiliarity with relevant helping approaches, seems to have kept helping of the elderly at a developmental standstill for years (Hern & Weis, 1991). How can you educate yourself about the elderly? How can you become familiar with approaches to helping older people within your own community?

According to Myers (1990), those in the mental-health professions are not exempt from such stereotypical thinking about the elderly, which discourages many helpers from working with older clients. Myers describes the interaction of negative societal perceptions and the psychological functioning of older people within the framework of the *social-breakdown syndrome*. This model holds that as people age, they become more vulnerable to perceptions and definitions of them by society. The social-breakdown syndrome involves a downward spiral in which older people increasingly internalize myths and negative perceptions, resulting in a view of themselves as incapable of experiencing a rich life. This self-perception leads to decreased attempts to control their environment. As they appear to have less control, negative input from society reinforces their shaky perceptions of self, and the downward spiral continues. Although during most of their adult years people may have had an internal locus of control, they may shift to an external locus when they are faced with crises of later life that they feel powerless to control.

Guidelines for effectively reaching older people. We do not think that there is one kind of person, one set of personal characteristics, or one style of helping that makes for effective involvement with older people. But effective helping of the elderly demands a knowledge of their special needs and the ability to form working relationships with them. Here are some guidelines that we think will increase your capacity for understanding and working with older people:

- Young people sometimes put older people in a very different category from themselves. In reality, there are more similarities than differences between older and younger people. Both age groups have a need for support and challenge, respect, understanding, and acceptance. A way to treat elderly people is to consider them as having the same feelings, wishes, and thoughts as many younger people.
- Elderly clients can activate the helper's recollections of parents and grandparents. At times, helpers avoid dealing with the elderly because of the stark reminders of their own inevitable aging and death. If helpers are unaware of the reactions that are being stimulated within them as they work with elderly clients, their efforts at helping will be thwarted.
- Realize that there is a continuity in life patterns, and help clients discern these themes. Individuals who are chronically unhappy in their youth also stand

a good chance of remaining unhappy as they age, unless they make a decision to do something to change certain patterns.

- Older people often have youthful feelings and wish they had a youthful body. Treat them as though they were young. Don't treat them as pitiable old people, and don't become overly focused on age. Believe in their capabilities rather than dwelling on their limitations.

- Babies have a need to be held; adolescents have a need to be let go of; older people have a need to be seen and heard. Typically, elderly people need to reminisce and reflect, and they need to be listened to and understood. Through talking and being heard, they are able to put facets of their lives into perspective. If you demonstrate a genuine interest in them, they will reveal a great deal of themselves through their stories. You can show respect by being patient and by accepting them through hearing their underlying messages.

- Don't get caught up in listening only to the content of what the elderly reveal, but listen for the deeper messages that they often convey nonverbally. Let them know how you are being affected as you listen to them.

- As a way of establishing rapport, remember that kindness goes a long way in building bonds. Touch is a meaningful way of contacting elderly people. A touch on the arm or shoulder can signify warmth. In their counseling groups with the very old, Hern and Weis (1991) found the use of touch to be one of the most effective forms of positive reinforcement. These elderly group members took delight in a pat on the hand or a quick hug, and this touching seemed to increase their sense of belonging. They also took pleasure in the joining of hands as one of the group members offered a prayer as a way to end a group session. Although hugging and touching may be meaningful, this contact should be used only when it is deemed acceptable by the older person (Myers, Poidevant, & Dean, 1991). In touching it is absolutely critical to be real. Do not use touching as a technique but only as an extension of concern you are feeling.

- Many elderly people suffer from confusion and forgetfulness. Strive to be patient, because their symptoms tend to worsen if you are impatient with them. They are probably frustrated with themselves over their symptoms. They have a need for self-pride, which is difficult to maintain as they face being dependent.

- Be open to understanding the ways in which older clients' cultural backgrounds continue to influence their present attitudes and behaviors.

- Your personal characteristics will influence the quality of your contact with elderly clients. Some of the qualities that are essential to cultivate are humor, a sense of playfulness, enthusiasm, patience, courage, endurance, hopefulness, tolerance, nondefensiveness, freedom from prejudices, and a willingness to learn. Your gift of presence and the understanding that flows from this presence can be powerful ways to make connections with the elderly.

- It is essential that you have an ability to be both gentle and challenging. It requires sensitivity to know when it is therapeutic to provide support and when to challenge.

Not everyone can work effectively with the elderly. However, before you too quickly decide that "I could never work with old people," test out your assumptions and any conclusions that you might have made. Just because you may be uncomfortable in relating to older people does not mean that you cannot change.

You do not have to be elderly to appreciate the difficulties of this time of life. Through your active caring, you can build a bridge between yourself and those who are considerably older. If you are open to your own feelings—over painful events, experiences of sadness, times of uncertainty, hopes and fears, and times of loneliness—these feelings can be your best tools in touching people who are older than you. As an adolescent you might well have struggled with finding meaning in your life. You might have felt stifled by your limited control at this time of your life. Many elderly people are also stifled in their attempts to realize their full potential, and they often struggle with finding meaning in the face of many losses. You can use your experiences as an adolescent to get a better sense of the nature of an elderly person's world. It is not necessary to share identical experiences with your clients but, rather, to find a way to tap into similar feelings over different life experiences. This principle is true not only in working with older people and those with disabilities but also in relating to individuals in other special client groups who are likely to differ from you in a number of significant respects. What is important is that you do what you can to learn about the world view of clients who are different from you and at the same time use your universal life themes as a way of building bridges between you and individuals and groups that differ from you.

HOW TO WORK
WITH OTHER CLIENT POPULATIONS

We encourage you to think about other neglected or unpopular client groups within your community and to apply our discussion about people with disabilities, elderly people, and people with AIDS to them. You need to know how to work *with* the community as well as *for* the community. Any program that you design must incorporate ways of reaching out to the target population as well as ways for potential clients to gain access to your services. How might you develop educational programs in your community to provide services to these client groups? Realize that education is only a first step and that important as it is it alone is not sufficient to bring about change. Educational efforts must be directed toward action programs that will bring about community improvement. How might you mobilize the community to take action that will improve the plight of certain at-risk groups? It is essential to identify the principles relevant for community action that we developed in the section on AIDS. Regardless of the client population, these questions illustrate principles that you can apply in understanding and working with a target group:

- What specific populations in your community are most in need of help? What kind of help do they need? To what degree do you understand the special needs of these target groups? What resources and capabilities of the community can be brought to bear on resolving the plight of a target group?
- What are your assumptions and attitudes toward this target group? What possible prejudices, biases, and stereotypes might you harbor toward this

group? Identify some of your fears or concerns in working with a client group. How will you deal with your own fears? How might you deal with the strong reactions of those within the community who may be shocked that you are working with such unpopular clients populations?

- In what ways might society stigmatize at-risk groups such as the homeless? substance abusers? veterans? children from alcoholic families? the unemployed? And in what ways might individuals within certain groups continue to stigmatize themselves? As a helper, how can you remove stigmas that block effective programs?
- How much do you know about the characteristics of a particular target group? Are you aware of what needs to be done and how you might begin? Are you aware of the resources within the community that can be utilized with this group?
- As a worker in the community, what can you do to empower a target group? What social and political channels are open to you and to your clients?
- How can you combine your talents and experience with others in the helping professions to improve a situation in the community?

We focused on the impact of the AIDS epidemic as an example of principles and strategies that you can employ in working with many groups in your community. You need to educate yourself about the characteristics of the client population and find ways to combine forces with other helpers and organizations so that you won't be a single voice in the wind as you attempt to bring about change within your community. Work with individuals and groups in a manner that will increase their chances of becoming empowered rather than depending on you for answers to their concerns. And remember, you don't need to operate as an individual. Seek help from experts within your community who can provide special knowledge and make suggestions for how you can best serve various client groups. For example, you may not have the specialized knowledge and skills to work directly with clients who have substance abuse problems, but you can recruit experts who are willing to consult with you and with small groups within your community.

CRISIS INTERVENTION IN THE COMMUNITY

For a few moments, think about some of the recent crisis situations you have read about in the daily newspaper or seen on television. Reflect on the direct impact that many of the crises on the international, national, and state levels have on the functioning of your community. Below is a sample listing of the kinds of crises that deeply affect the community in both direct and indirect ways:

- Floods kill hundreds and leave thousands homeless.
- Ravaging fire destroys an entire neighborhood.
- Gunman goes on shooting spree that leaves 27 people dead and many seriously injured.

- Two commercial jetliners collide in midair and fall in a heavily populated area, leaving residents in shock.
- Devastating earthquake levels much of the downtown area.
- War in the Middle East leaves families uncertain about their future.
- High school honor student takes his own life and leaves the school community stunned.
- Alcohol blamed in the death of six teenagers in car accident.

Modrak (1992) points out that newspaper headlines reveal tragedies that generate multiple victims and affect entire communities. As disasters have escalated, helping professionals have had to develop quick and effective intervention strategies to deal with the disruption in the community. Modrak cites the midair collision between a commuter plane and a helicopter that crashed into an elementary school, killing two children and injuring five others on the ground. The mental-health professionals in the area played a vital role in responding to the event, which devastated the community. Modrak also refers to the tragedy at the University of Iowa in 1991 when a graduate student, upset over not having received an award, shot and killed five people and critically injured another before killing himself. A crisis team at the university responded immediately by working first with those most immediately affected and then with those in the community who were more removed. The team of helpers provided crisis counseling for those affected by the event, assessed their needs, and then made appropriate referrals. There were open meetings of mourning three days after the shooting. People in the university community were invited to share their reactions in group sessions, which were held in the student union. This event jarred the community members into the realization of their own vulnerability. It also led to a cohesive sense of feeling that "we are all in this together."

In tragedies such as these, entire communities experience major disequilibrium and are in need of immediate and effective intervention to help them rally their resources. Modrak cites lessons that have been learned about the importance of being prepared to deal with tragedies. In some communities, crisis teams meet regularly to update information and work out procedures for responding. It is clear that those in the helping professions need to have the knowledge, skills, and training to provide immediate assessment, intervention, referral, and follow-up.

Our intention in this section is to introduce you to the nature of crisis intervention work, which might constitute the majority of your professional activity. The chances are that you will take at least one course in crisis intervention, will have opportunities to practice these skills, and will learn in your supervised field placements methods of dealing with a variety of crisis situations. The purpose of our discussion here is to explore various facets of the crisis intervention approach, such as ways of viewing a crisis; the phases involved; and the major assumptions, goals, clinical principles, and expected outcomes of intervention. A way to learn more about the practice of crisis intervention is to consult two excellent textbooks, Gilliland and James (1997) and Slaikeu (1990). Much of the following discussion is based on a modification of crisis intervention theory and practice as described by these authors and on ideas suggested by the late Daniel Saddler of Western Carolina University.

The Context of Crisis

Let's begin with a definition of crisis intervention as "a helping process aimed at assisting a person or a family to survive an unsettling event so that the probability of debilitating effects (e.g., emotional scars, physical harm) is minimized, and the possibility of growth (e.g., new skills, new outlook on life, more options in living) is maximized" (Slaikeu, 1990, p. 6). It should be stressed that the crisis model can be applied to working with the community as the "client" as well as working with individuals who are in crisis.

Crisis intervention is a short-term approach to helping that is the treatment of choice in cases where clients are experiencing a state of acute psychological disequilibrium. Individuals in crisis, or a community that is faced with a crisis, are temporarily disrupted cognitively, emotionally, and behaviorally, and they are in need of immediate and skilled help. This helping process should last as long as it typically takes people to bounce back to their precrisis level of functioning, which is generally up to six weeks.

Most of the clients who come to a community agency will be experiencing either a developmental or a situational crisis. A *developmental* crisis pertains to some expected difficulty at each stage of life. As you will see in Chapter 11, Erikson's eight developmental stages present opportunities for transformation and also represent a potential crisis. Some examples of developmental crises include the trauma of early childhood, getting married or divorced, the stresses of parenthood, coping with children's leaving home, finding meaning in life after retirement, and adjusting to the death of friends and family members. Events such as these do not necessarily lead to crises, for the person's interpretations and responses to these life transitions are the determining factors.

In crisis theory, the term *crisis* is not considered negative; rather, it is an essential ingredient in human growth and development. Crisis is a time in one's life for making choices. Situations do not merely happen to us. The stance we take toward life situations is what determines the quality of life. The word *crisis* is derived from the Greek word *krinein*, which means "to decide." The Chinese symbol for *crisis* represents both danger and opportunity. For example, being confronted by a serious illness can result in a reevaluation of one's priorities and a major change in the way one is living. How people respond to these critical turning points is what makes the difference. A utopian existence is not one without any crises, for crisis is an essential element in human development. The crises that we face at the various phases of life are frequently catalysts that awaken us to the richer possibilities awaiting us if we have the courage to go through a transformation.

In addition to the expected developmental crises that are associated with the various stages of life, we also must endure unexpected events that can have the impact of paralyzing our will to act or can result in new directions for living once the crisis situation is over. Such *situational* crises can include sexual assault, discovery of a serious illness in oneself or a loved one, the breakup of an intimate relationship, a serious financial setback, or a natural disaster. As a helper employed in a community agency, you may be called on to counsel suicidal clients, deal with posttraumatic stress disorders, help those with severe physical limitations, and offer strategies for those who abuse drugs and alcohol.

The Process of Crisis Intervention

There are two levels of crisis intervention. First-order intervention can be thought of as psychological first aid. This level of intervention is carried out by mental-health professionals and a network of others such as ministers, judges, police and fire personnel, nurses, paramedics, physicians, school counselors, parole officers, teachers, and a wide range of human-services workers. The other form of crisis intervention is second-order intervention, or crisis therapy, which requires considerably more specialized training and expertise.

First-order intervention involves immediate assistance and often takes only one session. The major goal of this level of intervention is to reestablish an individual's immediate coping capacity. To accomplish this goal, helpers offer support, do what they can to reduce the chances of death, and link people in crisis to other helping resources. There are many settings where the staff must be equipped to handle a wide range of crises, such as the hospital emergency room or the crisis intervention hot line. Staff members and paraprofessionals can be given training to respond quickly and effectively when they initially encounter people in crisis.

Helpers understand that the outcomes of a crisis can be for better or worse. As a result of a crisis, a person can return to an old level of coping, assume a new way of dealing with life, or ultimately decide on suicide. The task of helpers who offer psychological first aid is to help individuals tap any resources available to them to restore a sense of equilibrium, which will eventually allow them to work through their reactions so that they can meet future challenges.

Helpers create support through their attitudes and behaviors. Perhaps what helpers most have to offer is their gift of presence. This is the capacity to "be fully there" for individuals in crisis as they tell their story and seek human connection to guide them to some sense of stability amid the temporary chaos they are experiencing. In your initial encounter with a client in crisis, you can give the gift of presence partially by what you say but even more by a genuine manner that reflects caring and a deep sense of compassion. You may often feel helpless to change a tragic situation, and you could burden yourself with thoughts that what you are *doing* is not enough. Yet presence is powerful and goes beyond what you can do to change a reality. Your willingness to be fully in contact with others as they strive to put their lives back together can be most healing and necessary.

It is important that your clients feel invited to tell their stories and also that you avoid assuming that you know exactly what they need or what is best for them. As they tell their stories, your task is to listen with as much understanding as possible. The real task is for you to encourage them to talk and for you to see what they are going through from their perspective. This role implies getting a sense of where your clients want to go and ascertaining what options are open for action. As clients express themselves, it is important that you also make an assessment of the immediate situation, especially of their coping resources. Throughout the process, your primary task is ensuring their safety. Some clients may feel so distraught and so unable to cope with the crisis that they see suicide as their only way out. Suicidal urges may last for a short time in the face of despair, and it is your job to intervene to prevent any deadly actions. People in crisis frequently give clues, which you need to catch. In making an assessment of the client's potential for taking lethal action, you must know the appropriate questions to ask as well as being aware of danger signs. You also need to develop contracts with clients who pose a danger to themselves, as well as specific methods of follow-up after a session. Arranging for referrals is a very important part of this work. It is well for you to ask yourself if you have enough knowledge and skill to assist your crisis clients. You need to know your limits, and you need to know about resources within the community that can serve as a lifeline for those working through a crisis.

The first-order level of crisis intervention often entails a short-range plan of what to do next. People in crisis may overwhelm themselves with feeling that everything has to be attended to at once. You can help them get some focus on what must be done now and what can wait until later. Clients often feel immobilized to the degree that they cannot see any options or have difficulty knowing which are the best options. You can calm them and help them identify a network of resources available to them, such as family, friends, and community.

Through the process of receiving psychological first aid, people often get the understanding, support, and guidance they need to avoid harm to themselves or others. At this level, one of your tasks is to help clients identify and examine possible routes they can later use to work through a crisis. This initial level of intervention does not resolve their crisis, for the effects of the crisis linger, and vestiges must be worked through. This is where second-order intervention, also known as *crisis therapy*, becomes necessary. This is a short-term therapeutic process that goes beyond immediate coping and aims at crisis resolution and change. The main goals of this level of intervention are to help people in crisis better face their future and to minimize the chances of their being a psychological casualty. It is critical that clients learn from the crisis and that they be given opportunities to work through unfinished business. Ideally, they will be given the assistance that will result in their remaining open to life and to new choices, rather than closing themselves off to the vast range of future possibilities.

In crisis therapy, clients are encouraged to express and deal with feelings, some of which may have been locked up. It can be very freeing for clients to let go of trapped feelings, which can be converted into positive emotional energy that can be used constructively. Typically, the feelings that are denied expression (such as guilt or anger) are the ones that cause people grave difficulties. Venting pent-up feelings in itself often facilitates psychological healing.

Another task of second-order crisis intervention consists of helping clients attain a realistic perspective on the crisis event. There is a need to develop an understanding of how the event has affected them, including the meaning of the crisis in their lives. Clients typically must rebuild cognitions that have been damaged by a crisis. Part of the process of crisis therapy involves clients' learning how their thought patterns have resulted in certain behaviors. Clients are helped to cognitively reframe events, which allows for a new range of behavioral possibilities. As can be seen, this advanced phase of crisis work demands greater expertise than does the beginning phase. Crisis therapy is provided by helping professionals who have specialized knowledge and skills.

How Crisis Work Can Affect the Helper

In Chapter 12, we examine the demands and stresses of professional work, which can ultimately lead to burnout. In Chapter 4 we discussed how a helper's old wounds are opened in the process of getting involved in clients' lives and how this reactivation of earlier experiences can collide with the helper's personal and professional life. Both burnout and countertransference can particularly affect those helpers whose primary work is with client populations in some type of crisis. One young social worker we know did crisis intervention primarily with the family members of murder victims. Although she showed concern and empathy for her clients, the nature of her work was "getting to her," to the extent that she was planning to change jobs.

In our earlier discussion on AIDS, we mentioned that one helper, Steven Lanzet, organized and led AIDS support groups for four years in his community. In writing about how his work affected him personally, he indicated that dealing with the crises of others had led to a sense of burnout tapping on his shoulder. As a helper working with the crises of others, he learned how to take care of himself by reducing the frequency of the groups he led and by taking periodic breaks from facilitating groups. He dealt with his personal reactions to his work by joining a support group with fellow counselors (see M. Corey & G. Corey, 1997).

Perhaps getting involved in a group with peers who are also doing crisis intervention is one of the best ways of dealing with the emotions that surface as a result of your engagement with clients. If you are carrying around excess psychological baggage, the crises of your clients can soon become your crises. It is absolutely essential that you retain your sensitivity to the ways in which this work is affecting you personally and that you pay attention to what is emerging within you. If you forget to take care of yourself or if you delude yourself into thinking that you don't have time for yourself, you can be certain that you will not be able to function very long in the demanding work of helping others through their crises. You will have become stuck in the quagmire of your own crisis.

BY WAY OF REVIEW

- The community perspective emphasizes social change rather than merely helping people adapt to their circumstances.
- It is not useful to focus on individual client treatment and neglect the institutional or social conditions that contribute to an individual's problems. A process that considers both the internal conflicts within the individual and the social factors within the community will provide a balanced perspective for helpers.
- It is essential that training programs prepare students to assume a proactive stance toward community intervention, especially with reference to early prevention approaches for at-risk groups in the community.
- A comprehensive community counseling program has these four aspects: (1) Direct client services focus on outreach activities for at-risk groups in the community. (2) Direct community services in the form of preventive

education are geared to the population at large. (3) Indirect client services consist of intervening actively for an individual or a group. (4) Indirect community services focus on influencing policymakers and bringing about positive changes within the community.

- One way to meet the mental-health needs in the community is for professionals and paraprofessionals to work cooperatively.
- The AIDS crisis challenges professional helpers to acquire basic information about the disease and also to develop strategies for helping those who are infected.
- Your values will influence your stance toward AIDS education and counseling.
- Crisis intervention is one of the main modalities in community agencies. Many at-risk groups are in need of immediate and short-term help in working through both situational and developmental crises.

WHAT WILL YOU DO NOW?

1. We recommend that you contact the national HIV and AIDS hot line (800-342-AIDS) for free written material about the disease as well as answers to your questions. This hot line functions 24 hours a day in every state. The information specialists are well trained, and they respect privacy. In addition to giving information, they provide referrals to appropriate sources among the more than 8000 entries in the hot-line database. Informational materials are also available from the National AIDS Clearinghouse (800-458-5231). More information about AIDS and AIDS-related illnesses can be obtained from your state or local health department and your local chapter of the American Red Cross. Call one of the sources above and ask for pamphlets that will provide you with the latest available information. As a class project, you and several classmates can make a brief presentation in class about the various facets of AIDS and what can be done to mobilize community action to prevent the spread of the disease.

2. Imagine that you are doing an intake interview with a man who has just found out that he tested HIV-positive. He is seeking counseling to deal with his high anxiety over fears of death and is in a crisis state. What might you feel? What might you say to this individual? How well prepared are you to listen to this man and help him through this crisis? If you do not feel adequately prepared to take this person as a client, consider going to an AIDS center and asking for information. Talk with someone about this disease, especially its social and psychological aspects. Find ways to challenge any of your biases, misconceptions, assumptions, and values that could render you ineffective in helping HIV-positive individuals who are in crisis.

3. Select an at-risk population in your community. As a class project, you and several classmates can explore strategies for dealing with a particular client population by using a community approach. What can be done to awaken people in your community to the needs of the at-risk group that you've identified?

4. Investigate the services available in your community for people in crisis. Look into what is offered in your own college or university. Ask about the crisis

services provided by one of your community agencies. Inquire about what is being done by way of training volunteers for crisis intervention, such as working on a telephone hot line. You might consider doing volunteer work in your community as part of a crisis team. You could ask about training programs and the possibilities of serving as an "on-call" worker in times of special need.

5. If you are interested in working with the elderly, it would be valuable to become involved not only with older people but also with their families. Consider taking any of these steps to better prepare yourself to work with the elderly:

- Take courses and special workshops dealing with the problems of the aged.
- Get involved in fieldwork and internship experiences with the elderly.
- Investigate institutes and conferences that provide training for helpers who work with the elderly.
- Explore your feelings toward your own aging and toward the older people in your life.

6. Spend some time thinking about how you might get involved in your community by doing some kind of volunteer work or selecting a field placement that will get you directly involved in community projects. Brainstorm possible ways of making even small changes in some facet of your community. How can you involve yourself in projects that are already underway or with fellow students who are doing some form of work in the community? Write ideas in your journal of how you can use your interests and talents in the service of others in your community.

7. For the full bibliographic entry for each of the sources listed below, consult the References and Reading List at the back of the book.

Homan (1994) views the community as the client and offers the basic knowledge and skills needed to face the challenge of community change. For a treatment of multicultural social work practice with culturally diverse clients in family service centers, hospitals, and mental-health centers, see Lum (1996). Three useful books about HIV and AIDS are Kain (1996), Jones (1996), and Kübler-Ross (1993). Refer to Tice and Perkins (1996) for prevention of mental-health problems of older persons and methods within a community-based practice. See Lewis and Lewis (1989) for a comprehensive description of the community counseling perspective. For an excellent resource outlining the theory and practice of crisis intervention, see Gilliland and James (1997).

Chapter 9

WORKING WITH GROUPS

FOCUS QUESTIONS

1. Have you participated in any kind of group? If so, what was this experience like for you? What did it teach you about groups? about leading groups? about being a member? about yourself?
2. What value do you see in group work for meeting the needs of the various client populations that you hope to serve?
3. If you were to organize a group, what kind of group would you most like to get started? What would you most want to accomplish?
4. In designing a group, where would you begin? What specific actions would you take to start your group? What colleagues or other sources might you consult in getting this group going?
5. How prepared do you think you are to lead or co-lead a group? What personal qualities do you have that might help or hinder you as a group leader? What experiences have you had that you can draw from in working with people in groups? What knowledge and skills do you possess that will enhance your ability to lead groups? What do you still most need to learn?
6. If a supervisor or the director of the agency where you work approached you and encouraged you to start groups in your agency, how would you respond? What are the supervisory and consultation issues you would need to resolve with your supervisor?
7. How would you decide if a co-leader was necessary or appropriate? If you were to select a colleague to co-lead a group with you, what kind of person would you select? What characteristics would you look for?
8. What characteristics of a group would you look for to differentiate between a productive and a nonproductive group?

AIM OF THE CHAPTER

As a part of your training program, you will probably take at least one course in group processes, and you may also participate in an experiential group. As you assume the role of a helping professional, the chances are that you will be asked to design or facilitate some type of group, for group work is becoming an increasingly popular therapeutic modality. Your supervisor or the director of your agency may ask you to start a group for a particular at-risk population, and you are likely to feel anxiety over not knowing where to begin. If you are like many other helpers, you may feel unprepared to organize and lead a group, or you may be uncertain about the value of groups for special client populations. The purpose of this chapter is to introduce you to the distinct values of group work in general, to the advantages of specialized groups, and to the merits of your becoming involved as a member in groups. Our intention is not to teach you how to lead groups, for this is too ambitious for a single chapter. Instead, we aim to present a perspective on ways of helping people through various approaches to group work. You will be introduced to the characteristics that make groups productive and powerful. Guidelines are given for deriving the maximum benefit from a group experience. Some key ethical and professional issues are outlined, as are suggestions for acquiring the basic skills required for effective group leadership. We also present a rationale for co-leading groups. You are encouraged to think about how to get the skills you need to organize and facilitate groups for some of the diverse client populations that you will serve.

GROUP WORK AS THE TREATMENT OF CHOICE

During the 1960s and the 1970s, groups reached their zenith; then, group fever declined for a decade. In the 1990s group work has enjoyed a resurgence of interest. In the 1960s encounter groups and personal-growth groups were considered one pathway for making human connections and for moving toward greater self-actualization. Today the focus has changed, and the groups that have been springing up in all settings are short-term groups designed for specific client populations and remediation of specific problems.

In the American Psychological Association's *Monitor* (Sleek, 1995), the lead article describes an expanding array of group techniques that are affordable and effective in overcoming a range of psychological and medical problems. The crux of the article is that group therapy fits well into the managed care scene because groups can be designed to be brief, cost-effective treatments. Sleek summarizes studies giving evidence that, in general, group therapy is as effective as individual therapy in bringing about change. In addition, groups provide for a sense of community, which can be an antidote to the impersonal culture in which many clients live. However, the focus of these groups is definitely time-limited, and they have fairly narrow goals. Many of the time-limited groups are aimed at symptomatic relief, teaching participants problem-solving strategies and interpersonal skills. The interpersonal learning that occurs in groups can accelerate a person's changes.

Some helpers view groups as a second-best treatment modality. They are convinced that interventions for individuals, couples, and families are the most valuable and appropriate strategies. If groups are used in their work setting, these helpers believe that cost factors are the primary consideration. When budgets are tight and personnel are overworked, the economics of group treatment could seem paramount.

From our perspective, groups are the treatment of choice, not a second-rate approach to helping people change. We hold this view, not just because the dollars are stretched but because inherent values in the group process result in self-understanding, healing, and change on the part of participants. Most client populations can benefit from a properly designed group with a qualified leader or co-leaders. Consider the fact that many of the problems that bring people to counseling are interpersonally rooted. Many people seek professional assistance because of difficulties forming or maintaining intimate relationships. Clients often feel that their problems are unique and that they have few options to get out of deadening ruts. They may be at a loss in knowing how to live well with the ones they love. Groups provide a natural laboratory that demonstrates to people that they are not alone and that there is hope for creating a different life. Groups are powerful because they allow participants a chance to experience some of their long-term problems being played out in the group sessions. At the same time, the group gives members opportunities to design and try out more effective ways of behaving.

Groups have immense power to move people in creative and more life-giving directions. If a group is hastily thrown together, or if it is led by someone without proper training, there is also the potential for the group to be more damaging than beneficial.

Values of Group Work

We do not wish to suggest that groups represent the "only approach" or the "best way" of helping clients understand and cope with their problems. In some cases, groups may be the most appropriate intervention in a client's life. In other cases, they may be used as a supplementary form of treatment or as the next step a client takes after completing some individual counseling. In our own practice, we find groups to be powerfully effective and to offer unique advantages for new learning.

What are some of the main values of a group experience? Let us begin with the assumption that the group has been carefully designed. The purpose of the group is clear in the leader's mind, and much thought has been given to bringing people together who can profit from the group experience. The leader has the personal qualities, knowledge, and skills to facilitate members' work and to promote communication. Operating on this set of assumptions, this group offers a number of advantages to both the participants and the leader. Through the unfolding of the group process, the members can observe how others interact, and they can learn something about themselves by joining in the interaction. The group experience serves as a living laboratory, for it becomes a mirror in which members see themselves as they are. For instance, Luigi tends to keep himself isolated in the group, and in many ways he makes it difficult for others to get close to him. Through the feedback of other members and the leader, he has a chance to learn about his part in contributing to his own isolation, not only in the group but also in his everyday life. The safety of the group affords him opportunities to experiment with being different. Instead of holding in his feelings, he can begin to let them out. Rather than being quickly defensive, he can open himself to really hearing others. He can try reaching out to others and asking for what he wants, to see what happens. Others in the group profit from Luigi's work, because it allows them to see how they are like him in certain ways.

People who are beginning to deal with their problems often feel that they are alone in the way they think and feel. Groups offer a forum in which members share their confusion, anger, helplessness, guilt, resentment, depression, and panic. By sharing their feelings, they feel less alone. If some members in the group have difficulty expressing their feelings, they are likely to find comfort in listening to others who are able to express the range of their emotions. For example, Carola has adopted a stoical attitude, thinking that her situation will be more tolerable if she contains her feelings. She may not realize the stress to which she is subjecting herself by denying her emotions. Generally, as she begins to share her concerns, she will probably realize that others also experience some of her pain and that she is not alone in what she feels. Her sharing can help tear down some of the walls that keep her isolated.

Some universal human themes typically become apparent through a group experience. It is true that clients are separated by differences in age, gender, sexual orientation, social and cultural background, and experience. Yet as people risk revealing their deeper concerns and express feelings that they might have kept within themselves, they typically comment on how they are more alike than different. Although the circumstances leading to pain over disappointment may be different for each person, the emotions associated with certain events have a universal quality. In groups composed of people with a common struggle, such as a support group for women who have been victims of incest, the sharing of feelings is often even more intense. Before joining the support group, they probably felt alone in their feelings of hurt, sadness, fright, guilt, resentment, and anger. As each woman reveals her story and her feelings about her situation, others are able to identify and come to understand a pattern that unites them. The bonding that builds within the group creates an atmosphere in which women can see more clearly how they have been affected by incest. It also leads to insights into how their earlier experiences have set the stage for the way they now think, feel, and behave.

Another value of groups is the hope they offer to members that a new life is possible. For example, groups for people who admit that their lives are out of control when they use alcohol offer steps leading to recovery. When these clients were caught in drinking patterns, they were convinced that they were powerless to change and that they were hopeless. But the modeling of others who are learning to take control of their lives one day at a time is living proof that there is hope for a better life.

The caring and acceptance that develop in a group are a powerful healing force. In a group for children of divorce, compassion and support are given not only by the leader but also by other children. Individuals within this group are able to risk being vulnerable as they sense that what concerns them has importance to others.

A distinct advantage of groups is the opportunity for learning from the feedback of many others. If reactions are given with sensitivity, members come to realize the ways in which their behavior affects others. The process of interpersonal feedback shows people how they contribute to both favorable and unfavorable outcomes, and it also gives them new possibilities for relating to others.

How Groups Can Help You

Take a few moments to reflect on how open you are to being a group member. How willing are you to define goals that will enable you to participate actively and fully in learning about yourself and others? Are you willing to recognize your own vulnerabilities and to share them in the context of the group? As you think about yourself as a group member, let yourself imagine that you are leading a group in which all the members are very much like yourself. What might it be like for you to lead such a group?

If you participate in experiential groups as a part of your training, you can use your experience for personal change and also for working on concerns you have as a helper. Other members can help you take an honest look at yourself, which can also teach you how to confront yourself. Your own honesty about who and what you are is the most significant factor in your ability to change. We would encourage you to do what you can to make any group you enter as personally meaningful as possible.

In Chapter 4 we went into detail about dealing with the transference reactions your clients may have to you, as well as ways of recognizing any countertransference reactions you may have to them. A group is an ideal place to explore your feelings toward clients and the effects that clients' behavior has on you. The group can be useful in bringing about an awareness of blind spots that make it difficult for you to be objective. A group experience that is connected with your training program may not be an appropriate place to work through unfinished business from your past, but it can serve you by sensitizing you to how your vulnerabilities could interfere with your work as a helper. For instance, assume that you discover that you act somewhat like a child seeking approval of your parents when you are in the company of certain older persons. You will probably need to work outside of the group, such as in your own therapy, on early wounds associated with your parents. However, the group can reveal when you tend to revert to less mature ways of responding. In a group you can learn a great deal about your resistance when you feel vulnerable, and this awareness of your own defenses can be extremely useful in teaching you how to work with clients who exhibit resistant behaviors.

In several previous chapters, we alluded to thought and feeling patterns with which many helpers struggle during their training. For instance, you may have a sense of not knowing enough to really help others. You may be overly cautious lest you make mistakes that your clients will see. Or you may find yourself overly sensitive to anything that sounds like criticism. Refer to some of the common concerns of helpers that we examined in Chapter 4 for other examples of places where you might get stuck yourself. Again, being in a group as a part of your program affords you an avenue for talking about the feelings, fears, and uncertainties that characterize the developing helper you are becoming.

Remember that you don't have to be sick or seriously disturbed to profit from a group experience designed for personal growth. Instead, your willingness to seek input from others and to consider feedback can start a pattern that will allow you to continue seeking others out when the demands on you in your helping role are great. Your capacity to receive support and challenge from others can enable you to give quality service to clients. If you are a reluctant client yourself, you will probably have trouble inspiring others, especially clients who seem reluctant.

How can you get the most from a group experience? How can you maximize your learning? If you are able to become an active group member yourself, you can use this experience later in teaching members in the groups you lead how to make the most of their group experience. We are convinced that those who participate in groups will get more from the experience if they are given some instructions. After all, the norms that govern group process are somewhat different from the norms of some other social situations. We offer some recommendations below that you can apply both to yourself as a member and to teaching others about groups. If you'd like a more detailed discussion, we refer you to M. Corey and G. Corey (1997) and Corey, Corey, Callanan, and Russell (1992).

- Recognize that trust is not something that "just happens" in a group but that you have a role in creating this climate. If you are aware of anything getting in the way of a sense of safety, share your hesitations with the group.
- Commit yourself to getting something from your group by focusing on your personal goals. Before each meeting, make the time to think about how you can get involved, what personal concerns you want to explore, and how to use the time in the group meaningfully.
- Rather than waiting to be called on, bring yourself into the interactions at the beginning of each session by letting others know what you want from this particular meeting. Although it is useful to have a tentative agenda of what you want to discuss, don't cling inflexibly to your agenda if other issues surface spontaneously within the group. Be open to pursuing alternative paths if you are affected by what others are exploring.
- Realize that if the work other members are doing is affecting you, it is crucial that you let them know. If you are able to identify with the struggles or pains of others, it generally helps both you and them to share your feelings and thoughts.
- Decide for yourself what, how much, and when you will disclose personal facets of yourself. Others will not have a basis for knowing you unless you tell them about yourself. If you have difficulty sharing yourself personally in your group, begin by letting others know what makes it hard for you to self-disclose.
- Don't confuse self-disclosure with storytelling. Avoid getting lost and overwhelming others with mere information about you or your history. Instead, express what is now on your mind and in your heart. Reveal the struggles that are significant to you at this time in your life, especially as they pertain to what others in the group are exploring.
- Express your persistent feelings about what is emerging in the group in the here and now. For example, if you are intimidated by other people in the group, announce that you feel this way. If you feel somewhat isolated, say so. Be willing to assume responsibility for what you feel rather than blaming others for it.

- Realize that others will not know you if you do not speak up about issues that are important to you, nor will they know that you identify with them or feel close to them unless you tell them.
- Practice your attending and listening skills. If you can give others the gift of your presence and understanding, you are contributing a great deal to the group process.
- Don't worry too much about taking too much group time for yourself. If you become overly concerned about measuring how much you are taking and receiving, you will inhibit the spontaneity that can make a group exciting and productive.
- Use your group as a place to experiment with new behaviors. Allow yourself to try out different ways of being to determine how you may want to change. Carry out any new ways of thinking, feeling, and acting into your outside life. Between sessions, practice the skills you are learning in your group. Give yourself your own homework assignments, and let other members know how you are applying what you learn in the group to your behavior with family, friends, and associates.
- Understand that making changes will not be instantaneous. You can also expect some setbacks. Keep track of any progress you are making, and remember to give yourself credit for your efforts and the subtle changes that you are making.
- Avoid giving others advice, giving intellectualized interpretations of their behavior, or using questioning as your main style of interacting with them. You may find yourself questioning others or offering them advice while keeping yourself distant in the process. If you are inclined to ask a question, let others know why you are interested in hearing their answer. Or if you want to give advice, reveal to others what your investment is. Learn to speak *for* yourself and *about* yourself.
- Concentrate on making personal and direct statements to others in your group. Direct communication with a member is more effective than "talking about" that person through the leader.
- In giving feedback to others, strive to avoid categorizing or labeling them. Instead of telling others who or what they are, tell them what you are observing, and let them know how they are affecting you. Rather than judging them as persons, focus on how you respond to some of their specific behaviors in group.
- Pay attention to any consistent feedback you receive. If you hear that others perceive you as being somewhat judgmental and critical, don't be too quick to argue and convince others that you are open and accepting. Instead, take in what you are hearing, and determine the degree to which what they are saying might fit you.
- Respect your defenses, and understand that they have served a purpose for you. When you become aware of feeling or acting defensively in your group, however, challenge your defenses by seeing what will happen if you strive to be less guarded. At least identify out loud that you are feeling defensive, and begin exploring what you might be resisting.
- Provide support for others by expressing your care for them, but don't quickly intervene by trying to comfort them when they are experiencing

feelings, such as expressing pain over an event. Realize that they need to experience, share, and work through certain feelings; they do not need reassurance that "all will turn out for the best." Let them know how their pain may be touching you, but don't attempt to "cure" them of their pain.

- Take responsibility for what you are accomplishing in your group. Spend some time thinking about what is taking place in these meetings and evaluating the degree to which you are attaining your goals. If you are not satisfied with your group experience, look at what you can do to improve it.
- Be aware of respecting and maintaining the confidentiality of what goes on inside your group. Even though you may not maliciously breach others' confidences, recognize how easy it might be to talk inappropriately to people who are not in the group about what others have revealed. The way that you handle confidentiality says a great deal about your professional character. If you have any concerns that what you are sharing is staying within the group, be willing to bring this matter up in a session.
- Be prepared if friends and loved ones do not always understand or accept you, especially as you make changes. Some people may not support the new directions in which you choose to travel, and your changes may be threatening to them.
- Consider keeping a personal journal in which you record impressions of your own explorations in the group. The journal is also a good place to enter your reactions to your fieldwork experiences or any work with clients.

WHAT MAKES FOR A PRODUCTIVE GROUP?

The differences between a productive and a nonproductive group depend to a large extent on the group's basic purpose. In general, we use the following characteristics to identify the level of effectiveness of our groups.

A productive group is one in which the goals are clear to all and are determined jointly by the members and the leader. The level of trust within the group allows members to take risks by sharing personally meaningful material. If trust is lacking, members are at least willing to express what makes it difficult for them to feel safe in the group. Communication among members is open and direct and involves an accurate expression of what they are thinking and feeling. There is a focus on what is occurring here and now within the group. Members talk about their reactions to one another rather than limiting their discussion to out-of-group concerns. There is a willingness to engage in significant and appropriate self-disclosure, but without getting lost in detailed stories.

Through mutual sharing, those in a group develop cohesion and feel a kinship to one another. In their identification, members are willing to risk dealing with threatening material. Most members feel a sense of inclusion in the group, and if someone feels excluded, there is an invitation to the member to do what is needed to feel included.

Feedback is given freely and accepted without defensiveness. Although members are willing to share the struggles they have in common, they do not merely give others advice. There is a respect for promoting independence, which implies that all members are supported in their efforts to find the answers to their problems within themselves.

If conflict emerges in the group, it is recognized, and there is a willingness to work through differences that could block progress. When confrontation occurs, the confronter reveals his or her reactions to a person's behavior rather than judging or labeling. Members are willing to both support and challenge one another. They feel hopeful that constructive change is possible if they are willing to work to bring about such change. Individual and cultural differences are recognized and respected. The norms that govern the group are clear and are designed to help the members attain their goals.

The members are willing to experiment with new ways of thinking, feeling, and behaving both within the group and in their everyday lives. They carry out homework assignments, they evaluate the degree to which they are achieving their goals through participation in the group, and they take responsibility for contributing to the enhancement of the group process. They use time outside the group to work on problems raised in the sessions. They also use one another as resources and show mutual interest.

This discussion of the nature of a productive group fits most groups that you will lead. As you form a group, it would be a good idea to think about the desired norms and outcomes so that you can develop specific criteria to assess its progress.

THE ETHICAL AND PROFESSIONAL GROUP LEADER

In our view, the best way to ensure that your groups will be productive for your clients is to strive to follow ethical and professional standards in your practice of group work. What follows is an overview of some of the qualities that we think reflect such standards.

You first spend time thinking about what you most want to accomplish through a group format. If you intend to co-lead your group, you arrange to carve out time before you even meet potential members to discuss with your colleague general group goals and an overall plan for getting your group into motion. You will not be getting a group together simply because groups are fashionable but because you believe that your group has real potential for making a difference to those who join.

You then provide information to prospective group candidates. Realizing that some of the people who need your group the most may be reluctant to seek your services, you are willing to make some provisions for outreach work and getting the word out to a particular target population that could most benefit. You make arrangements for some orientation sessions where potential members can find out more about the group and decide whether it is what they need. You also make some provision for screening prospective group members. In the screening sessions, you give consideration to selecting members whose needs and goals are compatible with the goals of the group, those who will not impede the group process, and those whose well-being will not be jeopardized by the group experience. You explore with the members the risks of potential life changes, and you help them explore their readiness to face these possibilities. In short, before your group ever meets, you will have spent time laying a foundation and preparing members for a successful learning experience.

Once the group begins to meet, you assess the degree to which its purposes are being met. If you are co-leading the group, you arrange to meet with your colleague regularly so that your efforts are coordinated. Ideally, these meetings take place both before and after each group session.

Because you are aware that confidentiality is the cornerstone of any group, you make sure that the participants know what it implies, and you encourage them to bring up any concerns they might have about maintaining confidences. You make some effort to teach the members how to become active participants so that they can get the most from the group sessions and also how to apply their newly acquired interpersonal skills in everyday living.

If you have an open group, one characterized by changing membership, you help members who are ready to leave the group integrate their learning, and you allow those who are staying to talk about their feelings about losing a member. As new members join, you attend to them so that they will be able to make use of the group resources. Although members ultimately have the right to leave a group, you discuss with them the possible risks of leaving prematurely, and you encourage them to discuss their reasons for wanting to quit. If your group is made up of involuntary members, you take steps to enlist their cooperation and their continuation on a voluntary basis.

Just as you take care not to impose your values on those clients you see individually, you are also sensitive to the ways in which your own values and needs have an impact on the group process. You exert care not to coerce participants to change in ways they have not chosen. Although you avoid imposing your values on members, you are willing to expose your beliefs and values if doing so is likely to benefit the members. Although you are able to meet your needs through your work, you do not do so at the members' expense. You also protect members' rights against coercion and undue pressure from other participants. You teach the members that the purpose of the group is to help them find their own answers rather than yielding to pressure from others.

For the duration of the group, you monitor your own behavior and become aware of what you are modeling to the members. You recognize the importance of teaching members how to evaluate their progress in meeting their goals, and you also design follow-up procedures.

You recognize and respect diversity within the group. You also encourage members to be sensitive to cultural, racial, religious, lifestyle, age, disability, and gender differences. The techniques that you employ are appropriate to the needs of diverse client populations. Depending on the type of intervention, you are aware of the limits of your competence. You avoid using potentially powerful techniques unless you are trained in their use under supervision. You are willing to seek out consultation or supervision when encountering ethical concerns that could interfere with the functioning of the group.

Just as you prepare members for entering a group, you also prepare them for termination from the group in the most efficient period of time. You also help members pull together what they have learned from their experience and assist them in developing an action plan for the period after they leave the group. If possible, you arrange for some method of follow-up with individuals or with the entire group to assess the outcomes. You are knowledgeable about the resources within your community that can assist members in their special needs, and you help members seek any professional assistance they need. As the group comes to an end, you encourage members to find resources that will enable them to continue the growth they've begun through the group.

TRAINING AND SUPERVISION IN GROUP WORK
Competence in Leading Groups

Many institutions now use a variety of groups as their primary therapeutic approach in helping clients resolve their problems. If these groups are led by practitioners who are not competent in group work with a given population, more harm than good will result. One of the most important ethical helping principles pertains to obtaining the necessary knowledge and skills to lead groups effectively. As we mentioned, supervised training is an indispensable element in becoming a competent leader of groups. Unfortunately, some who lead groups are uncertain about what they are doing and have not had adequate course work or training in group process. You are faced with an ethical dilemma if a supervisor asks you to design or lead a group when you have not had the proper professional preparation. In talking with both students and professionals, we frequently find that they have not had even minimal training in group work. The only group experiences to which some of them have been exposed are activities as part of a required group course. This group experience is often led by students, and sometimes there is very little supervision or direction. Not infrequently, we find that professionals who attend our workshops recall negative experiences with their one and only group course. This experience sometimes sours them on wanting to conduct groups themselves or makes them skeptical about the value of groups.

Developing the Skills for Leading Groups

In Chapter 3 we described some of the helping skills that are basic to interviewing, assessing, and counseling individuals. Some of these skills include active listening, providing support, challenging clients when appropriate, responding with empathy, clarifying feelings and thoughts, helping clients formulate goals, reflecting feelings, reframing problems in a new light, and helping clients develop action plans. All of the skills that are needed for individual counseling are also required of group workers. Your knowledge of the major theories and techniques of counseling, as well as your familiarity with what it is like to be a member of a group, will be most useful as a background for developing group skills. Effective group leaders are aware of group processes and know how to tap the special forces within a group. It is clear that leading a group is far more complex than merely counseling individuals in a group setting. In addition to the basic skills for individual counseling, group-leadership skills include helping members create trust, linking members' work, teaching members how to give and receive feedback, facilitating disclosure and risk taking, intervening to block counterproductive group behavior, identifying common themes, setting up role-playing situations that help members dramatize their struggles, and preparing members for closure. Being a successful facilitator of groups requires these and other group-leadership skills and the ability to carry out appropriate leadership functions. Although it may seem beyond your reach to know enough and be skilled enough to lead a group, you can learn a great deal about how groups function by participating in them, as we discussed earlier. Course work in group processes, opportunities to co-lead groups under adequate supervision, and participation in training groups will give you many opportunities to acquire, practice, and hone the essential skills needed to lead groups.

A summary of group skills is provided in Table 9-1. These helping behaviors are part of the repertoire of practitioners who work with individuals, couples, and families as well as of group practitioners.

Standards for Training

One way to acquire the knowledge and skills required for effective group leadership is by obtaining training and supervision in group work. The Association for Specialists in Group Work (ASGW) has developed and published the *Professional Standards for the Training of Group Workers* (ASGW, 1991), which are a specific set of core competencies in general group work. The training standards make it clear that mastery of the core competencies does not qualify a group worker to independently practice in any group work specialty. Practitioners must possess advanced competencies relevant to a particular area of group work.

The current trend in training group workers focuses on learning group process by becoming involved in supervised experiences. Certainly, completion of one graduate course in group theory and practice does not equip you to competently lead groups. Both direct participation in supervised small groups and clinical experience in leading various groups under careful supervision are needed to equip leaders with the skills to meet the challenges of group work.

Different kinds of groups differ with respect to goals, techniques used, the role of the leader, training requirements, and the people involved. The following definitions of each group work specialization are given by the ASGW (1991) and by Conyne, Wilson, Kline, Morran, and Ward (1993).

Task/work groups. The task/work group specialist assists task forces, committees, planning groups, community organizations, discussion groups, study circles, learning groups, and other similar groups to correct or develop their functioning. The focus is on the application of group dynamics principles and processes to improve practice and accomplish identified work goals.

Group workers who specialize in promoting the development and functioning of task and work groups help these groups enhance or correct their performance. In addition, this group specialist might develop skill in organizational assessment, training, program development, consultation, and program evalua-

Table 9.1
Overview of Group-Leadership Skills

Skill	Description	Aims and desired outcomes
Active listening	Attending to verbal and non-verbal aspects of communication without judging or evaluating.	To encourage trust and client self-disclosure and exploration.
Restating	Saying in slightly different words what a participant has said to clarify its meaning.	To determine if the leader has understood correctly the client's statement; to provide support and clarification.
Clarifying	Grasping the essence of a message at both the feeling and the thinking levels; simplifying client statements by focusing on the core of the message.	To help clients sort out conflicting and confused feelings and thoughts; to arrive at a meaningful understanding of what is being communicated.
Summarizing	Pulling together the important elements of an interaction or session.	To avoid fragmentation and give direction to a session; to provide for continuity and meaning.
Questioning	Asking open-ended questions that lead to self-exploration of the "what" and "how" of behavior.	To elicit further discussion; to get information; to stimulate thinking; to increase clarity and focus; to provide for further self-exploration.
Interpreting	Offering possible explanations for certain behaviors, feelings, and thoughts.	To encourage deeper self-exploration; to provide a new perspective for considering and understanding one's behavior.
Confronting	Challenging members to look at discrepancies between their words and actions or body and verbal messages; pointing to conflicting information or messages.	To encourage honest self-investigation; to promote full use of potentials; to bring about awareness of self-contradictions.
Reflecting feelings	Communicating understanding of the content of feelings.	To let members know that they are heard and understood beyond the level of words.
Supporting	Providing encouragement and reinforcement.	To create an atmosphere that encourages members to continue desired behaviors; to provide help when clients are facing difficult struggles; to create trust.
Empathizing	Identifying with clients by assuming their frames of reference.	To foster trust in the therapeutic relationship; to communicate understanding; to encourage deeper levels of self-exploration.

Table 9.1
(continued)

Skill	Description	Aims and desired outcomes
Facilitating	Opening up clear and direct communication within the group; helping members assume increasing responsibility for the group's direction.	To promote effective communication among members; to help members reach their own goals in the group.
Initiating	Promoting group participation and introducing new directions in the group.	To prevent needless group floundering; to increase the pace of group process.
Goal setting	Planning specific goals for the group process and helping participants define concrete and meaningful goals.	To give direction to the group's activities; to help members select and clarify their goals.
Evaluating	Appraising the ongoing group process and the individual and group dynamics.	To promote better self-awareness and understanding of group movement and direction.
Giving feedback	Expressing concrete and honest reactions based on observation of members' behaviors.	To offer an external view of how the person appears to others; to to increase the client's self-awareness.
Suggesting	Offering advice and information, direction, and ideas for new behavior.	To help members develop alternative courses of thinking and action.
Protecting	Safeguarding members from un-necessary psychological risks in the group.	To warn members of possible risks in group participation; to reduce these risks.
Disclosing oneself	Revealing one's reactions to here-and-now events in the group.	To facilitate deeper levels of group interaction; to create trust; to model ways of revealing oneself to others.
Modeling	Demonstrating desired behavior through actions.	To provide examples of desirable behavior; to inspire members to fully develop their potential.
Linking	Connecting the work that members do to common themes in the group.	To promote member-to-member interactions; to encourage the development of cohesion.
Blocking	Intervening to stop counter-productive group behavior.	To protect members; to enhance the flow of the group process.
Terminating	Preparing the group to close a session or end its existence.	To help members assimilate, integrate, and apply in-group learning to everyday life.

Note: The format of this chart is based on Edwin J. Nolan's article "Leadership Interventions for Promoting Personal Mastery," *Journal for Specialists in Group Work*, 1978, 3(3), 132–138.

tion. The training for task/work groups involves course work in the broad areas of organizational development, consultation, and management.

Guidance/psychoeducational groups. Education and prevention are critically important goals for the contemporary counselor. The guidance/psychoeducational group specialist strives to educate group members who are relatively well-functioning individuals but who may have a deficit of information in a certain area. The specialist uses the group medium to educate group participants who are "at risk" but are presently unaffected by a potential threat (such as AIDS), who are facing a developmental life event (such as a transition point), or who are experiencing an immediate life crisis (such as suicide of a loved one). The goal is to prevent an array of educational and psychological disturbances from occurring.

The specialist training for guidance/psychoeducational groups involves course work in the broad areas of community psychology, health promotion, marketing, consultation, group training methods, and curriculum design. These specialists should have content knowledge in the topic areas in which they intend to work (such as substance abuse prevention, stress management, parent effectiveness training, assertion training, AIDS).

Counseling/interpersonal problem-solving groups. The group worker who specializes in counseling/interpersonal problem solving seeks to help group participants resolve the usual yet often difficult problems of living. An additional goal is to help participants develop existing interpersonal problem-solving competencies so they may be better able to handle future problems of a similar nature. Nonsevere career, education, personal, social, and developmental concerns are frequently addressed.

The specialist training for counseling/interpersonal problem-solving groups should ideally include as much course work in group counseling as possible but at least one course beyond the generalist level. Group counselors should have knowledge in the broad areas of human development, problem identification, and treatment of normal personal and interpersonal problems of living.

Psychotherapy/personality reconstruction groups. The group worker who specializes in psychotherapy/personality reconstruction seeks to help individual group members remediate in-depth psychological problems. This specialist's scope of practice is focused on individuals with acute or chronic mental or emotional disorders that evidence marked distress, impairment in functioning, or both. Because the depth and extent of the psychological disturbance are significant, the goal is to aid each individual to reconstruct major personality dimensions.

The specialist training for psychotherapy groups consists of courses taken in the area of abnormal psychology, psychopathology, and diagnostic assessment to assure capabilities in working with more disturbed populations.

GROUPS FOR SPECIAL CLIENT POPULATIONS

The range of groups designed to help people cope with specific problems or those aimed at particular client populations is limited only by a practitioner's imagination. We find that such special groups are mushrooming and that they frequently arise from the needs of a particular group or from the interests of the professional who is designing them. Many groups have both an educational and a psychotherapeutic dimension. These groups are often short term, have some degree of structure, deal with a particular population, and focus on a specific theme. They can serve a number of purposes, such as giving information, sharing common concerns, teaching coping skills, helping people practice better ways of interpersonal communication, teaching problem-solving techniques, and assisting people once they leave the group.

Eventually, as a part of your job as a professional helper employed in a public or private agency, you may be asked to set up and lead one or more groups. Depending on the age and population with which you work, you are likely to find yourself looking for resources that will help you design a group. You may be expected to form a group to help children in your community. Many creative groups are designed to meet the special needs of children. These groups are generally structured by focusing on a theme such as surviving divorce, controlling acting out, dealing with abuse or neglect, enhancing self-esteem, or coping with terminal illness.

For adolescents, you may be asked to organize a group program for alcohol and drug rehabilitation, a growth group to meet normal developmental needs, a group for young women with eating disorders, a group for school dropouts, or a group to help young people cope with the aftermath of some crisis. For adults, there are groups for single parents, for middle-aged people contemplating a career change, for couples who hope to improve their relationship, for people who have tested HIV-positive, for people who are diagnosed with cancer, for incest victims, and for the physically handicapped. Increasing in popularity are groups for women and groups for men, which allow for the exploration of gender-identity concerns and issues pertaining to gender-role conditioning. There are many different groups designed for specific skills training or learning to manage particular problem areas.

Structured groups appear to be growing in popularity. They fit well into managed care systems that stress short-term interventions aimed at specific problems. Structured groups generally have an educational focus in that they are designed to teach participants coping skills. These groups, which tend to focus on a particular theme, are being increasingly used by agencies, schools, and college counseling centers. Generally, the sessions are about two hours each week for 4 to 15 weeks. Depending on the population, some group sessions may be as short as 30 to 45 minutes, especially with children or clients with a short attention span.

At the beginning of these structured groups it is common to ask members to complete a questionnaire on how well they are coping with the area of concern. Such groups make use of structured exercises, readings, homework assignments, and contracts. When the group comes to an end, another questionnaire is often used to assess the members' progress.

This list will give you some idea of the scope of topics for structured groups:

- Stress management
- Assertion training
- Eating disorders (bulimia and anorexia)
- Women in transition
- Dealing with an alcoholic parent

- Learning coping skills
- Groups for re-entry students
- Managing relationships and ending relationships
- Parenting skills groups
- Groups for the elderly
- Support for incest victims
- Support groups for victims of crime
- Support groups for persons with AIDS

In reality, the kinds of groups you might design are limited only by your ingenuity. For most client populations, a support or structured group can be organized that combines educational and therapeutic aims. Once you determine some areas of need within the community or at the agency where you work, you and your co-workers can launch short-term groups to address these needs. In this short space it has not been possible to provide in-depth descriptions of different kinds of groups for various client populations. If you would like more information on group process and setting up groups for various age groups, see *Groups: Process and Practice* (M. Corey & G. Corey, 1997).

WORKING WITH CO-LEADERS

In our practice of group work, in teaching and supervising group practitioners, and in conducting group-process workshops for students and professionals, we favor working as a team. Each of us teaches group courses and conducts groups and workshops, yet we often co-lead groups or workshops because of the benefits to both our clients and ourselves. We very much enjoy co-leading and continue to learn from each other, as well as from other colleagues with whom we co-lead. Although our preference is for the co-leadership model, this is not the only acceptable model of leadership. Many people facilitate a group alone quite effectively.

There are a number of advantages to co-leading groups for all concerned: the group members can gain from the perspectives of two leaders; depending on their styles, the co-leaders can each bring a unique focus to the session and can complement each other's facilitation; and the co-leaders are able to consult before and after a group and learn from each other.

In conducting training workshops with university students, we continually hear how they value working with a partner, especially when leading a group for the first time. Organizing and conducting a group seem less overwhelming if trainees can work with a co-leader whom they trust and respect. In our workshops for group workers, we find it useful to observe them as they co-lead so that we can discuss what they are actually doing as they facilitate a group. Then, during our feedback to them, we frequently ask them to talk with each other about how they felt as they were co-leading and what they think about the session they have just led. The feedback between these co-leaders can be both supportive and challenging. They can make constructive suggestions about each other's style, and the process of exchanging perceptions can enhance their ability to function effectively together.

Careful selection of a co-leader is essential. A major factor should be mutual respect. Two leaders working together may have differences in leadership style, and they are not likely always to agree or share the same perceptions or interpretations. If there is mutual respect and trust, however, they will be able to work cooperatively instead of competitively, and they will be secure enough to be free of the constant need to prove themselves. If the two leaders are incompatible, their group is bound to be negatively affected. For example, if one is jealous of the other and tries to discount the other's interventions, the group members will sense the tension, and their cohesion will suffer.

We cannot stress enough the importance of co-leaders' making a commitment to meet regularly. We encourage those who co-lead groups to spend some time both before and after each session discussing their reactions to what is going on in the group as well as their working relationship.

Not infrequently, a group session is characterized by the expression of intense emotions. If you or your co-leader is strongly affected by what occurred in a session, your own meetings allow for the exploration of any feelings, impressions, or reactions. The two of you can use each other as sounding boards, can check for objectivity, and can offer useful feedback. However, it is often necessary for leaders to express and deal with such feelings in the session itself. For example, if you are aware that you are consistently feeling put off by a particular member, it would be best for you to deal with your reactions to this person in the group itself. In certain cases a group member's concerns may touch your own "unfinished business," and you may explore your personal issues, either within or outside of the group, depending on which would be more appropriate. This is a time when a competent and trusted co-leader is especially important.

You can see that one of the advantages of co-leading is that it can help you identify and work with countertransference that emerges within the group. As you recall from our earlier discussion of countertransference in Chapter 4, this phenomenon can distort your objectivity to the extent that it interferes with effective counseling. For example, your co-leader may typically react with great impatience to men who are reluctant to express their feelings. You may be better able to make contact with such a man. You can also help your co-leader identify his or her reactions and attachments to a certain member.

There are other benefits to the practice of co-leading. One important one is that your relationship with your co-leader can be nourishing, both personally and professionally. The chances of burnout can be reduced, especially if you are working with a demanding and draining client population.

Even with a co-leader you choose, whom you respect and like, there are likely to be occasional disagreements. These differences in perspective and opinion need not necessarily pose a problem; rather, they can keep both of you professionally alert. Moreover, if you deal with your differences constructively during the session, you are providing excellent modeling on how to work with conflicts. Most of the disadvantages in co-leading groups have to do with poor selection of a co-leader, random assignment to a co-leader, or failure of the two leaders to meet regularly.

Although we like a co-leading model, we think it is important that the two leaders have some say in deciding to work as a team. Otherwise, there is a potential for harm for both members and leaders. In addition to the values we've mentioned, co-leading can keep your work interesting, and it can also be fun.

By Way of Review

- Groups are not an inferior approach to working with clients but rather, for many populations and for certain purposes, are the treatment of choice.
- Inherent values in the group process lead to self-acceptance, deeper understanding of oneself, and change. Some of these values are learning that one is not alone, receiving feedback from many sources, gaining opportunities for experimenting with new behavior, and using the group as an interpersonal laboratory.
- As a student in a training program, you have a great deal to gain from groups in your personal and professional development.
- Leaders are expected to follow ethical guidelines in forming and conducting groups.
- It is important to know your limits of competency if you are asked to lead a group. If you expect to make group work a part of your profession, training and supervision are essential.
- Group leadership skills can be acquired and refined. They can be applied to working with a wide array of groups and special populations.

What Will You Do Now?

1. After reading the section dealing with groups for special client populations, investigate which of these or other groups are offered in a local community agency or facility. Ask about how the groups are organized, what services are available to special client groups, and what outcomes these groups have had. If you are doing fieldwork in an agency now, inquire about its groups. How do people find out about these groups?

2. If a group experience is not part of your training program, seek out what is available in your college or university, in the community, or through private practice. Even if you decide not to join a group, this exercise can be useful in learning about community resources.

3. If you are working in an agency or if you have a fieldwork placement, see whether you can observe a group. Of course, both the group members and the leader would have to agree before you could visit a session. The purpose of this visit is to acquaint you with the potential of groups for meeting the needs of various client populations.

4. If you are currently involved in a group, or have been in a group in the past, in your journal describe the kind of group member that you are (or were). What might this teach you about your ability to lead or co-lead groups? You might also write about your concerns or fears in doing group work. Let yourself brainstorm as you write about the possible advantages to working with people in groups. Think about your interests, and see if you can identify some general

ideas for ways to employ small groups as a vehicle for branching out from your interests.

5. For the full bibliographic entry for each of the sources listed below, consult the References and Reading List at the back of the book.

For a practical handbook on the evolution of a group and key group process issues at each stage, see M. Corey and G. Corey (1997). For a manual on ways of creating, implementing, and evaluating techniques for therapeutic groups, see Corey, Corey, Callanan, and Russell (1992). For an excellent discussion of conducting groups for higher-functioning hospital patients and for more regressed individuals, see Yalom (1983). Consult Yalom (1995) for an in-depth treatment of theoretical and practical issues dealing with interpersonal therapy groups. For an overview of ten major theories of group counseling, with practical applications to various groups, see Corey (1995). For a description of the interactive nature of systemic groups that demystifies the workings of groups, see Donigian and Malnati (1997).

Chapter 10

WORKING WITH THE FAMILY

FOCUS QUESTIONS

1. How much do you know about your family of origin? What do you know about the life experiences of your parents? your grandparents? other relatives?
2. To what degree do you think your experiences with your family of origin have affected your other current relationships?
3. Do you think that a course in the family of origin should be required of students in a counseling program? Why or why not?
4. How might your family experiences either help or hinder you in your role as a professional helper?
5. Can you identify any unresolved issues between you and your family that are likely to make it difficult for you to work with certain problems? What steps can you take to resolve such issues?
6. What growth experiences do you seek? Do you value travel? reading novels? personal psychotherapy? exploring your family patterns by reviewing your family's history? involvement in family therapy? being a member in a therapy group? What importance do you place on self-exploration as part of your development as a helper?

AIM OF THE CHAPTER

In this chapter we provide a brief overview of a systems approach, building on the two previous chapters that dealt with working with the community and with groups. We identify the themes that characterize a family systems perspective and show how this view differs from an individual counseling perspective. Key concepts of family therapy are also described, providing a clearer picture of how practitioners work with a family systems perspective. We continue this theme of self-exploration, applying it to understanding how your family of origin may influence your present relationships and how your early background influences your work with both individuals and families. All of your clients come from families, and many of the problems they bring to counseling are grounded in events and learnings as children growing up in their families.

When you work with a couple or a family, or with an individual who is sorting out a family-of-origin issue, your perceptions and reactions are bound to be influenced by your personal experiences as you were growing up. If you are unaware of your sensitive areas, you are likely to misinterpret your clients or steer them in a direction that will not arouse your own anxieties. If you are aware

We express our appreciation to James Bitter, of East Tennessee State University, for his role in critiquing and contributing to this chapter.

of emotional issues that activate your resistances, however, you can avoid getting entangled in the problems of your clients. The material we present is personal and is designed to assist you in examining as many dimensions of your family as possible so you will not be overly susceptible to countertransference.

The purpose of this chapter is not to teach you how to do family therapy or to give you a comprehensive view of the field but to provide you with an introduction to the concepts of a family systems perspective. Here we invite you to unravel the mystery of your connection with your family of origin so you may develop a richer appreciation for the many ways you continue to play out patterns established during childhood. In helping you review your family history, we present the perspective we use in our professional work. In doing so, we draw from numerous approaches and methods that we have found helpful in giving clients a focus for their work.

Chapter 11 will build on the family-of-origin material addressed in this chapter, linking early childhood influences and family patterns to present developmental concerns. Both chapters are designed to stimulate self-exploration that will help you reflect on how you can increase your effectiveness as a helper by exploring your personal issues.

A SYSTEMS APPROACH

Much of the practice of marital and family therapy rests on the foundation of a systems perspective, which views psychological problems as arising from within the individual's present environment and the intergenerational family system. (We refer to "a" rather than "the" systems approach to indicate that there are different forms of this theory.) In a family systems approach, symptoms are viewed as an expression of a dysfunction within a system, with dysfunctions often passed across several generations.

Family therapy involves a conceptual shift from individual dynamics to interaction within the system. A systems perspective views the family as a functioning unit and as an entity unto itself that adds up to more than the sum of its members. The family provides the context for understanding how individuals behave. Actions by any individual family member will influence all the other members, and their reactions will have a reciprocal effect on the individual.

An assumption of the systems approach is that change in any one part of the system affects all parts of that system. For example, a couple devote most of their energy to their acting-out son. They form an alliance to save him. Once he leaves home and they no longer have control over his actions, they begin to fight with each other. A short time later they file for divorce because of their differences. This example illustrates that a change in one part of the family affects the actions of other family members.

Another systems principle is that each family member is part of a whole pie, even though it is easy for the members to think of themselves as merely separate pieces of the pie without an integral connection. The system assumes its own personality. You cannot pluck yourself out of your family system, for you are dynamically related to it. If you restrict yourself exclusively to your internal dynamics, without considering your interpersonal dynamics, you are not getting a full picture of yourself. From a systems perspective, being a healthy person involves both a sense of belonging to your family system and a sense of separateness and individuality. As you read the material that follows, think about how you have been influenced by your family system and how you have influenced others in your family.

One of our colleagues, Jim Bitter, who teaches in a graduate program in counseling, emphasizes that helpers who work with families need not be perfect people with perfect families but that they do need to be as vitally interested in the connections between people as they are in problem-solving skills. He believes that in addition to learning techniques and theory, helpers need to be committed to their own personal and professional growth.

A Family Systems Perspective

The family systems perspective holds that individuals are best understood through assessing the interactions of the entire family. Symptoms are viewed as an expression of a dysfunction within the family; these dysfunctional patterns are thought to be passed across several generations. It was revolutionary to conclude that the identified client's problem might be a symptom of how the system functioned, not just a symptom of the individual's history and psychosexual development. Today, much of the practice of family therapy rests on the foundation of a systemic perspective. This perspective is grounded on the assumptions that a client's problematic behavior might: (1) serve a function or purpose for the family; (2) be the result of the family's inability to function productively, especially during developmental transitions; or (3) result from dysfunctional patterns handed down transgenerationally. All these assumptions challenge traditional individual therapy frameworks for conceptualizing human problems and their formation.

All family therapists subscribe to the basic notion that families are systems. Therefore, a treatment approach that comprehensively addresses the other family members as well as the "identified" client is required. Goldenberg and Goldenberg (1996a) point to the need for therapists to view all behavior, including the symptoms expressed by the individual, within the context of the family and society. The Goldenbergs add that a systems orientation does not preclude dealing with the dynamics within the individual, but that this approach broadens the traditional emphasis. Because a family is an interacting unit, it has its own set of unique traits. It is not possible to accurately assess an individual's concerns without observing the interaction of the other family members as well as the broader context in which the person lives. Focusing on the internal dynamics of an individual without adequately considering interpersonal dynamics yields an incomplete picture of that individual. Because the focus is on interpersonal relationships, Becvar and Becvar (1996) maintain that *family therapy* is a misnomer and that *relationship therapy* is a more appropriate label.

Family therapy is more than an approach to working therapeutically with a family; it is a perspective that sheds light on the individual's and the family's development over time. It also provides a lens through which to view connections in the world. It takes into consideration the influence of an individual's neighborhood, community, church, work environment, school, and other systems. Indeed, the family systems perspective holds that significant change within an individual is not likely to be made or maintained unless the client's network of intimate relationships is taken into account. Systems practitioners assume that even if an individual makes changes they are not likely to endure if there is little support for, or if there is opposition to, these changes from the individual's family and other social relationships.

Family therapists view individuals from a relational, developmental, cultural, and gender perspective. Although systems theory does not ignore the importance of an individual's intrapsychic dynamics, attention is not limited to the individual and individual problems. Instead, a broader view is taken, and the focus is on relationships and relationship issues. The best vantage point for understanding an individual's personality is by paying attention to what is occurring within the many layers of systems that touch the individual.

An individual's level of functioning can be seen as a manifestation of the way the family is functioning. For example, a young girl who develops ulcers may be signaling not only her own pain but the unexpressed pain of the family. If individual change is a goal of therapy with the daughter, it is essential to understand how the family influences her and how any changes she makes are likely to affect other members of her family. It should also be noted, however, that an individual can have a symptom that may exist independent of the family structure. For example, clinical depression could be caused by a biochemical imbalance; it is not necessarily a result of some family dynamic.

Key Concepts of Family Therapy

Family therapy is a diverse field with respect to concepts, techniques, and approaches. This chapter is only a beginning; for a more complete picture of the theory and practice of family therapy, you will need to do further reading. The key concepts presented here detail some of the themes that unite the many schools of family therapy and look at some of the variations that exist among these theoretical orientations.

View of the family. Family therapy approaches shift the focus from the individual to the system. Rather than viewing an individual as being the focus of a problem, family therapists view all parts of the system as contributing to an individual's problem. The individual's presenting problem is a symptom of the disturbance within the family system. In the case of an acting-out adolescent son, his symptoms express a wider issue than his own internal struggles. Although individuals are considered, the focus is on a relational context. The "client" is the family system rather than one individual with a presenting problem in this system.

Focus of family therapy.   Most of the family therapies are brief, as families who seek professional help typically want resolution for some problematic symptom. In addition to being short-term, solution-focused, and action-oriented, family therapy tends to deal with present interactions. One way family therapy differs from many individual therapies is in its emphasis on the way current family relationships contribute to symptom development and maintenance. Virtually all the family therapies are concerned with here-and-now interactions in the family system.

Another focus that characterizes family therapy is the attention paid to communication. All family therapy orientations emphasize verbal and nonverbal communication. Some approaches to family therapy assume that the central aim of communication is attaining power in interpersonal relationships. Symptoms are seen as ways of communicating with the aim of controlling other family members. For instance, a child who fears going to school might be expressing his or her insecurity in dealing with the world alone. In this case, strategic therapists would not generally attempt to teach the parents what the child's symptoms mean but would attempt to provoke the parents to communicate with the child in a different way, which would make the symptom unnecessary (Nichols & Schwartz, 1995).

Role of the therapist.   Family therapists function as models, teachers, and coaches. What most approaches have in common is their commitment to helping family members learn new and more effective ways of interacting. All family therapists have a keen interest in the process of family interaction and in teaching patterns of communication.

Goals of family therapy.   The main goal of most traditional orientations of helping is to bring about changes within an individual in the realms of thinking, feeling, and behaving. These changes often have repercussions on the system of which the client is part. In contrast, the goal of most approaches to family therapy is change in relationships and system change, predicated on the assumption that if a system changes so will the individuals within the system. Family or relationship therapy is aimed at helping the members change the patterns of relationships that are not working well and helping the family create new ways of interacting.

Most family therapists adhere to some general goals, but specific goals are determined by the practitioner's orientation or by a collaborative process between the family and the therapist. Global goals include intervening to enable individuals and a family to change in a way that relieves their distress. Tied to the question of what goals should guide a therapist's interventions with a family is the question of the therapist's values. Ultimately, every intervention a therapist makes is an expression of his or her values. It is critical for therapists, regardless of their theoretical orientation, to be aware of these values and to monitor how they influence their practice with families.

How families change.   An integrative approach to the practice of family therapy must include guiding principles that help organize goals, interactions, observations, and ways to promote change. Theories of family therapy can be grouped into two categories: (1) those that focus on change within the therapy sessions, and (2) those that deal with the occurrence of change outside the therapeutic context in the natural world (Hanna & Brown, 1995). Some theories focus on perceptual and cognitive change, others deal mainly with changing feelings, and others emphasize behavioral change.

Techniques of family therapy. Diverse techniques are available to family therapists, but the intervention strategies they employ are best considered in conjunction with their own personal characteristics. It is essential that therapists use skills and techniques that fit their personality and that are appropriate for the goals of therapy. Goldenberg and Goldenberg (1996a) and Nichols and Schwartz (1995) emphasize that techniques are tools for achieving therapeutic goals, yet these intervention strategies do not make a family therapist. Personal characteristics, such as respect for clients, compassion, empathy, and sensitivity, are human qualities that influence the manner in which techniques are delivered. Faced with the demands of clinical practice, practitioners need to be flexible in selecting intervention strategies that will meet specific therapeutic objectives and contribute to specific outcomes. The central consideration is what is in the best interests of the family.

Contributions of family systems approaches. A key contribution of the systemic approaches is that neither the individual nor the family is blamed for a particular dysfunction. The family is empowered through the process of identifying and exploring interaction patterns. If change is to come about in a family or between individual members of a family, the family must be aware of the systems that influence them. Contemporary approaches to family therapy emphasize understanding the individual within the systems that influence him or her. This sheds an entirely different light on assessment and treatment of individuals and families. In the remainder of the chapter we invite you to understand yourself more fully by coming to a deeper understanding of your family of origin.

WORKING WITH YOUR FAMILY OF ORIGIN

Some writers suggest that training programs provide family-of-origin work for students as part of growth group experiences (Lawson & Gaushell, 1991; Wilcoxon, Walker, & Hovestadt, 1989). Other authors discuss how family-of-origin work can be used for personal growth training of marriage and family counselors (Getz & Protinsky, 1994), ways that early childhood family influences are related to counselor effectiveness (Watts, Trusty, Canada, & Harvill, 1995), and ethical considerations when using the family autobiography in training counselors (Goodman & Carpenter-White, 1996). Most hold that a practitioner's mental health, as defined by relationships with his or her family of origin, has implications for professional training. Trainees can benefit from exploring the dynamics of their family of origin because it enables them to relate more effectively to the families they will meet in their clinical practice.

Getz and Protinsky (1994) take the position that personal growth is an essential part of training counselors and that knowledge and skills cannot be separated from a helper's internal dynamics and use of self. Getz and Protinsky point to growing clinical evidence that a family-of-origin approach to supervision is a necessary dimension of training helpers who want to work with families. They contend that the reactions of helpers to their clients' stories tend to reactivate helpers' old learned patterns of behavior and unresolved problems. By studying their own families of origin, students are ultimately able to improve their ability to counsel families.

Lawson and Gaushell (1991) recommend that training programs address candidates' family issues before admitting them to a program. They suggest requiring a family autobiography as part of the application materials. This would yield useful information concerning intergenerational family characteristics that would have a relationship to a helper's ability to work with families. Lawson and Gaushell emphasize these intergenerational family characteristics of counselor trainees:

- Clinicians who have resolved negative family experiences are better able to assist their clients, especially those with whom they have issues in common.
- It is essential that trainees be given assistance in identifying and addressing their own problematic family issues to enhance their psychological functioning and their effectiveness as helpers.
- Unmet needs in early family experiences later manifest themselves in intense and conflicting ties with these family members.
- Helpers' early roles as peacemakers create later ambivalence regarding intimacy with significant others.
- Counselor trainees' experiences in their families of origin can lead to difficulties in their current relationships.

Identifying Your Issues in Your Family of Origin

If you lack awareness of ways that particular members of your own family may trigger strong emotional reactions in you, it is likely that you will react too quickly to clients in the context of family therapy. When clients in families evoke your instant and intense reactions, it is well for you to reflect on unfinished business with significant people in your past. If you do not, your perceptions will be colored and distorted by your history, which means that you will probably not be objective or open to understanding certain clients. Family therapists generally assume that it is inevitable that they will meet parts of their family in every other family with whom they have a professional relationship. If you do not understand the patterns of interpersonal behavior learned in your family of origin, you will repeat these patterns with clients (Getz & Protinsky, 1994; Goodman & Carpenter-White, 1996; Lawson & Gaushell, 1988).

Virginia Satir, one of the pioneers in family therapy, used to say that if she walked into a room with 12 people she would meet everyone she ever knew. When you are counseling a couple or a family, a roomful of people are participating in this interaction. In other words, you are not always perceiving individuals whom you meet with a fresh and unbiased perspective. The more you are aware of your patterns of interacting with your own family members, the greater is the benefit to your clients. It is crucial that you know to whom you are responding: to the individual in front of you or to a person from your past.

Try this exercise that Satir used to demonstrate that people are constantly revisiting friends and loved ones in their lives. Stand in front of someone (Person A) in your current life who interests you or with whom you are having some difficulty. This individual might be a client, an associate, a family member, or a friend. If the person is not present, you can imagine him or her. Take a good look at this person and form a picture on the screen of your mind. Now, let a picture of someone in your past come forward (Person B). Who comes to mind? How old are you, and how old is Person B? What relationship do you, or did you, have with this individual you are remembering? What feelings are linked with this relationship? What did you think about Person B? Now, examine again your reactions to Person A. Do you see any connection between what Person A is evoking in you and the past feelings evoked by Person B? You can apply this exercise by yourself through the use of imagery when you have intense emotional reactions to other people, especially if you do not know them well. This exercise can help you begin to recognize how your past relationships may sometimes affect here-and-now responses. Perhaps what is most important is simply to be aware of ways in which you are carrying your past into present interactions.

In this section we invite you to identify as many family-of-origin experiences as possible and also to reflect on how these life experiences are likely to have an influence on *who* and *what* you are at this point. Goldenberg and Goldenberg (1996b) have written a workbook designed to provoke students into thinking about how their roles in their family of origin and their current family continue to play out in maintaining their attitudes, values, and behavior patterns. In the preface they write: "By learning more about yourself, especially by adopting a family perspective, . . . you can help others, including future clients, see themselves within the contexts of their families" (p. iii). You are not necessarily determined by your earlier experiences, and they do not have to serve as the template for your current significant relationships. You can make shifts in your perspectives, but only if you have recognized and dealt with your experiences. If you are working with a family, moreover, you will have an experiential starting point to invite them to look at their functioning as a system and as individuals within the family.

Much of the remainder of this section is based on our perspective on family history, which is a modification and integration of material taken from several sources: (1) Adlerian lifestyle assessment methods (see Corey, 1996a; Dinkmeyer, Dinkmeyer, & Sperry, 1987; Mosak & Shulman, 1988; Powers & Griffith, 1986, 1987; Sherman & Dinkmeyer, 1987; Shulman & Mosak, 1988); (2) Satir's communication approach to working with families (Satir, 1983, 1989; Satir & Baldwin, 1983; Satir, Bitter, & Krestensen, 1988; see also Bitter, 1987, 1988); (3) concepts of family systems (see Goldenberg & Goldenberg, 1996a, 1996b; Nichols & Schwartz, 1995); (4) genogram methods (see McGoldrick & Gerson, 1989); and (5) family autobiography methods (see Lawson & Gaushell, 1988). As you read the following material, we encourage you to personalize the information. We are primarily providing you with ways to understand and work with your own family material and secondarily offering you a basis for understanding the individuals and families in your professional work.

Your family structure. The many patterns of family life include nuclear, extended, single-parent, divorced, and blended. The term *family structure* also refers to the social and psychological organization of the family system, including factors such as birth order and the individual's perception of self in the family context.

- In what type of family structure did you grow up? It might be that the structure of your family changed over time. If so, what were these changes? What were some of the most important family values? What most stands out for you about your family life? How do these experiences continue to influence who you are today?
- What is your current family structure? Are you still primarily involved in your family of origin, or do you have a different family structure? If you do, what roles do you play in your current family that you also enacted in your original family? Have you carried certain patterns from your original family into your current family? How do you see yourself as being different in the two families?
- Draw a picture of your family of origin. Include all the members, and identify their significant alliances. Identify the relationships with each person that you had as a child and your relationships with each member now.
- Make a list of the siblings, from oldest to youngest. Give a brief description of each (including yourself). What most stands out for each sibling? Which sibling(s) is (are) most different from you, and how? Which is most like you, and how?
- Review some key dimensions of your experiences as a child growing up in your family. How would you describe yourself as a child? What were some of your major fears? hopes? ambitions? What was school like for you? What was your role in your peer group? Identify any significant events in your physical, sexual, and social development during childhood.
- Identify one of your personal problems. How has your relationship with your family contributed to the development and perpetuation of this problem? Besides blaming your family for this problem, what options are open to you for making substantial changes in yourself? What are a few ways in which you can be different in your family?

Parental figures and relationships with parents. Your parents were central figures in your development, and your interactional patterns with them have set the stage for many of your present relationships. A father or mother may have been absent from your early family life. If so, did any substitute figures emerge? If you grew up in a single-parent family, did this one parent play the roles of both mother and father? What did your parent or parents teach you, mainly through the behavior they modeled, about marriage and about family life? Spend some time thinking about your parental figures and your relationships with them. Focus on what you learned from observing and interacting with your parents, on what you observed in their interactions with each other, and on how each parent interacted with each sibling. Remember how each of the siblings viewed and reacted to your parents. Reflect on your parents separately:

1. Describe your father (or the person who substituted for him). What is he like as a person? What are his ambitions for each of the children? How did you view him as a child? How do you view him now? How are you like him? How are you unlike him? What does your father say when he compliments you? when he criticizes you? What was his main advice to you as a child? What is his main advice to you now? What could you do to disappoint him? What can you do to please him? What was his relationship to his children? What is his current relationship to the siblings? What sibling is the most like your father, and in what ways? What did your father tell you (either directly or indirectly) about you? life? death? love? sex? marriage? men? women? your birth?

2. After describing your father, go back over the above list of questions and ask each of them about your mother (or the person who substituted for her). Give a sketch of how you viewed your mother.

Your parents have been the "air-traffic controllers" of your life. They launched you, guided you, and helped you survive. They are the people on whom you depended for survival, and you may feel less than grown up in relation to them. You may find yourself acting the way you did as a child when you are with them as opposed to functioning as a psychological adult. It is important to remember that for many people the last relationships they work out are those with their parents.

Becoming your own person.   An assumption of the systems approach is that a healthy person has achieved both a psychological separateness from and a sense of intimacy with his or her family. The late Murray Bowen, a distinguished family systems therapist from Washington, D.C., believed that differentiation of self was the hallmark of health and was a necessity for counselors and family therapists. Our discussion of several key concepts in this section is based on his perspective. For good presentations of Bowenian family therapy, see Goldenberg and Goldenberg (1996a, 1996b) and Nichols and Schwartz (1995).

Becoming your own person entails acquiring a separate and individual identity. This process of *individuation* involves the aforementioned balance between belonging to and separating from your family of origin. The increasing differentiation from the family allows you to accept personal responsibility for your thoughts, feelings, perceptions, and actions. Individuation, or psychological maturity, is not a fixed destination that you reach once and for all; rather, it is a lifelong developmental process achieved through reexamination and resolution of internal conflicts and intimacy issues with loved ones.

If you are moving in the direction of autonomy, you are aware of the ways in which your "inner parent" exerts control over you. Although you can never free yourself of parental influence, it is possible to assume responsibility by doing for yourself what you expected others to do for you as a child. Instead of looking outside yourself for your direction and focusing on what others expect, you are clear about your own expectations. This process of individuation does not mean that you are indifferent to what others need or want from you, nor does it imply an exaggerated sense of independence. Indeed, if you are devoting much energy to reacting against your parents and striving to prove that you are your own person, it could be a sign of your deeper fears of being dependent or of being engulfed by your parents. Thus, if you are becoming a separate being, you are also concerned with maintaining connections, reaching out to others, sharing with them, and giving yourself in your relationships. Being an integrated person implies that you recognize the many and varied aspects of your being, that you accept both positive and negative sides, and that you do not disown parts of yourself.

These notions of individuation, independence, autonomy, and self-determination are Western values, and not all cultures pay this homage to such values. This emphasis on independence and self-determination tends to reduce the importance of the family of origin. Sue and Sue (1991) point out that in Chinese-American families the notion of filial piety is a strong determinant of how children behave, even as they move to adulthood. Obedience, respect, obligation to parents, and duty leave little room for self-determination. For example, allegiance to one's parents is expected from a man, even after he marries and has his own family. The concept of individuation and separation from his family can easily lead to conflicts in his family relationships. For example, a son may have difficulty with the notion of being his own person beyond the limits of his family role. He may always think of himself as first a son and in the line of his family tree. For such a person, individuation is neither ideal nor particularly functional. He will discover who he is more easily within the family context than outside of it. It is quite clear that cultural values play a key role in adopting behaviors that reflect an individualistic or collectivistic spirit. At this point, reflect on these questions:

- What cultural values influenced the degree to which you have striven toward autonomy? Are there any values that stem from your culture that you want to retain? any that you want to challenge or modify?
- In what significant ways, if any, do you see yourself as having a distinct identity and as being psychologically separate from your family of origin? And in what ways, if any, are you psychologically fused with your family of origin? Are there any aspects of this relationship that you want to change?
- The concept of *boundaries* is used in family therapy to refer to emotional barriers that protect and enhance the integrity of members of a system. It also refers to a delineation between members that is governed by implicit or explicit rules. Apply the notion of boundaries to your development. In growing up in your family, what boundaries existed between you and your parents? between your parents and the siblings? among the siblings? between your parents? What did you learn about boundaries? Do you have any problems with boundaries today?

Triangular relationships.   Reflect for a moment on some relationships that you have primarily allowed others to define. Can you think of situations in which you have felt "dragged into" some conflicting triangle? A triangular relationship refers to the anxiety and emotional tension that exist when at least one person is pulled between the other two. For example, in seeking a balance between their needs for closeness and separateness, a wife and a husband may experience considerable stress and anxiety. One attempt at resolving the emotional tension that results within a family is for the couple to bring in another family member to form a three-person interaction. Thus, instead of the couple dealing with the conflicts between themselves, each may talk to one or more of the children about these tensions. The process of triangulation seems to reduce the stress experienced by the couple, but the basic conflict remains frozen in place. Another example of a triangle is the daughter who tells her mother how awful her father is to her. The mother can become entangled in this three-way relationship if she fosters indirect communication by encouraging her daughter to tell detailed stories about him. The mother can also refuse to triangulate by saying to her daughter: "You are speaking to the wrong person. What you are telling me is what I hope you will let your father know directly." This response reinforces the value of direct communication and avoids a collusion of the mother and daughter against the father.

Nichols and Schwartz (1995) point out that emotional triangles are not limited to three separate individuals but can involve any three-sided system. In a family triangle, a father may be distant from the mother. In turn, the mother may seek closeness with her children and may also pit them against their father. Relationships are not static, for participants go through cycles of closeness and distance. Triangles are most likely to develop when there is distance.

This presentation about triangles leans on the Bowenian point of view, which suggests that triangular relationships are problematic. There are other views of triangles, however. From Satir's perspective there are also nurturing triads. For example, the basic family triad consisting of the mother, father, and child can be constituted of loving, supportive, and cooperative forces. In these nurturing triads the individuals have high self-esteem, congruent communication, and an interest in others as well as themselves. This view is similar to Adler's notion of social interest, which refers to a sense of identification with humanity, a feeling of belonging, and an interest in the common good. According to Satir, in functional family triangles the mates have a high degree of self-esteem and are confident in their relationship, which allows for different relationships to bloom. As Satir (1983, p. 73) puts it:

- The mother is able to allow the child a father/child relationship.
- The father is able to allow the child a mother/child relationship.
- Yet both mates make it clear to the child that he or she can never be included in their relationship as mates.

Satir contrasts this functional family triangle to the dysfunctional family triangle. In the latter, one or both of the mates have low self-esteem, and they are not confident about their marital relationship. The partners feel a sense of disconnectedness with each other and look to the child to satisfy their unmet needs in the relationship.

In thinking about the concept of triangles in relationships, reflect on these questions:

- In growing up in your family, do you recall seeing any triangular relationships? On a continuum of functional to dysfunctional family triangles, how would you describe some of the relationships you observed in your family of origin? Where were you in the process? What did you learn about relationships?
- Do you see any signs of triangulation taking place in your present family? If so, what are some examples of this process? How do they affect you?
- To what degree did your family communicate openly? Did family members speak directly to each other about their concerns, or did they talk to a family member about another person? How would you identify your own communication style at this point? Are you able to be direct in making requests or in establishing your own limits?
- How were feelings expressed and dealt with in your family? Were they expressed directly or indirectly? What feelings were not expressed?

Coping with conflict in the family.   If you have difficulty dealing with conflict in your current relationships, one reason may be that conflict was not addressed in direct ways in your family of origin. Perhaps you were taught that conflict was something to be avoided at all costs. If you observed that conflict had no resolution in your family of origin or that people would simply not speak to each other for weeks after a conflict, you are bound to be intimidated when conflicts emerge. Conflicts belong to the whole family, although parents often make their children into scapegoats. The key to successful relationships lies not in the absence of conflict but in recognizing its source and being able to cope directly with the situations that lead to conflict. Conflicts that are denied tend to fester and strain relationships. Reflect on what you learned about conflict in your family. How was it expressed and dealt with? What were its sources? What was your role? Were you encouraged to resolve conflict directly with your antagonist? Did you feel safe in recognizing and dealing directly with disputes between you and members of your family?

The family as a system.   Families have certain rules governing interactions. These *family rules* are not simple commandments, such as what time children need to be home after a date. They also include unspoken rules, messages given by parents to children, injunctions, myths, and secrets. These rules are often couched in terms of "dos" or "don'ts." When parents feel worried or helpless, they tend to dictate rules in an attempt to control any situation. These family rules initially assist children in handling anger, helplessness, and fear. They are intended to provide a safety net for children as they venture into the world (Satir et al., 1988). It is impossible for children to escape growing up without such rules or injunctions, and on the basis of them, children make early decisions. They decide either to accept family rules or to fight against them. Examples of rules are: "Never be angry with your father." "Always keep a smile on your face." "Don't confront your parents, but do what you can to please them." "Don't talk to outsiders about your family." "Children are to be seen but not heard." "Have fun only when all the work is finished."

Rules or messages that were delivered by our parents and parent substitutes are often couched in terms of "do this or that." Consider the following "do" messages: "Be obedient." "Be practical at all times." "Be the very best you can be." "Be appropriate." "Be perfect." "Be a credit to your family." "Be better than we are."

Consider some of the major dos and don'ts that you heard growing up in your family and your reactions to them:

- What are a few messages or rules that you accepted?
- What are some rules that you fought against?
- What early decisions do you deem most significant in your life today? In what family context did you make these decisions? If you grew up in your family thinking "I am never enough," how has this conclusion played out in your current relationships?
- Do you ever hear yourself giving the same messages to others that you heard from your parents?
- Consider for a moment the overall impact of the messages that you have received, both from your parents and from society. How have these messages influenced your self-worth? your view of yourself as a woman or as a man? your trust in yourself? your ability to be creative and spontaneous? your ability to receive love and give love? your willingness to make yourself vulnerable? your sense of security? your potential to succeed?

As children we receive rules in a less than clear manner, often learning by observing the behavior of our parents. When rules are presented without choice and as absolutes, they typically present problems for us. For example, you may have accepted a family rule that "I must never get angry." The "must" limits choice completely, and the "never" is an absolute that proves impossible to live by. As a small child, you may have decided to accept this rule and live by it for reasons of both physical and psychological survival. When you carry such a pattern into your adult interactions, it can become self-defeating and dysfunctional. When you live by an absolute rule that "I must never get angry!" it loses its functional nature and inevitably breaks down, and stress in the family goes up.

Rather than trying to get people to give up these survival rules in their lives, Satir suggests helping people transform rules that were not useful into something useful and functional. For example, if Satir were working with your rule that "I must never get angry!" she would broaden the range of choice and challenge you to rid yourself of the impossibility of living up to "always" and "never" standards. She would ask you to first try the statement "I can never get angry." Although this rule still isn't realistic, the word *can* implies more choice than the word *must*. Then she would ask you to try "I *can sometimes* get angry." This statement has both choice and possibility. To make the element of choice more salient, Satir would ask you to think of three situations in which you could imagine getting angry. Through this process, a dysfunctional survival rule can be transformed rather than being attacked.

In healthy families the number of rules is small, and rules are applied consistently. The rules are humanly possible, relevant, and flexible (Bitter, 1987). According to Satir and Baldwin (1983), the most important family rules are those that govern individuation (being unique) and sharing of information (communication). These are the rules that influence the ability of a family to function in open ways and to allow all members the possibility for changing. Satir notes that many people develop a range of styles as a means for coping with stress resulting from the constrictions of family rules.

Bitter (1987) contrasts a functional family structure with one that is dysfunctional. In functional families each member is allowed to have a separate life as well as a shared life with the family group. Different relationships are given room to grow. Change is expected and invited, not viewed as a threat. When differentiation leads to disagreements, the situation is viewed as an opportunity for growth rather than an attack on the family system. The structure of the functional family system is characterized by freedom and flexibility and by open communication. All the family members have a voice and can speak for themselves. In this atmosphere, individuals feel support for taking risks and venturing into the world.

By contrast, dysfunctional families are characterized by closed communication, by the poor self-esteem of one or both parents, and by rigid patterns. Rules serve the function of masking fears about differences. They are rigid and are frequently inappropriate for meeting a situation. In unhealthy families, the members are expected to think, feel, and act in the same way. Parents attempt to control the family by using fear, punishment, guilt, or dominance. Eventually, the system breaks down because the rules are no longer able to keep the family structure intact.

When stress is exacerbated because of the breakdown of the family system, members tend to resort to defensive stances. Satir (1983) and Satir and Baldwin (1983) identify four universal communication patterns that express these defensive postures or stress positions: *placating, blaming,* being *overly reasonable,* and being *irrelevant.*

- Individuals who use *placating* as a style for dealing with stress pay the price of sacrificing themselves in their attempt to please others. Because they do not feel an inner sense of value and feel helpless without others, such people say and do what they think others expect of them. Out of their fear of being rejected, they strive to be too many things to too many people.
- People who adopt a *blaming* posture will sacrifice others to maintain their view of themselves. As they point the finger of blame at others, they avoid dealing with the deeper issues of their lack of self-worth and meaninglessness. They frequently say "if it weren't for you . . . ." They attribute responsibility to others for the way they are.
- People who become *overly reasonable* tend to function much like a computer. They strive for complete control over themselves, others, and their environment. In their attempt to avoid humiliation and embarrassment, they keep their emotions tightly in check. Of course, they pay a price of isolation and distance from others for being overcontrolled.
- *Irrelevant* behavior is manifested by a pattern of distractions in the mistaken hope that pain will diminish. Such people appear to be in constant motion. Because they are frightened of stress, they avoid taking a clear position lest they offend others.

Is there an alternative to dealing with family rules other than taking one of the four defensive postures described above? How does a healthy person deal with the stress of meeting family rules? Bitter (1987) describes how congruent people cope with this stress. They do not sacrifice themselves to a singular style in dealing with it. Instead, they transform stress into a challenge that is met in a useful way. Such people are centered, and they avoid changing their colors like a chameleon. Their words match their inner experience, and they are able to make direct and clear statements. They face stress with confidence and courage, because they know that they have the inner resources to cope effectively and to make sound choices. They feel a sense of belongingness and a connectedness with others. They are motivated by the principle of social interest, which means that they are not interested merely in self-enhancement but are aware of the need to contribute to the common good.

We encourage you to think about this discussion of how family rules are manifested in both functional and dysfunctional family structures. Rather than labeling your own family as "functional" or "dysfunctional," think about specific aspects within your family system that may not have been as healthy as you wish. Also think about those aspects of your family life that were helpful, functional, and healthy. Apply the discussion of family structures and family rules to your own experiences. We recommend several books that will provide you with more detailed information on this topic: Satir (1983), Satir (1989), and Satir and Baldwin (1983).

It is a mistake to assume that once decisions have been made they are cemented forever. Even children are not completely helpless in responding to the messages sent to them. If there are two children in a family, for example, each may react very differently to the same message of working hard that is modeled by their parents. The daughter decides to have more fun in her life than her parents and places little value on work. The son decides to outdo his parents and work even harder, becoming a workaholic. Children are not passively programmed, although they frequently develop patterns in reaction to what they see their parents doing. On some level, children cooperate in making the early decisions that direct their lives, which means that they have the capacity to make new decisions that are appropriate to changing life circumstances. Apply the notion of early decisions and making new decisions to yourself. How have some of your early decisions served you? And how have they interfered with your present significant relationships? Can you think of any early decisions that you have modified? If so, what are some new decisions that you made, and how has this redecision process affected your life today?

At this point, reflect on the rules that were apparent in your family. What were some unspoken rules between the adults in your family? Was your father rational and objective, especially when your mother was emotional and nurturing? What rules did you learn about appropriate sex-role behavior? What did you learn about femininity? about masculinity? To what degree did you abide by all these rules? Were there any that you challenged? How did these unspoken rules affect you?

Various family members take on roles that influence the interactions within that family. For instance, your youngest brother may have assumed a role of victim, whereby he typically felt picked on and was constantly seeking protection. It could be that you assumed the role of keeping peace within the family. Even at an early age, others in your family may have looked to you as their counselor or expected you to take care of family difficulties. Your father may have taken on the role of the stern taskmaster and disciplinarian, whereas your mother may have assumed a nurturing role. What roles did you play in your family as a child? as an adolescent? And what are some key roles that you are playing today in your family and in your work?

Family secrets can also influence the structure and functioning of a family. Secrets can be particularly devastating, because that which is hidden typically assumes greater power than that which is out in the open. Generally, it is not what is openly talked about that causes difficulty in families but what is kept hidden. If there are secrets in the family, children are left to figure out what is going on in the home. Did you suspect any secrets in your family? If so, what was it like for you to perpetuate the secrecy? to divulge the secrets? What do you think that secrecy did to the family atmosphere?

Significant developments in your family.   You might find it useful to describe your family's life cycle. Chart significant turning points that have characterized the family's development. One way to do this is to look at family photo albums to see what the pictures reveal. Let them stimulate memories and reflections. As you view pictures of your parents, grandparents, siblings, and other relatives, look for patterns that can offer clues to family dynamics. In charting transitions in the development of your family, reflect on these questions:

- What were the crisis points for your family?
- Can you recall any unexpected events?
- Were there any periods of separation due to employment, military service, or imprisonment?
- Who tended to have problems within the family? How were these problems manifested? How did others in the family react to the person with problems?
- In what ways did births affect the family?
- Were there any serious illnesses, accidents, divorces, or deaths in your family? If so, how did they affect individual members in the family and the family as a whole?
- Was there a history of physical, sexual, or emotional abuse?

Stages in Learning about the History of Your Family

One of our daughters is enrolled in a doctoral program in clinical psychology that requires a course on the family of origin. The state mandates such a course as a requirement for licensure as a marriage and family therapist. We hope other training programs will follow this lead.

In a colleague's graduate training program in marital and family therapy, students are required to engage in experiential work with their family of origin. This exploration is presented to students in four graded phases with some supervision. These four phases correspond to the family autobiography method used by Lawson and Gaushell (1988) as a tool to promote the personal growth of students in the helping fields. The goal is to provide counselor trainees with opportunities to examine the influence of their family of origin on their current functioning. This method allows students to expand their perceptual and behavioral choices as they interact with family members, peers, supervisors, and clients. The process of pulling together material for a family history encourages trainees to recall, reexperience, explore, and rethink their beliefs and relationships in their family of origin. This sketch of one's family history is accomplished in a graduated way, by going from objective data collection to interpreting the personal meaning of key events.

1. First of all, students collect data from immediate and extended family members, and they begin organizing this information in the form of a genogram. McGoldrick and Gerson (1989) describe the genogram as a symbolic diagram that presents graphic pictures of the family's history and chronicles information about the basic structure, demographics, and functioning of family members over at least three generations. A genogram is a shorthand depiction of family patterns and provides rich material for following the family's evolution. Because our space is limited and does not allow more than a mention of the value of genograms, we recommend consulting McGoldrick and Gerson (1989) for a detailed discussion.

2. After students begin organizing their genogram, they collect family demographic data and develop a time line that chronicles the specific years of significant events, such as births, deaths, marriages, and divorces. Even though this phase mainly consists of collecting data, it can bring up emotional issues, such as feelings associated with a death in the family.

3. In the next phase trainees identify important events and turning points in their lives. This process involves an interactional description of their family, along with an examination of sibling positions. The focus now is on what is subjectively important for the students as they uncover significant material that has played a role in the formation of who they are.

4. The final phase involves the students sketching an emotional diagram of their family, from their own perspective. As they create this diagram, the emphasis is on understanding the impact of certain events and processes and how it is translated into their everyday living. Students describe their perceptions of their family interactions and other relationship patterns over a period of time, and they explore how they have been personally affected by these events. It is stressed that students do not have the task of changing their family. Instead, they are asking themselves questions about their earlier experiences and are seeking information from other family members to assist them in this understanding.

Proceed with Caution

Simply reflecting on the questions we've raised that deal with your family history can be therapeutic by itself, even though it may be accompanied by turmoil. If you decide to carry the process a step further and interview members of your family, or if you get involved in the four-stage process of putting together a family autobiography, this can be an anxiety-provoking exercise not only for you but also for members of your family and extended family. Although Goodman and Carpenter-White (1996) highly recommend family autobiography assignments, they identify ethical concerns that need to be addressed in using this excellent teaching tool. Doing a family autobiography involves self-disclosure, not only on the trainee's part but also on the part of family members. Interviewing family members could unearth sensitive areas that could be harmful to a family member if privacy were to be breached in some way. Once family secrets are brought out in the open, all family members are likely to have reactions, which could affect a family's dynamics, for better or for worse. Goodman and Carpenter-White recommend that instructors who use the family autobiography assignment also present cautions along with the benefits of the assignment. Students need guidelines in dealing with areas such as family requests to read the completed report, dealing with disclosed information that is potentially sensitive to self or others, and anticipating family reactions that cover a range of emotions and behavior.

We want to offer a few other cautions that we hope will reduce the chances of your meeting with resistance and alienating members of your family. In Chapter 7 you learned that it is essential to be sensitive to cultural themes in the lives of your clients and that you might lose certain clients if you do not demonstrate an understanding of how their culture affects their choices and actions. Apply this general principle as you approach members of your family. Be sensitive of the manner in which you seek personal information. Tell family members you are interviewing your reasons for wanting the information. If they think you are giving them the third degree, they may clam up. Furthermore, you need to be aware of the cultural rules operating in your family structure, and you need to be aware of family systems concepts such as triangles, roles, rules, myths, and rituals. In some families, a mother or father would feel offended if a child were to seek information from an aunt or uncle. A Japanese graduate student approached his father to interview him as part of his family autobiography assignment. The father was reluctant to engage in any significant sharing of family material despite the student's insistence that getting this knowledge was important for him.

In doing a review of your family history, be prepared for the possibility of a crisis erupting, either in you or within your family. One student discovered that she had been adopted. She was faced with dealing with anger and disappointment over not having been told. Doing this level of work may lead to a number of surprises and discoveries for which you are not prepared. You may learn of family secrets, or you may learn that your "ideal family" is not as perfect as you thought. You may well find that your family has both functional and dysfunctional aspects. Many of the students who were enrolled in a personal-growth group with one of us (Marianne) became anxious or depressed by what they were learning about both themselves and their family system and felt a need to talk about how they were being affected.

It is important to remember that doing a genogram involves tracing historical events for at least three generations. If you have access to such sources, it would be a good idea to look for patterns that seem to have been passed down from generation to generation. Look especially at your interactions with your current family to discern any ways in which you might be repeating these patterns in your relationships now.

You may well find out that the sources of information are scarce, even about your grandparents. For example, I (Jerry) know precious little about my father's life before he and my mother married. From my father, I have some knowledge about his difficult beginnings in this country. At the age of 7, he and his brother came from Italy to New York. His father (whom I know almost nothing about) brought the two children to this country after his wife died. Again, there is scant information about my father's mother. I don't even know how she died. Apparently, my grandfather's intentions were to have a relative in this country care for his boys, yet she was unable to do so because of her own family responsibilities. This led to my father's placement in an orphanage. I recall some stories he told me about the loneliness of his childhood in the institution and how difficult it was coming to this country not being able to speak a word of English. What is striking to me is how little I do know about my father's side of the family, and this in itself reveals how much material was denied and was kept secret. Because my father died 30 years ago, I have had to look for bits of information that my mother remembers about my father's history and also to relatives who knew something about his life.

In contrast, Marianne's family history is easily traced back to the early 1600s. For many years, I (Marianne) have heard rich stories that formed the tapestry of my family's history. As I grew up in an extended family in a German village, many relatives and townspeople revealed information about several generations. I did become aware of one pattern from my father's side. Someone in the family would typically get angry, and an emotional cutoff would result in which certain people would never speak to each other again. It saddens me to see how this pattern unfolds even with one of my brothers, who, in spite of my efforts to form a closer relationship, seems to be following the tendency of keeping himself distant. This experience is teaching me that family patterns repeat themselves and that we cannot change another person. But we do have power over how we allow ourselves to be affected by the actions and decisions of others.

Doing this level of self-exploration is a must if you intend to work with families. Committing yourself to this arduous task will better enable you to appreciate what client family members go through when they are in therapy with you. We encourage you to stick with the process of discovery, preferably under supervision. It helps to be able to talk to someone about what you are learning.

A related matter is our belief that being involved in a training program as a helper involves some risks to your current relationships. We have emphasized throughout this book that growth is not without some pain and can be anxiety-producing. Moreover, your commitment to exploration and change may bring discomfort to significant people in your life. Your parents, siblings, husband, wife, children, or other relatives may well be threatened by some of your changes. You may believe in the value of recognizing pain and dealing with it, and as a result of your changed perspective you may want your parents or siblings also to adopt a new outlook and change their ways. Perhaps they have avoided pain and are not interested in disturbing the conditions they've settled for. Even if facing their situation could lead to basic changes and a fuller existence, it is not for you to decide that they should be any different than they are.

As a result of what you are learning about human relationships in your program, along with positive changes you are making in your life, it is bound to be difficult for you to witness people you love settling for a dull existence, if not a destructive lifestyle. You might ask, "How can I help other families in trouble if I cannot help my own family?" If you burden yourself with the thought that it is your mission to change members of your family, you are bound to wind up feeling frustrated.

A graduate student in a counseling program approached one of us and said he felt burdened in putting to use in his own family what he was learning in his courses. Asked what he hoped to accomplish for a weekend therapeutic group aimed at self-exploration, he said: "I feel an urgency to clean up all my problems with my family by the end of this weekend workshop. After all, how can I help my future clients solve their problems if I have problems within my family?" Although this student was to be encouraged in his attempt to deal with his problems, he was setting himself up for failure by trying to meet an unrealistic expectation. Even more of a burden was his belief that it was his place to get significant people in his life to change. He needed to realize that no matter how talented he was, if people within his family were not motivated to make certain changes, he would never be able to do it for them. What he could do was to focus on himself and tell them about himself, which in itself could be an invitation for them to change. He could talk about the changes he had made and what they meant to him. He could also let others know how he was affected by some of their behaviors and, as well, what kind of relationship he would like with them.

The point is to avoid adopting a zealous attitude that others should be different and then attempting to convert them to your way. Above all, patience is critical. To make changes in your life, you probably had to get through layers of your own resistances that masked your fears. It took both time and patience for you to allow yourself to become more vulnerable and open to new possibilities. Allow this space for others in your life to consider your invitations.

Avoid Blaming, and Keep the Focus on Yourself

As you learn about the effect that your family of origin has had on the person you have become, there is a danger of getting stuck in a blaming stance. If you are not careful, you could get sidetracked by believing "If only you had done ____ , I would be different." A blaming posture will keep you frozen in your attempt to make significant changes, both in yourself and in your relationships. Regardless of the quality of your experiences in your family and no matter how horrible your childhood years may have been, you do not have to remain a victim of your circumstances. It may well take your involvement in personal therapy to work through some of your feelings, so that you can eventually make peace with your past and more freely choose a new direction.

Through our work in group counseling, we have learned time and again that the tendency of many who participate in our groups is to put the focus on the other person in the relationship rather than emphasizing their own role. For example, a college student is quick to tell his mother that she should change and that then they would get along better. He puts considerable energy into searching for her faults, judging her for what she did to him or failed to do for him, and trying to get her to think, feel, and act in ways that he thinks she should. He does his best to control her, so that he is more comfortable in his relationship with her. Luciano and Merris (1992) have shown in their book *If Only You Would Change* how couples become trapped in this rigid way of thinking, which creates a myriad of troubles in their marriage. It is almost impossible for one partner to control how the other will behave, but there is a wide range of possibilities when it comes to controlling your own life.

When we warn clients about the dangers inherent in blaming people and setting out to change others, they invariably resist changing their perspective. For many, focusing on others does serve the purpose of preserving their self-image. Paradoxically, however, many of our clients find that when they do stop trying to change another person and concentrate more on revealing themselves, the other person is more open to change.

If you are caught up in blaming others for the way that you are, in your counseling you will probably allow clients to blame others for their misery. From our perspective, a mistake that many helpers make is to listen endlessly to their clients recounting stories about how others have mistreated them. Helpers actually form a coalition with such clients, keeping them in a powerless position instead of confronting them on the ways in which they are avoiding taking responsibility for themselves.

Helpers promote growth by challenging clients to recognize their projections and disowned material. People who are very judgmental and critical of traits in others often fail to see those qualities in themselves. In *The Promise of a New Day*, Casey and Vanceburg (1985) beautifully capture this idea of owning one's projections:

> Our negative judgments about others very frequently inform us of our own shortcomings. In other words, what we dislike in others are often those things we hate about ourselves. Much better than criticizing another's abhorrent behavior is a decision to look inwardly at our own collection of traits and attitudes. Our desire to criticize, to pass judgment, offers an excellent mirror of who we truly are. And the image we see reflected can guide our movements toward becoming healthier, happy individuals. (Meditation of January 24)

When individuals devote a great deal of energy to denying aspects of their being that are not ego-enhancing, they are vulnerable to becoming possessed by the side that they refuse to recognize in themselves. A task of helpers is to provide a climate that invites clients to become excruciatingly honest, which allows them to recognize in themselves what they are projecting outward. This process helps clients focus on what they can do for themselves, as opposed to expecting others to adapt to their expectations. As you will see in the next section, effective therapy helps clients assume this stance.

THE VALUE OF
SELF-EXPLORATION FOR THE HELPER

If you expect to work with couples and families, experiencing family therapy yourself would be ideal. We consider it essential that you at least engage in the self-exploration of your family of origin that we raised earlier. If it is not possible to be in therapy with your family, individual counseling or psychotherapy is an appropriate element in your process of becoming a helper. Many of the patterns you acquired as a child may still be problematic for you today. For instance, you could do useful work in individual or group therapy on any unresolved issues you have with your parents, with family rules that you have accepted, or with places where you feel stuck.

We do not assume that therapy—be it individual, group, or family—is just for treatment purposes or for curing deeply rooted personality disturbances. We see therapy as an avenue for continuing to deepen your self-understanding and for looking at the ways in which your needs are related to your work. Becoming involved in some form of intensive self-exploration or therapy can stimulate you to assess your motives for becoming a helper, which were outlined in Chapter 1. Through the process of self-exploration, which constitutes the essence of personal therapy, you can get firsthand knowledge of what your clients are likely to experience. This process will enable you to respect your clients as they do what it takes to face their fears, vulnerabilities, inner conflicts, and psychological wounds. It will be difficult to teach others about the joys and pains of growth that result from a therapeutic relationship if you have not experienced what it is like to be on the receiving end of this process. If you expect to provide family counseling, we hope that you can be in therapy with your family. If you want to lead therapy groups, it would certainly be advantageous to have been a member of a group.

One study appears to lend support to the idea that overcoming negative family experiences may positively affect the facilitation skills of helpers in training (Wilcoxon et al., 1989). Resolving unfinished business related to the family of origin is essential if individuals hope to establish relationships that do not repeat negative patterns of interaction. Facing and working through psychological wounds sustained in the family seem to be related to a helper's effectiveness during the initial stages of training. If helpers are encumbered by the excess psychological baggage of unresolved conflicts, this burden is bound to interfere with their ability to create different relationships in their personal lives and to help a family work through its conflicts.

You probably have certain blind spots, unfinished business, and old conflicts that could hamper your attempts to work effectively with clients. As you reviewed your family history, you no doubt gained some insights into unresolved conflicts and patterns that you have "adopted" from your family of origin. Therapy can aid you in seeing how these past conflicts are affecting you in the present. Furthermore, it can illuminate your own areas of transference and countertransference, which we discussed in Chapter 4. If you have fears about your own dying or the aging and death of your parents, for example, you can expect to encounter difficulty in working with older people. The struggles of these clients can activate unconscious processes in you, which if left outside your awareness will be likely to interfere with your ability to be fully present for clients who remind you of your pain. You will recall the example of the supervisee who was blocked in working with a family because of her unfinished business over the death of her father. Her contact with her supervisor helped her see her own part in getting bogged down with the family. But it was necessary for her to get involved in her own therapy to work through her unresolved feelings about her father. Counseling can assist students in situations like these to identify the source of their pain and to work through places where they may be psychologically stalled.

You too will find that working with individuals or families resurrects themes in your life, some of which have lain outside your conscious awareness. If you are not in touch with issues stemming from your family experiences, you will find ways to avoid potentially painful areas with your clients. The chances are that your tendency will be to make a quick referral. As your clients confront events that trigger their pain, memories of your own pain will come forth. For example, you may still have a great deal of hurt over your parents' divorce. It may be that you are struck with thinking that the divorce was your fault and that you could have done something to keep them together. Thus, if you are counseling a couple considering divorce, one of your tendencies may be to steer them toward remaining married for the sake of their children. You are giving them solutions that originate from your reservoir of hurt. On some level, you could be protecting the children from the pain of your situation that you have yet to fully realize or appreciate. It is important for you to recognize that your capacity to facilitate the healing forces in others lies in your willingness to experience your own wounds and to do what is needed to bring about healing for yourself.

Many situations in a family can plant the seeds of potential countertransference: growing up in a home with the unpredictability of violence, conflicts that were never addressed, secrecy that was protected at all costs, fears surrounding incest, absence of any boundaries, and significant events (such as grave illness or the death of a family member) that were ignored on a psychological level. If you felt that no matter how much you did, it was never quite enough to win your mother's approval, for example, you may now be very finely attuned to the judgments of women who remind you of your mother. If you allowed your father to completely affirm or deny your value as a person, you may be very sensitive to what male authority figures think about you. You may give them the power to make you feel either competent or incompetent. As a child, if you often felt rejected and on the outside, you may now create situations in which you feel like the one who is left out and just does not fit.

In your own therapy you will be able to explore some of the ways in which you unconsciously set up situations that repeat past situations that have been a source of pain to you. A woman who was rejected by her mother, for example, finds that in every relationship with a woman the end result is that she feels rejected. Thus, she is recreating an old, familiar scene with every significant woman she meets. In her therapy she can come to understand her role in the continuation of this pattern of rejection, and she can then begin to establish new and more satisfying ways of relating to women. A man who perceived his mother as a chronic complainer might have done everything in his power to lighten her load so that she could eventually have some peace. Yet no matter what he did, he always ended up feeling that nothing he could do would make her happy. How might this man react to a female client who had many of his mother's dynamics?

As a helper you can perhaps learn nothing more important than the ways in which you carry old feelings from the past into present situations. It is illuminating for you to consider that you are living out unfinished scenarios from the dance enacted by your parents, both as individuals and in their relationship with each other and their children. You are not free of the vestiges of what you experienced in your family. You have a set of convictions that structure your life, and you may be intent on confirming these assumptions even though some of them are self-defeating and no longer functional.

When someone in your family was angry, for example, people got hurt, either physically or emotionally. As a child you made a decision that anger was a useless emotion, that you would never show this feeling, and that you would not even allow yourself to feel angry. This decision could have protected you at the time, when you felt helpless and did not know how to cope with destructive expressions of anger. But your extreme denial of anger now interferes with your significant relationships at home and at work. People find it difficult to trust you, because you never express negative reactions to anything. If you have this trouble accepting your own anger, you will have difficulty allowing your clients to express their anger and deal constructively with it.

Many professional training programs recognize the value of some form of self-exploration for the trainees. Whether this personal-growth experience is conducted one-to-one, in simulated family-therapy sessions, or in a group setting, the focus can still be on the helper as a person. We have found that many beginning helpers would rather look at the dynamics of their clients than at themselves. Although there is nothing wrong in wanting to understand better ways of working with clients, you can best learn how to do this by allowing yourself to be as open as possible to your own life experience. Thus, whenever you take measures to understand yourself more fully, you are at the same time preparing yourself to help others in their quest for self-understanding.

Professional help is useful not only for trainees but also for practicing professionals. At times, experienced practitioners can use the challenge to reevaluate their beliefs and their behaviors. Furthermore, they may experience a crisis or an impairment for a period of time. For impaired helpers, getting professional help is both an ethical and a legal mandate. Mental-health professionals who themselves are in the midst of a psychological morass and who are still attempting to carry on their normal client caseloads are breaching a basic ethical code that states that the welfare of the client is supreme. Impaired professionals are not in a position to render high-quality service, which also makes them vulnerable to a malpractice suit.

We encourage both beginning helpers and those with many years of experience to pay attention to what they are giving to their work and getting from it. We find it hard to understand why so many helping professionals see themselves as beyond getting any help for themselves, even in times of personal crisis. It is as though some helpers think that they should be able to work out any problem they have by themselves. Although helpers claim to value the therapeutic process for others, they do not attribute the same value to receiving help from others. In Chapter 13 we focus on the lifelong challenge that helpers face in taking care of themselves as persons and as professionals so that they will have something of value to give clients who seek their services.

BY WAY OF REVIEW

- A systems approach forms the basis for understanding an individual's behavior within any system. Changes within the system will affect the individual, and individual changes influence the system. This perspective illuminates our understanding of interaction within families.
- The family systems perspective holds that individuals are best understood through assessing the interactions of a dysfunction with an entire family. Symptoms are viewed as an expression of a dysfunction within a family; these dysfunctional patterns are thought to be passed across several generations.
- Most family-therapy approaches tend to be brief, solution-focused, and action-oriented. This model of working with families fits well in the managed care concept that is a basic part of most agencies.
- One of the major contributions of the systemic approaches is that neither the individual nor the family is blamed for a particular dysfunction. Blaming others rarely leads to growth. Rather, it tends to cement the individual into a pattern of helplessness. Family therapy helps each family member change relationship patterns that are not working well and helps the family create new ways of interacting.
- Some training programs offer family-of-origin work for students as a way for them to come to a fuller appreciation of how their family experiences have influenced who and what they are. This training enables helpers to relate more effectively to the families they will meet in their clinical practice.
- To increase your effectiveness when working with families, it is essential that you unravel the mystery of your connection with your family of origin and that you become aware of ways you continue to play out patterns established during childhood.
- When interpreting the meaning of your experiences growing up in your family, it is useful to think about the structure of your family, your relationships with your parents and siblings, key turning points for your family, and the messages your parents conveyed.
- Personal counseling is of value in increasing a helper's self-awareness. Healthy individuals who want to help others can profit from professional assistance, especially in gaining increased insight into personal issues that could intrude in their work.

- Family therapy and personal therapy can illuminate your own areas of transference and countertransference and broaden your vision of how your family-of-origin experiences have served as a template for later interpersonal relationships. Your experience with the therapeutic process can increase your awareness of certain patterns of thinking, feeling, and behaving.

WHAT WILL YOU DO NOW?

1. As a basis for discovering more about your family of origin, interview your parents and any others who knew you well as you were growing up. You can ask each of these people a specific list of questions about yourself. The point of this exercise is for you to gather events or situations that can assist you in getting a fuller picture of your childhood. What does each person remember the most about you? Are you able to detect any themes in what the people you interview recall about you?

2. In an exercise similar to the one above, develop a list of questions to help you understand what it was like for your parents as they were growing up. For example, you might ask your parents what their relationships with their parents were like at ages 6, 14, or 21. The aim of the exercise is not to put them on the spot or to get them to divulge secrets, but to better understand the hopes, goals, concerns, fears, and dreams your parents had as children, adolescents, and young adults. You might talk with your parents about how their early experiences influenced them as parents. Discuss with them any patterns you see between them and yourself.

3. Consider interviewing your grandparents. Again, in thinking about questions you would like them to address, be sensitive to how they might respond to sharing personal facets of their lives. You might simply ask them to share any events or memories that they would feel comfortable disclosing. Rather than simply asking them questions, consider sharing with them significant memories you have of them as you were growing up. What did they teach you? What similar patterns do you see that have been handed down from your grandparents to your parents to you and to your children, if any?

4. Consider making a personal journal that will compile significant information about your family of origin. In putting this journal together, focus on the self-exploration questions raised in this chapter. You might even have short chapters illustrating turning points in your life. In doing this project, it would be useful to include pictures of you and your parents, siblings, grandparents, other relatives, and friends. Include any input from your parents, grandparents, and other relatives that will provide details of your family-of-origin experiences. Look for themes and patterns that will give you a clearer picture of the forces that still influence you today.

5. On the left side of a sheet of paper, write what specific things you'd most want from your supervisor. Imagine that you were to seek out a therapist for per-

sonal and professional growth, and write down on the right side what you'd most want from your therapist. Compare your lists.

6. Much of this chapter provides you with material for reflection about how your family-of-origin experiences influence the person you are today. Spend some time thinking about what you learned about yourself *personally* by reading this chapter. Are there any personal issues that you see as being unresolved and are committed to exploring? If so, in your journal write about this unfinished business. How might your own unresolved personal issues affect your ability to work with individuals who are struggling with concerns pertaining to their family?

7. For the full bibliographic entry for each of the sources listed below, consult the References and Reading List at the back of the book.

The following textbooks provide an overview of the major theories of family therapy: Becvar and Becvar (1996); Carlson, Sperry, and Lewis (1997); Goldenberg and Goldenberg (1996a); Hanna and Brown (1995); Nichols and Schwartz (1995). Goldenberg and Goldenberg (1994) deals with effective interventions for a range of traditional and nontraditional families that helpers will encounter. Satir (1983) elaborates on communication theory as it applies to working with families. One of the best sources of information for doing a lifestyle analysis is Powers and Griffith (1987).

Chapter 11

Understanding Life Transitions

Focus Questions
Aim of the Chapter
Helper, Know Thyself
Developmental Themes and Life Choices
By Way of Review
What Will You Do Now?

FOCUS QUESTIONS

1. From which of your life experiences can you draw as you attempt to understand the diverse range of client problems you will encounter?
2. At this point in your life, how well do you think you know yourself? What can you do to increase your range of self-knowledge?
3. Your current life is largely a result of the earlier choices you have made. What choices have particularly affected the person you are now?
4. As you think about your childhood and adolescent years, how do you see those experiences as continuing to influence your present behavior?

AIM OF THE CHAPTER

Meeting the challenges of life transitions, whether your own or your clients', entails making an assessment of personal assets (strengths) and liabilities (weaknesses). If helpers expect their clients to make an honest self-assessment, they themselves must be committed to this same quest for self-awareness.

In this chapter we include a detailed discussion of major life themes at the stages of human development from infancy through old age. Our hope is that you will reflect on critical turning points in your own life along with significant decisions that you've made at those junctures. This can also be a time to review any personal crises you may now be facing to assess how well you are using both your internal and external resources to meet the challenges of ending one stage of life and moving into the next phase of your development.

Personal transformation demands an awareness of how you dealt with developmental tasks in the past and how you are now addressing these issues. By drawing on your own life experiences, both past and present, you are likely to be in a better position to appreciate the struggles of your clients. To help you explore your personal struggles, we provide many case examples that illustrate problems clients are likely to bring to you. We focus on how awareness of your own life experiences can be a useful instrument when you intervene to help your clients.

HELPER, KNOW THYSELF

In applying to an educational program in the helping professions, you may well have been asked to write a brief autobiography, addressing questions such as: "What are your reasons for pursuing work in this program? What have been some of the most significant turning points in your life? How have you dealt with any crises you might have encountered? What did you learn about yourself from dealing with these crises? In terms of working with clients, what personal experiences can you draw on?" These programs take note of the fact that your life struggles will greatly affect your capacity to deal effectively with clients.

When you decide to come to terms with a crisis in your personal life by reaching out to others, either to a friend or loved one or to a professional, you are doing in your life what you will support in your clients. If you face and deal with your crisis will all the resources within you and around you, you will learn lessons about the value of working through your responses to demanding situations. Remember that the word *crisis* means both peril and opportunity. Your crises not only represent some danger but also present opportunities for a life transformation. It takes courage to work through an upheaval such as marriage or divorce, the birth or death of a child, losing a job, or retiring. All of these turning points test your ability to tolerate uncertainty, to leave what is known and secure, and to begin a new course in life. A transformation to a more mature level of personal growth entails your willingness to suffer and to learn life-giving lessons through that suffering. If you are tethered to personal comfort at all costs, you will miss rich opportunities to become more of the person you were meant to become.

One way we train beginning helpers is to assist them in focusing on their own development as a person. We assume that helpers must first know themselves if they hope to be instrumental in aiding clients to learn about themselves. Another of our assumptions is that helpers cannot take clients any further than they have gone in their own life. As a result, we structure our training sessions for group counselors around personal issues. We ask the trainees to read about certain life themes, to think about their own development and turning points, and to recall key choices they have made. Some of these themes include dealing with childhood, adolescent, and adult struggles; love and intimate relationships; loneliness and solitude; death and loss; sexuality; the choice of a lifestyle; and the meaning in life. These are also some of the main themes clients will bring into counseling sessions. Helpers will be affected by the problems clients discuss in these areas. If helpers themselves have limited awareness of their own struggles with these themes, they are not likely to be very effective. In training workshops the participants can discover what impact their life experiences have on their clients and, in turn, how their clients' life experiences affect them. We ask you to reflect on how the themes we discuss pertain to your life.

DEVELOPMENTAL THEMES AND LIFE CHOICES

We assume that you have had, or will have, a course in human growth and development that spans infancy through old age. This section deals with developmental themes at these various phases of life. Our idea here is not to teach you about the stages of development but to use key concepts of these stages as illustrations of problems you are likely to encounter with clients. Our emphasis is on you and your earlier life experiences and how they are likely to influence the way you work with people who come to you with their problems.

We describe the eight stages of development from infancy to old age by pointing out the psychosocial tasks for each phase. We also briefly describe potential problems in personality development if these tasks are not mastered. With each stage of development we present a case illustration to give you some practice in thinking about how to approach given clients. We also encourage you to recognize how your own development in each of these areas can be either an asset or a liability as you help others. How well have you mastered some of the major psychosocial tasks at each period of your development?

One of the more useful models of the stages of human growth and development is Erik Erikson's (1963, 1982) psychosocial perspective. Erikson describes human development over the entire life span in terms of eight stages, each marked by a particular crisis to be resolved. For Erikson, *crisis* means a turning point in life, a moment of transition characterized by the potential to go either forward or backward in development. These moments point to both dangers and opportunities. From a positive perspective, crises can be viewed as challenges to be met rather than as catastrophic events that simply happen to you. It is also possible to fail to resolve the conflicts and thus regress. To a very large extent, an individual's current life is the result of earlier choices. Life has continuity.

From Erikson's perspective each transition stage represents a psychosocial crisis, or a turning point when individuals are faced with fulfilling their destinies. Each of these developmental stages builds on the psychological outcomes of earlier stages. In Stage 1 infants develop a sense of trust if traumatic events do not halt this process of growth. This basic trust paves the way for children to expand their range of experiences, leading to autonomy in Stage 2. With a trust in self and environment, children are able to take the initiative in Stage 3 that results in widening their social circle and achieving a sense of competence. If these earlier tasks have been successfully accomplished, children are ready to begin meeting the challenges associated with formal schooling in Stage 4. The search for an identity that is characteristic of Stage 5 is made possible by the foundation of trust, autonomy, initiative, and industry that has been formed during childhood. Many of the tasks of Stage 6 involve the young adult's establishing and nurturing intimate relationships, which can be done to the extent that the individual knows who he or she is and feels a sense of self-worth. Stage 7 represents the crisis of middle adulthood, which relates to living a productive life and to showing care and concern for others. How one ends life has a lot to do with how he or she has dealt with the life challenges presented at earlier phases. Stage 8 brings with it the possibility of achieving a sense of integrity if one can look back without getting stuck in regrets. This brief overview demonstrates that each of these developmental stages is influenced by earlier psychosocial tasks.

We have drawn from Hamachek's (1988, 1990) conceptualization of evaluating self-concept and ego development within Erikson's psychosocial framework. Hamachek has identified a list of comparative behavioral characteristics that highlight the differences between individuals who have mastered the psychosocial task at each of Erikson's eight stages of development and those who have not. According to Hamachek, Erikson's psychosocial stages shed light on understanding how the self develops over time, why one's self-concept is more psychologically intact in some areas than in others, and why individuals differ with respect to variables such as ego strength and emotional resiliency. Erikson's model is holistic, for it views humans as biological *and* social *and* psychological beings.

Infancy

Trust versus mistrust. In infancy (the first year of life) the basic task is to develop a sense of trust in self, others, and the environment. The core struggle at this time is between trust and mistrust. If the significant persons in an infant's life provide the needed warmth and attention, the child develops a sense of trust. This sense of being loved is the best safeguard against fear, insecurity, and feelings of inadequacy. Children who receive love from parents or parental substitutes generally have little difficulty accepting themselves.

Some characteristic behaviors of people who have a high sense of basic trust include asking others for emotional help when it is needed, a tendency to focus on the positive aspects of others' behaviors, having a generally optimistic worldview without being naive or unrealistic about it, and preferring a balance between giving and receiving (Hamachek, 1988).

If there is an absence of security in the home, personality problems tend to occur later. Insecure children come to view the world as a potentially hostile place. They have a fear of reaching out to others, a fear of loving and trusting, and an inability to form or maintain intimate relationships. Rejected children learn to mistrust the world and view it largely in terms of its ability to do them harm. Some of the effects of rejection in infancy include tendencies in later childhood to be fearful, insecure, jealous, aggressive, hostile, and isolated.

Case example. Imagine that a child with a history of being abused is brought to you for counseling. As a result of her experiences, she is frightened and distrustful of the world. Some of her experiences stir up your own memories of difficult periods in childhood. Although you were never physically abused, you suffered much psychological cruelty from two alcoholic parents. Your reason for becoming a helper was to make the world a better place. In working with children like this, you become aware that some of your old cynicism and distrust of the world, which you thought you had successfully dealt with, is resurfacing. You find it increasingly difficult to counsel abused children.

This case illustrates how your personal involvement can render you ineffective in working with a child's pain that reminds you of your own pain. This is especially true if you have not resolved your early conflicts between trust and mistrust. However, such early experiences do not necessarily have to be a liability. If you are aware of your vulnerability in trusting and have worked through this negative conditioning to the point that you are now able to trust, your experiences can be an asset. By drawing on your own experiences, you can empathize with abused children and assist them in learning to trust the world.

Reflections and application. As you reflect on the developmental tasks during this stage, think about the foundation you had during your earliest years and how these experiences either prepared you or handicapped you for the tasks you now face in your life. Particularly consider what you learned about trusting the world. Most of the decisions you made in infancy were unconscious and preverbal. Nevertheless, such decisions were powerful shapers of the way you viewed the world later. Consider these questions: "Do you have difficulty trusting others? Are you able to trust yourself and your ability to make it in the world? Do you have fears that others will let you down and that you have to be very careful about how much you show of yourself?"

Early Childhood

Autonomy versus shame and doubt. The most critical task of early childhood (ages 1–3) is to begin the journey toward autonomy by progressing from being taken care of by others to being able to care for one's own needs. Some characteristic behaviors of people who have developed a sense of autonomy include making their own decisions about matters that are important to them, resisting being dominated by people who want to control them, working well by themselves and with others, listening to their own inner voice when deciding on a right and appropriate course of action, and feeling at ease in group situations (Hamachek, 1988).

Children who fail to master the task of establishing some control over themselves and coping with the world around them develop a sense of shame and feelings of doubt about their capabilities. Parents who do too much for children hamper their proper development. If parents insist on keeping them dependent, these children will begin to doubt the value of their own abilities. During this period it is essential that feelings such as hostility, anger, and hatred be accepted rather than judged. If these feelings are not accepted, children may not be able to accept their feelings later on. They will become adults who feel they must deny all of their negative feelings.

Case example. Your supervisor has asked you to co-lead a group of involuntary clients. Much anger is being expressed in the room. You find that you are working very hard to deflect this anger. At one point you tell a client that he doesn't have to get so angry. He responds by shouting "You don't understand me, so why don't you just shut up!" You feel scared and instinctively leave the room.

Reflections and application. If you were the helper in this situation and thought about why it was so hard for you to be the recipient of intense anger, you might come up with several answers. You grew up in a sheltered and protected environment. Since your parents made all of your decisions, you never had to struggle with deciding for yourself. You experienced your parents as very loving and kind. In your family nobody ever got angry. Even when your parents unexpectedly divorced, no one expressed anger or hurt. Basically, you were taught messages such as "Be happy and look at the brighter side of things." "Don't get angry." "We will always be there for you." "If you can't say something nice, don't say anything at all."

Some helpers have trouble recognizing or expressing angry feelings. Thus, they also have trouble allowing their clients to have these "unacceptable" feelings. They might talk their clients out of these feelings. If any of this situation fits you, are you able to see any alternatives besides withdrawing from anger? One way you could behave differently is to remain in the room and deal with the fears that are evoked in you as a client directs his anger toward you. A situation such as this confronts you with some feelings and attitudes that get in the way of your dealing with clients.

Preschool Age

Initiative versus guilt.   During the preschool years (ages 3–6) children seek to find out what they are able to do. They imitate others, they begin to develop a sense of morality, they increase the circle of people who are significant to them, they learn to give and receive love and affection, they learn basic attitudes regarding sexuality, they begin to learn more complex social skills, they take more initiative, and they increase their capacity to use and understand language. According to Erikson, the basic task of the preschool years is to establish a sense of competence and initiative. If children are allowed realistic freedom to choose their own activities and make some of their own decisions, they tend to develop a positive orientation characterized by confidence in their ability to initiate and follow through. Some characteristic behaviors of people who have a sense of initiative include having a high energy level, being a self-starter, being able to complete tasks at hand, having a strong sense of personal adequacy, being able to set goals and to accomplish them, accepting new challenges, and having a sense of ethics without being overly moralistic (Hamachek, 1988).

If children are unduly restricted or not allowed to make decisions for themselves, they develop a sense of guilt and ultimately withdraw from taking an active stance toward life. Parental attitudes toward children are communicated both verbally and nonverbally. Thus, children often develop feelings of guilt based on negative messages from their parents. Strict parental indoctrination tends to lead to rigidity, severe conflicts, remorse, and self-condemnation. Children may pick up subtle messages that their body and their impulses are evil, for example, and thus they soon begin to feel guilty about their natural impulses and feelings. Carried into adult life, these attitudes can prevent them from enjoying sexual intimacy.

During this period the foundations of sex-role identity are laid. Children begin to form a picture of appropriate masculine and feminine behavior. The models that children have are important in determining whether their self-concepts are healthy. Many people seek counseling because of problems they experience in regard to their sexual identity. Some men have a lot of confusion about what feelings and behaviors are appropriate for them. Some men resist doing anything that resembles feminine behavior. Some women have submerged their identity totally in the roles of mother and housewife. At some point they may want to broaden their conception of what is appropriate for them as women. Yet their early conditioning may make the expansion of their self-concept somewhat difficult.

Case example.   You are doing an intake interview with Paula, age 14, who was sent to you by her parents. She has had an abortion, is sexually promiscuous, is regularly abusing drugs, and is failing in school. You gather information about her developmental history, and it appears that many of her problems originated during her preschool years. The parents tell you that she was a model child who never gave them any trouble. They were strict disciplinarians. The children she was allowed to play with were all selected by her parents. Since she was an unusually pretty child, the parents worried about her sexual development. They basically communicated a distrust of boys. During the preschool years, when most children are given some freedom and some room for making decisions, Paula was highly controlled by her parents. She had no room to maneuver. Since no freedoms were granted to her, she never had the opportunity to develop self-responsibility. Her mother went to work when Paula was 12 years old, and she immediately began to take advantage of being on her own several hours a day. It was then that she made friends of whom her parents disapproved. With time she became increasingly rebellious toward the rigid climate in her home. She seemed determined to become everything her parents did not want her to be.

On the basis of the above knowledge about Paula's situation, there are a number of directions in which you might proceed as her counselor. You could become an ally of her parents and take the role of attempting to "straighten her out." You can see that she is heading down a destructive path, and you could attempt to influence her to give up her irresponsible ways of behaving.

From another perspective, you could become Paula's ally. You have empathy for her situation in that you see her oppressive background as largely contributing to her present behavior. You could decide to bring in the family, since you see the problem as being related to the parents' need to control. Do you think you could make sure that everybody in the family was being listened to? Would you be tempted to take sides?

Reflections and application. As you reflect on the case of Paula, how do you think you'd fare as a helper in this situation? What do you think you would do? Might you focus on the parents? on Paula? on both? Are you aware of any of your attitudes that would influence your interventions? How might your own struggles for independence with your parents affect you? If you have children, how might your relationship with them influence the way you'd work with Paula or her parents?

As you read and apply the developmental tasks of this stage to your own life, look for patterns in your present attitudes and behavior that could be traced to your preschool years. Pay special attention to how these preschool patterns operate today in your life, either positively or negatively. Also, note how your life experiences either contribute to or detract from your ability to be helpful to Paula. Consider some of these questions: "Do you have a clear sense of your own sex-role identity? Are you the kind of woman or man you want to be? Where did you acquire your standards of femininity or masculinity? Are you comfortable with your own sexuality? with your body? with giving and receiving in a sexual relationship? Are there any unresolved conflicts from your childhood that affect you today? Do your present behaviors and current conflicts indicate areas of unfinished business?"

Middle Childhood

Industry versus inferiority. For Erikson, the major struggle of middle childhood, or the school years (ages 6–12), is between industry and inferiority. The central task is to achieve a sense of industry; failure to do so results in a sense of inadequacy. Children need to expand their understanding of the world and continue to develop an appropriate sex-role identity. The development of a sense of industry includes focusing on creating goals, such as meeting challenges and finding success in school. Some characteristic behaviors of people who have a sense of industry include enjoyment in learning about new things and ideas, being excited by the idea of being a producer, having a sense of pride in doing at least one thing well, taking criticism well and using it to improve one's performance, and tending to have a strong sense of persistence (Hamachek, 1988).

Children who encounter failure in their early schooling often experience major handicaps later in life. Those children with early learning problems may begin to feel worthless. Such feelings often dramatically affect their relationships with their peers, which are also vital at this time. Problems that can originate during middle childhood include a negative self-concept, feelings of inferiority in establishing and maintaining social relationships, conflicts over values, a confused sex-role identity, dependency, a fear of new challenges, and a lack of initiative.

Case example. José and Maria are a middle-aged couple who come to you for marital counseling. One issue that has caused trouble in their marriage is the fact that José continually changes jobs, and as a result they are always financially strapped. Maria insists that her husband seeks jobs that are far below his capabilities. José basically agrees with Maria. During the interview you learn that he had many academic difficulties in elementary school. His parents were migrant farmers, and as a result he attended many different schools. When he started school, he did not speak English, and he recalls that his teachers were not understanding of him. Most of the time he felt like a failure and an outcast, he hated school, and he decided that he was unintelligent. As the years went on, his feelings of inadequacy progressed. He always reacted with surprise when some of his teachers told him that he was performing below his abilities. Even though he realizes that he is not stupid, he has decided that it is too late to overcome some of these earlier obstacles. Out of his fear of failure and limited self-confidence, he avoids pursuing jobs that are more challenging and that could be potentially more satisfying.

Assume that you are a white, upper-middle-class counselor. You are impatient with José, for you see him blaming the system and making chronic excuses for his failures. You have a hard time understanding why he has not overcome the obstacles that he faced so long ago. If this is your frame of reference, do you think that you would be able to provide him with encouragement to explore his deeper problems, such as self-doubt and inadequacy?

Now consider that you feel for José's situation and understand how his early experiences in grade school are continuing to affect his self-confidence. You could work with him on modifying his self-limiting assumptions and changing some of the decisions he made about himself as an early learner. With José you formulate a plan for change that includes participating in remedial courses in adult education. The crux of your work involves getting him to see that his early failures stemmed from unfortunate circumstances and not from the fact that he was unintelligent.

Reflections and application. If you had a client like José, how might your own life experiences either hinder or enhance your ability to counsel him? What were some of the highlights of the first few years in school for you? In general, did you feel competent or incompetent as a learner? Did you see school as an exciting place to be or as a place that you wanted to avoid? What were some of the specific ways in which you felt that you were successful or that you were a failure? What attitudes did you form about your competence as a person during your early school years? Think of some significant people in your life at this time who affected you either positively or negatively. Attempt to recall some of their expectations for you, and remember the messages they gave you about your worth and potential. What connections do you see, if any, between the assumptions you made then and the assumptions that influence your life today?

Adolescence

Identity versus identity confusion. Adolescence (ages 12–18) is the time for testing limits, and there is a strong urge to break away from dependent ties that appear to be restricting freedom. Although many adolescents feel frightened and lonely, they often mask their fears with rebellion and cover up their need to be dependent by exaggerating their degree of independence. Much of adolescents' rebellion grows out of the context of wanting to determine the course of their own lives. Adolescence is a critical time for integrating the various dimensions of one's identity. For Erikson, the major developmental conflicts of adolescents center on the clarification of who they are, where they are going, and how they are getting there. The struggle involves integrating physical and social changes. Adolescents may feel pressured to make career choices early, to compete in the job market or in college, to become financially independent, and to commit themselves to physically and emotionally intimate relationships. Peer-group pressure is a major force, and it is easy to lose one's self by conforming to the expectations of friends. With the increasing stress experienced by many adolescents, suicidal ideation is not uncommon.

During the adolescent period a major part of the identity-formation process consists of separation from the family system and establishment of an identity based on one's own experiences. The process of separating from parents can be an agonizing part of the struggle toward individuation. Although adolescents may adopt many of their parents' values, to genuinely individuate they must choose these values freely as opposed to blindly accepting them.

Some characteristic behaviors of people who have a sense of identity include having a stable self-concept that does not easily change, being able to combine short-term goals with long-range plans, resisting peer pressure, having a reasonably high level of self-acceptance, believing that they are responsible for what happens to them, feeling physically and emotionally close to another person without fearing the loss of self, and being able to make decisions without undue vacillation (Hamachek, 1988).

Case example. Adam is referred to you by the school counselor. When you ask him what brings him to your office, he first tells you abruptly that his counselor has made him come to see you. After overcoming his initial resistance, he eventually tells you this about his problems:

"I used to be a good student, but about a year ago I lost interest in school because I felt the pressure of having to get A's in all my classes. I want to go to college, but I'm afraid I won't make it because I've been failing some of my classes. My parents are very disappointed in me. We used to have a great relationship, but now I don't even want to talk to them. I'd much rather stay in bed than get up and go to school. My friends tell me I've become a bore to be around, and I don't want to be around them either. What really hurt me was when my girlfriend broke up with me. When I'm not at school, I spend most of my time alone in my room listening to music. I don't know anymore what I want to do. There's nothing I look forward to, and sometimes I wish I could go to sleep and never wake up."

Reflections and application. If you were Adam's counselor, how able would you be to hear his hopelessness, his feelings of desperation, and his possible suicidal intentions? Would you want to cheer him up and tell him that he is just going through a phase and that things are bound to get better? Would you get lost in his feelings of hopelessness by remembering some of your own unhappy adolescent years? If someone you know well has committed suicide, how might that affect your ability to work objectively with Adam? Did you ever feel a sense of hopelessness and a belief that your future would never be any better? Feelings of hopelessness and suicidal thoughts are among the most difficult issues that you will have to explore with your clients. It will probably be most difficult to remain objective and not get lost in the client's hopelessness. You may feel afraid when your clients express the depths of their despair and their desire to end it all. At these times you will feel much pressure and responsibility in wondering what to do to be helpful. At some point in your life you may have lost a sense of meaning and not seen much hope for change or reason to continue living. How you recognized and dealt with these feelings will greatly influence the way you intervene with clients who see little hope.

Take a few moments to review some of your adolescent experiences. How did you feel about yourself during this time? In reviewing these years, how might your experiences work for or against you in dealing with Adam? Think about your degree of independence from your parents during your adolescence. Focus on what gave meaning to your life. Also ask yourself questions such as: "At this time in my life, did I have a clear sense of who I was and where I was going? Were my values my own, or did I merely unquestionably accept the values of my parents? What major choices did I struggle with during my adolescent years?" As you review this period, focus on how your adolescent experiences affected the person you are today.

Early Adulthood

Intimacy versus isolation. According to Erikson, we enter young adulthood (ages 18–35) after we master the adolescent conflicts over identity. Our sense of identity is tested anew in adulthood, however, by the challenge of intimacy versus isolation. The ability to form intimate relationships depends largely on having a clear sense of self. One cannot give to another if one has a weak ego or an unclear sense of identity. Intimacy involves sharing, giving ourselves, relating to another based on our strength, and a desire to grow with that person. If we think very little of ourselves, the chances are not good that we will be able to give meaningfully to others. The failure to achieve intimacy often results in feelings of isolation from others and a sense of alienation. Erikson's concept of intimacy can be applied in any kind of close relationship between two adults. Relationships involving emotional commitments may be between close friends of the same or the opposite sex, and they may or may not have a sexual dimension.

Some characteristic behaviors of people who have a sense of intimacy include the ability to establish a firm sense of their own identity, tolerance and acceptance of differences in other people, trusting others and themselves in the relationships they form, establishing close emotional bonds without fearing the loss of their own identity, and being able to commit themselves to relationships that demand cooperation, sacrifice, and compromise (Hamachek, 1990).

During their 20s, young people are challenged to make many critical choices. They wrestle with the choice of clinging to security or leaving those things that bring a secure existence. They struggle with the costs and benefits of developing relationships with a few people. Career choice becomes an important part of this time of life. Whether to marry and to become a parent is another issue. Young people are creating dreams and wondering about how they can translate their dreams into real life. Because of the many areas of choice pertaining to work, education, marriage, family life, and lifestyle, it is not uncommon for them to wonder what it is they really want. At this time of life, some allow others to decide for them what their standards and choices will be.

The struggle toward autonomy. During early adulthood the central task is to assume increased responsibility and independence. Although most of us have moved away from our parents physically, not all of us have done so psychologically. To a greater or lesser degree, our parents will have a continuing influence on our lives. Cultural factors play a significant role in determining the degree to which our parents influence our lives. For example, in some cultures developing a spirit of independence is not given priority. Instead, these cultures place a prime value on cooperation with others and on a spirit of interdependence. In some cultures, parents continue to have a significant impact and influence on their children even after they reach adulthood. Respect and honor for parents may be values that are extolled above individual freedom by the adult children.

The struggle toward autonomy entails choosing for yourself and working for your own approval rather than living your life for the approval of your parents or others. Making decisions about the quality of life you want for yourself and affirming these choices are partly what autonomy is about. Autonomy also entails your willingness to accept responsibility for the consequences of your choices rather than looking for others to blame if you are not satisfied with the way your life is going. Furthermore, separating from your family and finding your own identity is not something you do at a given time once and for all. The struggle toward autonomy begins in early childhood and continues throughout life.

Transition from the 20s to the 30s. The transition from the late 20s to the early 30s is a time of changing values and beliefs. Inner turmoil increases for many during this period. However, many others choose to delay making a commitment about relationships and careers. It used to be quite common for young people in their late 20s and early 30s to have a family and to be firmly established in a career. Now, taking on these responsibilities is often delayed, and it is not uncommon for couples to begin having children in their later 30s.

During this transition people often take another look at their earlier dreams. They may reevaluate their life plans and make significant shifts. Some become aware that their dreams have not materialized, and they wonder what kind of future they want for themselves and others in their lives. Although this recognition often brings anxiety, it can spur the necessity of making new plans and working hard to attain them.

Case example.   Becky, 23, comes to you for counseling on the urging of a concerned friend. She tells you that she has been in a relationship with a young man for more than five years, yet she has never really been satisfied with it. Although she has tried to break off with him a number of times, she typically resumes seeing him when he begins to "treat her so nice" and when she begins feeling guilty. If she were to give him up for good, she fears she would have no man in her life. She concludes that having him is better than having nobody. In most aspects of her life Becky has allowed her parents to make her choices for her. Under parental pressure she pursued a teaching major and is currently in student teaching. She discovered that she really is not interested in teaching, yet she doesn't trust herself to follow her own interests. Becky has a great deal of talent in dancing, and she wanted to become a professional dancer. She abandoned this idea because she could tell that her parents did not support this choice. She is aware that she has been both financially and emotionally dependent on her parents. Although she would like to choose for herself, she stops herself from doing so out of her fear of making poor decisions. Many of her high school and college friends have gotten married, and she picks up signals from her family to find a "nice boy" to marry. At this time in her life she feels a great deal of pressure within herself to please her parents, yet she realizes that she cannot please both them and herself.

Reflections and application.   Put yourself in the position of being Becky's counselor. Imagine that although you are her age, you have had a very different kind of life from hers. You had few problems establishing goals and following them. You knew what you wanted to do, and you pretty much did it. With a minimum of help from your parents you attained most of your goals. If this were the case, do you think you'd be able to empathize with her? Would you be able to identify with any of her struggles and thus help her find a way to move ahead?

If you are a middle-aged or older person, what decisions did you make in early adulthood, and how do you think those decisions would influence the way you work with Becky? Do you have any regrets about the choices you made? If you are unhappy about some of these choices, might you be inclined to be another person who would influence her to move in a particular direction?

Think especially about what you want in close relationships. What do you expect of others in intimate relationships? What do you think you can contribute to these relationships to enhance them? From a career point of view, what have you most looked for in your work? How do you think your own struggles or lack of them would affect you in working with clients like Becky who have problems deciding for themselves what they want to do personally and vocationally?

Middle Adulthood

Generativity versus stagnation. Middle adulthood (ages 35–60) is a period when people reach the top of the mountain and become aware that they must begin the downhill journey. They might painfully experience the discrepancy between the dreams of their younger years and the harsh reality of what they have actually accomplished with their life so far. According to Erikson, the stimulus for continued growth during middle age is the core struggle between generativity and stagnation. Generativity includes more than fostering children. It includes being creative in one's career, finding meaningful leisure activities, and establishing significant relationships in which there is giving and receiving. During this time people become more aware of the reality of death, and they may reflect more on whether they are living well. It is a time for reevaluation and a time when people are at the crossroads of life. They may begin to question what else is left, and they may establish new priorities or renew their commitments.

Some characteristic behaviors of people who have a sense of generativity include being personally concerned about others, tending to focus more on what they can give to others than on what they can get, becoming absorbed in a variety of activities outside of themselves, leading productive lives and contributing to the betterment of society, manifesting other-centered values and attitudes, and expressing themselves creatively (Hamachek, 1990).

During middle age there is sometimes a period of depression. When people begin to see that some of their visions have not materialized, they may give up hope for a better future. Some women who married and made a family their main priority may begin to wonder if this is all there is to life. At this time many women will choose to return to college or to work full time or to combine the triple roles of homemaker, student, and worker. Some men begin to wonder if they want to stay in their career. They may have to cope with depression when they realize that they have not reached some of their important dreams.

As is true with any stage, there are both dangers and opportunities during this time. Some of the dangers include slipping into secure but deadening ruts and failing to take advantage of opportunities for enriching life. Many individuals experience a midlife crisis, when their whole world seems to be unstable. A few of the events that lead to such a crisis include the realization that youthful dreams will not come about; an illness or the onset of the aging process; the death of one's parents; the realization of one's ultimate aloneness in this life; the realization that life is not always fair and just; a marital crisis or the break-up of a long-established relationship; children leaving the nest; or losing one's job. A problem of this period is the failure to achieve a sense of productivity, which then leads to feelings of stagnation. What is important is that individuals realize the choices they have in their life and see the changes they can make rather than giving in to the feeling that they are victims of life's circumstances.

The 30s and the 40s. Sheehy (1995) identifies different decades of adulthood as the turbulent 30s, flourishing 40s, flaming 50s, and serene 60s. She refers to middle life as "the most unrevealed portion of adult life from the mid-forties to mid-sixties." Sheehy's first adulthood period is from 30 to 45, and the second adulthood period is from 45 to 85 and beyond. Second adulthood, which encompasses the broad span including both middle adulthood and late adulthood, includes what she refers to as the "Age of Mastery" (45 to 65) and the "Age of Integrity" (65 to 85+).

Sheehy compares life to a three-act play:

> It's as though when we are young, we have seen only the first act of the play. By our forties we have reached the climactic second-act curtain. Only as we approach fifty does the shape and meaning of the whole play become clear. We move into the third act with the intention of a resolution and tremendous curiosity about how it will all come out. (1995, p. 150)

Sheehy (1976) used to consider the mid-30s as the halfway mark and the prime of life. She referred to the period between 35 and 45 as the "Decline Decade," as if people had only until their mid-40s to resolve the crisis of midlife. Sheehy (1995) claims that it is a mistake to view the early 40s as a time when people drop off the edge of a cliff. Although many people believed that when they reached 40 their time was running out, more and more people are finding ways to avoid the restrictive identity that used to define middle age. In Sheehy's recent research involving life-history interviews with people in middle life, she found a new theme of rebirths permeating their stories. She writes:

> More and more people were beginning to see there was the possibility of a new life to live, one in which we could concentrate on becoming better, stronger, deeper, wiser, funnier, freer, sexier, and more attentive to living the privileged moments, even as we were getting older, lumpier, slower, and closer to the end. (p. xiii)

Indeed, we are retaining some of our youth for a longer period of time. The second half of life enlarges the boundaries of vital living, and it offers new opportunities for growth and change.

According to Carl Jung, we are confronted with major changes and possibilities for transformation as we begin the second half of life between 35 and 40. Jung's therapy clients consistently revealed signs of experiencing a pivotal middle-age life crisis. Although they may have achieved worldly success, they typically were challenged with finding satisfaction in projects that had lost meaning. Many of his clients struggled to overcome feelings of emptiness and flatness of life.

Jung believed that major life transformations are an inevitable and universal part of the human condition at this juncture in life. He maintained that when the zest for living sags, this can be a catalyst for necessary and beneficial changes. To undergo such a transformation requires the death of some aspect of our psychological being so new growth can occur that will open us to far deeper and richer ranges of existence. To strive for what Jung called *individuation*—a condition of integration of the unconscious with the conscious and of psychological balance—people during their middle years must be willing to let go of preconceived notions and patterns that dominated the first part of their lives. Their task now is to be open to the unconscious forces that have been influencing them all of their lives and to deepen the meaning of their lives.

For Jung, people can bring unconscious material into awareness by paying attention to their dreams and fantasies and by expressing themselves through such avenues as poetry, writing, music, and art. Individuals need to recognize that the rational thought patterns that drove them during the first half of life represent merely one way of being. At this time in life, they must be willing to be guided by the spontaneous flow of the unconscious if they hope to achieve an integration of all facets of their being, which is part of psychological health (Schultz & Schultz, 1994).

The 50s.   In the 50s people often begin the process of preparing for older age. Many are at their peak in terms of status and personal power. This can be a satisfying time of life, because now they do not have to work as hard as they did in the past, nor do they have to meet others' expectations. They can enjoy the benefits of long struggle and dedication rather than striving to continually prove themselves. It is likely that childrearing and work are moving toward a culmination. Adults at this stage often do a lot of reflecting, contemplating, refocusing, and evaluating of themselves so they can continue to discover new directions. Sheehy (1995) captures this period as a time of new opportunity:

> Millions of people entering their forties and fifties today are able to make dramatic changes in their lives and habits, to look forward to living decades more in smoothly functioning bodies with agile minds—so long as they remain open to new vistas of learning and imagination and anticipate experiences yet to be conquered and savored. (p. xvii)

Sheehy (1995) suggests that we look at the positive and creative dimensions of middle life, including the sources of love, meaning, fun, spiritual companionship, sexuality, and sustained well-being. Sheehy reports that this is an exciting time for women:

> As family obligations fade away, many become motivated to stretch their independence, learn new skills, return to school, plunge into new careers, rediscover the creativity and adventurousness of their youths, and, at last, listen to their own needs. (p. 140)

Although many women may experience this as an exciting time, they are often challenged to cope with both the physical and psychological adjustments surrounding menopause. Some women, fearing that menopause means losing their youthful looks, sink into depression. For many, menopause represents a crisis. In *The Silent Passage*, Sheehy (1992) tells us that, far from being a marker that signifies the beginning of the end, menopause is better seen as a gateway to a second adulthood. Sheehy's book breaks the silence of menopause that is caused by shame, fear, misinformation, and the stigma of aging in a youth-obsessed society.

For men, the 50s can be a time for the potential awakening of their creative side. Instead of being consumed with achievement strivings, many men are opening up human facets of themselves beyond their rational thinking that can result in a richer existence. But men, too, are challenged to find new meaning in their lives. Projects that once were highly satisfying may now lack luster. Some men become depressed when they realize that they have been pursuing empty dreams. They may have met goals they set for themselves, only to find that they are still longing for a different kind of life. For both women and men in their 50s, examining their priorities can often lead to new decisions about how they want to spend their time.

Case example.   Ernie, age 44, has been referred to you by his minister. Ernie, who has been married for 24 years, has done everything with his wife. They have never spent a night apart. He did not make any close friends, either male or female, because his wife is very jealous and is threatened by any attempts to do so. He has totally surrendered to his wife's exaggerated fear of his having an affair. Ernie says that until recently there were no grounds for her fears. Although he had not questioned his marriage and life before, he finds himself growing more and more disenchanted with the boredom and predictability of his life. He feels caught in a rut, yet he hesitates to get out. Although he has a good job, it, too, has lost its appeal. He feels a lack of excitement in his work in much the same way that he feels a dullness about his marriage. He hates to go to work, and he hates to come home. He complains about a lack of sleep, waking up in the middle of the night and ruminating about his life situation.

A few months ago he found that he enjoyed talking to one of the women at work. She listened to him, and they shared some common concerns. They developed a friendship, which he carefully kept a secret from his wife. Eventually Ernie and his friend became involved in a sexual relationship. Although he finds his time with her exciting and very much values her as a friend, he cannot imagine himself leaving his wife to live with her. She is also married, and she has several small children. He says that he still loves his wife, yet he is not ready to quit seeing the other woman. Although he feels caught in deadening ruts at home and at work, he is not ready to quit his job or seek a divorce. He is in much turmoil, for, as he puts it, he is going against his own values. He comes to you because he is in a great deal of pain and does not know what to do next.

Reflections and application.   If you were counseling Ernie, what life experiences of yours do you think might help you in understanding him? If he were to ask you what he should do, how might you answer him? Assume that you have been hurt by an affair, and consider your capacity for remaining objective as you work with Ernie. He wants someone to tell him what to do. Would you be willing to provide him with answers? Which of the following themes in his life would you tend to focus on: his affair? his marriage? his dissatisfaction with his job? the meaninglessness in his life?

If you have reached middle adulthood, what struggles and decisions could you draw on as a resource? If you have not yet reached middle age, what would you most want to be able to say that you have accomplished in your life by this time? What would you hope to have in your relationships? What would you want from your work? How might you go about keeping yourself alive and avoiding predictable ruts?

Late Adulthood

Integrity versus despair. During this period of life (about age 60 and beyond), Erikson sees the central struggle as one of integrity versus despair. People who succeed in achieving ego integrity are able to accept that they have been productive and that they have coped with whatever failures they faced. Such people are able to accept the course of their lives, and they do not endlessly ruminate on all that they could have done, might have done, and should have done.

Some characteristic behaviors of people who have a sense of integrity include believing that who they are and what they have become are largely the consequences of their own choices; accepting death as an inevitable part of the life cycle; looking back on their lives without regret but with a sense of pleasure and feeling of accomplishment and appreciation; being reasonably happy and satisfied with their lives; approaching the final stage of their lives with a sense of personal wholeness; and integrating their past experiences with current realities (Hamachek, 1990).

In contrast, some elderly people fail to achieve ego integration. These people fear death. They develop a sense of hopelessness and feelings of self-disgust. They are able to see all that they have not done, and they often yearn for another chance to live in a different way. These people may feel that they have let valuable time slide by.

The 60s have changed just as dramatically as the earlier stages of middle life. The vast majority of over-60s are quite able, both physically and mentally, to function independently. Most people in their 60s have reached a stage where maximum freedom still coexists with a minimum of physical limitations. Indeed, only 10% of Americans 65 and over have a chronic health problem that interferes with their daily living (Sheehy, 1995, pp. 350–352).

As is the case for each of these developmental stages, there is a great deal of individual variance. Many 70-year-old people have the energy that many middle-aged people have. How people look and feel during late adulthood is more than a matter of physical age; it is largely a matter of attitude. To a great degree, vitality is influenced by state of mind more than by mere chronological years lived.

Case example. Cedric was picked up by the police after he was found wandering around, lost and disoriented. He was brought to the geriatrics ward where you work as an intern. You notice that he is unkempt and is talking incoherently. After some time on the ward he improves to the point of being able to join a therapy group. In this group he recalls many sad times in his life. He talks about his regrets. About two years ago he lost his wife, who died after a long illness. He feels lost without her, and he says that most of his will to live vanished after she died. Her medical bills ate up his savings. Because the company he worked for went bankrupt, he is left with few benefits for his old age. He has five children and 15 grandchildren, but he has no contact with any of them because they are spread around the country. One of his major regrets is that he never really established meaningful ties with his children or grandchildren, and now he feels that it is too late. At age 74 he just does not see much sense in going on with his life.

He never took the time to develop hobbies or friends. He finds life at this time to be boring and meaningless.

What clues does Cedric provide that would call for an assessment of suicidal thoughts and intentions? What questions would you ask him to determine how serious he was about suicide? If you decided that he was suicidal, what course of action might you take? What help do you think you would offer him? Would you agree that his state was hopeless and that there was little he could do to change his life at this late stage? Or would you see hope for him? What alternatives might you pose to him about ways of finding meaning in his life?

How do you think you would be affected by working with people such as Cedric? If you experienced countertransference in working with this client, what steps would you take to work through your own reactions?

Reflections and application.   If you haven't reached old age, imagine yourself at that time of life. Think about what you would like to be able to say about your life. Focus especially on your fears of aging and also on what you hope you could accomplish by this time. What kind of old age do you expect? What are you doing now that might have an effect on the kind of person you will be as you grow older? What things would you like to do during your later years? Can you think of any regrets you will be likely to express? As you anticipate growing older, think about what you can do today to increase the chances that you will be able to achieve a sense of integrity as an older person. Are you cultivating interests and relationships that can become a source of satisfaction in later years? If you find yourself postponing many things that you would like to do now, ask yourself why. Assess the degree to which you are satisfied with the person you are becoming today. If you let valuable time slip by and do not act on opportunities, the chances are greater that you will experience despair during your later years. Finally, assess your present ability to work with elderly clients. If you yourself have not reached this age, what experiences could you draw on as a way of understanding the world of an elderly client? Even though you might not have had some of the same experiences, do you see how you can relate to some of their feelings that are very much like your own?

By Way of Review

- How you cope with crises in your own life is a good indication of your ability to help your clients work through theirs. If you face and deal with your problems with all the resources available to you, you can be present for clients who are in crisis.
- Each of the eight stages of life represents a turning point when individuals are challenged with the fulfillment of their destinies. Both helpers and clients need to realize that personal transformation entails the willingness to tolerate pain and uncertainty. Growth is not generally a smooth process but involves some degree of turmoil.
- At each stage of life there are choices to be made. Your earlier choices have an impact on the kind of person you are now.

- Specific tasks and specific crises can occur from infancy through old age. Review your own developmental history so that you have a perspective in working with the developmental struggles of your clients. You will be in a better position to understand your clients' problems and to work with them if you have an understanding of your own vulnerabilities.

WHAT WILL YOU DO NOW?

1. Write down a list of resources for personal growth and ways of increasing your self-awareness. Think of some avenues that would promote self-exploration on your part. Are you inclined to do something that will encourage you to reflect on the quality of your life?

2. Review the highlights of the section on developmental themes and life choices. Remember a time in your life that was either the most difficult (painful) or the most exciting (joyful). What did you learn from these experiences? If this time occurred during childhood, talk with someone who knew you well as a child about what he or she remembers of you. What are the implications of these experiences in your own life for you as a helper? How might some of your life experiences affect you as you work with others who are like you? different from you?

3. Reflect on some of your life experiences that you think will facilitate your work with clients. In your journal write about a few key turning points in your life. Can you think of one or two times when you were faced with making a major decision? If so, how might this turning point still have an influence on your life? What lessons did you learn from making this decision, and how might this experience better enable you to identify with the struggles of clients?

4. For the full bibliographic entry for each of the sources listed below, consult the References and Reading List at the back of the book.

See Erikson (1963) for a description of the psychosocial theory of development with a focus on the critical tasks of each of the eight stages of development. For an updated description of developmental themes of the stages of adulthood, see Sheehy (1995). For themes and choices dealing with childhood, adolescence, and adulthood, refer to G. Corey and M. Corey (1997).

Chapter 12

STRESS AND BURNOUT

Focus Questions

1. The assumption is often made that helpers are not good at asking for help for themselves. To what degree are you willing to seek help from others when you are experiencing difficulties?
2. What major stresses do you experience, both at home and at work? How well do you cope with them?
3. Are you concerned about burnout for yourself? If you have experienced burnout as a student, what have you done?
4. What key stresses do you expect to encounter in your work as a helper? How well prepared do you feel you are to deal with such stresses?
5. Becoming a helper is bound to open you up to some of your own unresolved conflicts and personal vulnerabilities. What are some examples of unfinished business in your personal life that you think could present difficulties for you in working with clients with a range of problems?

Aim of the Chapter

If you choose one of the helping professions, you will have to contend with hazards throughout your career. As you well know, the demands on you as a student often create stress. In addition, a fieldwork placement or a class that involves an emotional focus is likely to bring out your anxieties. Such stress, of course, is not necessarily negative. This painful awareness, which is a normal process, can be a vehicle for growth and self-understanding.

When you leave your program and get involved in practicing full time, new stresses will stem from the nature of your work and from the professional role expectations for caregivers. Unfortunately, practitioners in a training program are typically not warned about the hazards of the profession.

Most helpers begin their career with little or no information about what they will really experience when they enter the field. Nor are professionals generally prepared to assume the variety of difficult roles they will be expected to play. As a result, they find that they must cope with high levels of stress and failure. They feel great pressure to perform well. Frequently, the lives and welfare of human beings depend on the decisions and recommendations they make. All of this work-related stress can result in serious psychological, physical, and behavioral disorders.

Typically, helpers are not good at asking for help. Many of them have been socialized to think of others, and they have difficulty accepting their own needs. Thus, they often give to the point of depletion. This resistance to recognizing the need for help is put cogently by Kilburg (1986):

Professionals can be their own worst enemies. Trained to be independent, creative, assertive, and hard driving, they do not readily acknowledge that they are in trouble or need assistance. More often, their combination of socialization and personality characteristics leads them to struggle on with a problem long after many other people would have at least sought consultation from family members or friends. Solitary battles are the most destructive for anyone because of the ease with which one loses perspective. (p. 25)

If you are considering a career as a counselor, you may be looking forward to helping people find a resolution to the problems they face and deal constructively with pain in their lives. You are likely to be thinking about the expected satisfaction that comes with knowing that you can be an agent of change for your clients. Yet you may not be fully aware that the commitment to being a therapeutic agent for others is fraught with difficulties. As you saw in Chapters 4, 10, and 11, the process of working with clients may open you up to some of your own deepest personal struggles and unfinished business. It also seems impossible to us that you can work intensely with clients week after week and not be affected by their pain. When old pain surfaces and present struggles become overwhelming, it is essential that you seek help for yourself. There is a steep price for numbing yourself to this pain, and you need to recognize that the nature of your work makes it difficult to hide from yourself.

In this chapter we explore how stress can affect you as a helper and how prolonged stresses can lead to burnout. In the next chapter we look at ways to cope with stress, prevent burnout, and retain your vitality.

SOURCES OF STRESS FOR HELPERS

The sources of work-related stress for helping professionals fall into two categories: individual and environmental. To understand the dynamics of the stress you will experience as a human-services professional, you must understand both the external realities that tend to produce stress and the individual contribution that you make to stress by your perception and interpretation of reality.

Individual stressors can be discovered by examining your attitudes and personal characteristics as a helper. Kottler (1993) provides this list of self-induced stressors:

- Feelings of perfectionism
- Ruminating about cases
- Need for approval
- Self-doubt
- Physical exhaustion
- Unhealthy lifestyle
- Emotional exhaustion
- Assuming too much responsibility for clients

Think about client behaviors that would represent the most stress to you. Look over the following checklist of client behaviors, and rate them according to this scale: 1 = this would be *highly stressful* to me; 2 = this would be *moderately stressful* to me; 3 = this would be *mildly stressful* to me; and 4 = this would *not be a source of stress* to me.

_____ 1. I am seeing a client who seems unmotivated and is coming to the sessions only because he was ordered to attend.

_____ 2. One of my clients wants to terminate counseling, but I don't think she is ready for termination.

_____ 3. A client is very depressed, sees very little hope that life will get better, and keeps asking me for help.

_____ 4. One of my clients makes suicidal threats, and I have every reason to take his threats seriously.

_____ 5. One particular client is angry with me for not doing enough to help her situation.

_____ 6. With this client I feel a great sense of identification, almost to the point of overidentifying with him.

_____ 7. A client tells me that he (she) is sexually attracted to me, and I am not sexually attracted to him (her).

_____ 8. A client tells me that she (he) is sexually attracted to me, and I am sexually attracted to her (him).

_____ 9. My client is very demanding and wants to call me at home for advice on how to deal with every new problem that arises.

_____ 10. This client almost never expresses any appreciation to me, but she often lets me know that I am not doing enough for her and don't seem to care enough about her.

After you've made your ratings, assess the patterns that emerge. What specific behaviors seem to be the most stressful for you? How does stress affect your self-esteem, both on a personal and a professional level?

In addition to these personal, or internal, sources of stress, external factors can also create stress in helpers. *Environmental* sources of stress include the physical aspects of the work setting or the structure of the position itself. A major stressor is the reality of having too much to do in too little time. Other environmental stresses are organizational politics, restrictions imposed by insurance companies, an abundance of paperwork, and cutbacks in programs. Since managed care programs have come into existence, helpers experience the stress of addressing critical needs of individual clients and families within a few sessions. Yet six or fewer sessions may be far from adequate to effectively help certain clients who require more extensive care. Helpers oftentimes feel personally responsible to provide the level of care that is necessary, but they must work within highly restrictive parameters. Attempting to accomplish the impossible in an unrealistically short time can certainly be highly stressful.

Another potential environmental stressor is the quality of your working relationships with colleagues. Dealing with co-workers and supervisors can be a source either of support or of stress. Some events can be extremely stressful, such as legal actions, financial pressures, major life transitions, threats of layoffs, and change of job responsibilities. Certain client behaviors, such as suicidal threats or attempts and severe depression, are highly stressful. Other client-induced stresses include anger toward the helper, aggression and hostility, apathy or lack of motivation, a client's premature termination, and lack of client cooperation.

Stress Associated with Working in Organizations

Because you may well work for some kind of organization, it is useful to reflect on the major sources of frustration, dissatisfaction, and tension that are likely to be part of this work. A rehabilitation counselor who worked with veterans told us of the stress he experienced as a result of the demands placed on him by his agency to see more clients in a shorter amount of time. He felt pressured to "close a case quickly and efficiently," yet his clients often wanted more from him than he was giving. In fact, he reported that many of his clients saw him as uncaring in that he did not give them enough time. What he did not tell them was that he would have liked to spend more time with them. Instead, he took on full responsibility for how his clients were reacting, with the result that he typically felt unappreciated by both his staff and his clients. Had he said more to his clients about what he was thinking and feeling, they would have had a basis to perceive him differently.

During your initial years of employment as a professional helper in an organization, it is common to experience a high level of stress and anxiety. Many helpers report that they were frustrated and disappointed about their job's unexpected stressors and demands.

We asked former students who had entered the helping professions to identify some of the main frustrations and stresses they were facing. Most of them identified the slowness of the system, the resistance of administrators and fellow staff members to new ideas, and unrealistic expectations and demands. One woman in her mid-20s commented:

"I get frustrated with the slow process of the system. New ideas are often overlooked. My age is a source of frustration when working with other people who will not take me seriously. Because of my age, I sometimes have difficulty gaining credibility. My biggest source of dissatisfaction, however, is watching a child that I have worked with and have seen improve go back into the system (or family) and regress to where they started."

A young social worker observed: "My greatest frustration is with the administration and its lack of support, common purpose, or teamwork."

A woman who was managing a volunteer staff of student interns reported: "I am most frustrated when the staff is resistant to new ideas. Dealing with governmental bureaucracy is another major source of stress. They make it very difficult to get things done."

A social worker who was a consultant to senior managers of a bank said that she became frustrated with executives who wanted her to "fix" their employees but were not willing to see their part in the employees' problems.

Agencies often make demands that are unrealistic, especially an insistence that problems be solved quickly. For those who work with clients sent by the courts or those on probation, for instance, the helper is under pressure to see that behavioral changes take place in a specified time, so that more people can be seen, which means more funding.

Organizations tend to make too many demands on workers—by reducing their autonomy, by providing little positive feedback for their job performance, and by setting policies that they feel compelled to resist. Poor management and inadequate supervision are other factors that increase workers' stress.

Case example.   Agencies can easily be run in dehumanizing ways, and the battle to retain your integrity is often fierce. The following interview with a social worker in a community agency in a large city gives some flavor of how endless demands can wear down one's stamina and lead to feelings of futility:

"Seeing clients is my primary interest. I must make progress notes after each client. These notes include descriptions of treatment methods, proof of measurable results, and assessment. The agency expects me to write notes after each session. We are further expected to write specifically and behaviorally. There is a press for constant justification for seeing a client. On one hand, if your client improves, there is pressure from the agency to terminate work with the client. On the other hand, if the client regresses, then treatment is typically judged as ineffective. Thus, there is the hassle with the paperwork game. What some of us write may not be what we are actually doing. In the back of my mind there is the constant stress of unfinished paperwork. The expectation of the agency is that of short-term treatment. I have to deal with edicts from above, which I often find frustrating.

"There is also the need for professional consultation. The expectation is that an interview can be completed in an hour, yet this often takes one and a half hours. I attend staff meetings, where we talk about policies. I have to deal with staff issues about clients and case conferencing at these meetings. On top of this there are many unexpected tasks that endlessly come up. There are phone calls, checking up on clients, contacts, and networking. I have to contact parents, teachers, and school counselors in cases involving children. Quality work takes time. There is so much indirect time that does not get recognized by the agency. I spend some time in peer review and in supervising case presentations. Supervising interns is part of my job, which takes much time. I am ultimately responsible for all of the clients my interns are seeing. The push is toward direct service and for seeing many clients. The more clients seen, the more money for the agency.

"Part of my work involves community outreach. I must make referrals and then check up on these referrals. This involves talking with personnel at the probation department and at schools. Although much of my time is taken up by many of these indirect services, we don't get credit for these activities. For every client seen, there is much extra work. Listening to tapes of client sessions and to interns' tapes takes time. At times, there are unexpected meetings with the auditors.

"Because of the pressure of these unanticipated audits, we must keep current with our paperwork, which is not always realistic or possible. At times I feel overwhelmed by petty policies and procedures. Once I made a mistake on a date on a written report, and I was told that this represented a 5% level of inefficiency. This resulted in being monitored by my supervisor for a month.

"There are ethical issues in submitting to the demands of a system or transgressing the demands of the system. Many of us are guilty of creative lying and stretching the truth. This involves writing reports in ways that we know they will be accepted. Working in an agency involves knowing when and how to report clients. Yet reporting always means more work. Because of the extra work and time involved in the process of making reports and following up, some workers tend to avoid reporting in certain cases where they should do so."

After reading this account, consider how you can creatively and successfully cope with the demands that agencies will make on you. How can you do what you believe in and at the same time deal with the multiple demands of your job? What are your reactions to this social worker's personal account?

The Impact of Work on Your Personal Life

The sources of stress we have discussed seem to hinder helpers' ability to form spontaneous and comfortable relationships with friends and seem to decrease their emotional involvement in their own family. The stress associated with intense personal contact with clients apparently results in therapists' wanting to pull back from family and friends (Guy, 1987).

In talking with mental-health providers, we find that many of them are not able to separate themselves from their work. They find it difficult to make a clear distinction between their personal life and their professional life. One helper said:

"My work takes a toll on me personally at times. In sad and difficult cases, such as working with clients who have been sexually abused, there is the danger of getting overly involved. I find that if I get a series of severe clients, then stress builds up."

Although this helper's professional life spills over negatively into his personal life at times, there are also some constructive effects of his work on him personally. Working intimately with others is a catalyst for him to look at the things he is doing in his own life. As he put it:

"My work helps me feel that I'm out there contributing and helping people. I feel that I'm doing something worthwhile and feel a sense of accomplishment. My work helps me put my own struggles in perspective. I'm able to learn a lot about myself through my involvement in the lives of others."

The myth of the wounded healer.   The myth of the wounded healer sheds some light on the ways in which the helper is personally affected by the helping process. Jaffe (1986) argues that health professionals must see that they cannot simply give and remain detached from their feelings. Instead, they must look inward at their personal needs. Jaffe decries the notion that healers are not supposed to have needs, that personal feelings are not relevant, and that helpers should learn to cut themselves off from their own pain as they work with others' pain. He describes the Greek myth attributing curative powers to the wounded healer. Such healers were supposed to possess the wisdom of life and death, yet they were not able to heal their own incurable wounds. According to Jaffe, helping professionals need to recognize the impact on their own life of working with suffering people. They must become aware of their inner responses and learn to work through their own pain in a constructive manner if they hope to avoid burnout.

Kottler (1993) argues that most therapists understand that they are jeopardizing their own emotional well-being when they intimately encounter the pain of others. He observes that the client and the therapist change each other and that there are hazards to the therapist as a result of this intimate relationship:

> There are tremendous risks for the therapist in living with the anguish of others, in being so close to others' torments. Sometimes we become desensitized by human emotions and experience an acute overdose of feeling; we turn ourselves off. Other times we overreact to personal incidents as a result of lingering dissonance created during sessions. (p. 12)

Unless practitioners have identified their own sources of vulnerability and to some extent worked through experiences that may have left them psychologically wounded, they may be constantly triggered by the stories of their clients. Therapists are affected by their clients. Their old wounds are opened, affecting both their personal and professional lives. It is clear that therapeutic practice can reactivate a therapist's earlier experiences and reawaken unresolved needs and problems (Farber, 1983; Guy, 1987, Kottler, 1993).

Case example.   Nancy, a beginning counselor working in an agency, is asked to co-lead a group of adults who are in some stage of grief over a significant loss. Nancy feels that there is a real need for this work, and she is enthusiastic in accepting the co-leadership role. She lost her husband through a tragic death, yet she feels that she has allowed herself to fully experience the pain of his death and has accepted the loss. She works very well with the members in her group. She can be compassionate, supportive, and empathic, and she is able to help them work through some of their pain.

After a few weeks Nancy notices that she is no longer looking forward to going to the group. She feels somewhat depressed and finds herself becoming apathetic toward the members. What she does not realize is that even though some of her old wounds were healed, exposure to the intense pain of so many other people has reopened these wounds. Thus, the only way she could survive was to numb herself from feeling the others' pain. This numbing led to her depression and her inability to work effectively with her clients. What she has ignored is her vulnerability to the pain of her loss and her need to express and work through this pain as it is being reexperienced.

Simply because Nancy reexperiences her old pain does not necessarily mean that she will become ineffective in working with this type of group. Quite to the contrary, if she accepts the fact that she is still wounded and explores these feelings, she can heal her own wounds at the same time that she is facilitating the healing process in others. She can model the ongoing nature of grief work and teach the members that although the pain will never be completely erased, it can become less controlling. If at times her own pain feels overwhelming in the group, she can share it with the members. She can use her experiences as a bridge to connect with the struggles of others. Alternatively, Nancy can choose to seek personal therapy. If she repeatedly puts her own emotions "on hold," either in or out of the group, she is bound to become ineffectual as a helper, and if she continues this type of involvement over a long period, the chances are that she will burn out. The challenge for Nancy is to learn to pay attention to her inner experience and to use it as a road to her growth and as a way of making contact with others.

UNDERSTANDING STRESS AND BURNOUT

When stresses are not coped with effectively, the end result can be burnout. This is a critical problem in the helping professions. Burnout is the result of severe, prolonged, and mismanaged stress. People in many different careers experience burnout, but helpers are especially vulnerable because of the nature of their involvement with people in need. Although there is no guarantee that you will remain immune, if you increase your awareness of the early warning signs of burnout and develop practical strategies for staving it off (see Chapter 13), you will be better able to respond effectively to the situation.

The Nature of Burnout

Burnout has been described as a state of physical, emotional, and mental exhaustion that results from constant or repeated emotional pressure associated with an intense, long-term involvement with people. It is characterized by feelings of helplessness and hopelessness and by a negative view of self and negative attitudes toward work, life, and other people. Burnout leads to personal feelings of depression, loss of morale, feelings of isolation, reduced productivity, and a decreased capacity to cope. Because their well is dry, helpers who are both physically and emotionally depleted have little to give to others.

Burnout manifests itself in many ways. Those who experience this syndrome typically find that they are tired, emotionally drained, and without energy or enthusiasm. Other symptoms include a loss of idealism, trust, concern, and spirit. They talk of feeling pulled by their many projects, most of which seem to have lost their meaning. They feel that what they do have to offer is either not wanted or not received; they feel unappreciated, unrecognized, and unimportant. They go about their jobs in a mechanical and routine way and tend not to see any concrete results or fruits from their efforts. There is a negative shift in responses to others that is characterized by depersonalization, negative attitudes toward clients, a decline of idealism, and general irritability. Often they feel oppressed by the "system" and by institutional demands, which, they contend, stifle any sense of personal initiative. A real danger is that the burnout syndrome can feed off itself, leaving practitioners feeling more and more isolated. They may fail to reach out to one another or to develop a support system. Because burnout can rob us of the vitality we need personally and professionally, it is important to look at some of its causes, possible remedies, and ways of preventing it.

Burnout is not something that happens to you suddenly. Rather, it is an ongoing process with developmental stages. It might be helpful to think of burnout on a continuum, rather than in either/or terms. In the beginning of a helping career, the worker might have the motivation to "set the world afire." As you experience the inevitable frustrations and stresses of being a professional helper, this flame may be dampened, and the initial ideals may give way to a cynical and hard view of the world.

Kottler (1993) observes that therapists who tend to burn out have probably ignored the signs of their condition for months and even years. He lists a number of key symptoms of burnout: (1) when clients call to cancel, the therapist celebrates with a bit too much enthusiasm; (2) daydreaming and escapist fantasies are common; (3) there is a tendency to cope with prolonged stress by abusing drugs; (4) therapy sessions lose their excitement and spontaneity; (5) the therapist gets behind in paperwork and billings; (6) the therapist's social life suffers; and (7) there is a reluctance to explore the causes and cures of one's burned-out condition.

Professional helpers need to see that what they do is worthwhile; yet the nature of their profession is such that they often don't see immediate or concrete results. This lack of reinforcement can have a debilitating effect as counselors begin to wonder whether anything they do makes a difference to anyone. The danger of burnout is greater if they practice in isolation, have little interchange with fellow professionals, have demanding or disturbed clients, have few vital interests outside of work, or fail to seek an explanation of their feelings of deadness.

Professionals who limit their work to one type of activity are particularly susceptible to burnout. Many therapists who work alone in their own practice report that they often get caught in the routine of seeing client after client. They find it increasingly difficult to be fully present for their clients, especially when it seems that they are dealing with the same kind of problem over and over. After a while they may well find themselves responding almost mechanically. It may be difficult to rectify this situation if one's livelihood seems to depend on maintaining one's own private practice. Nevertheless, therapists need to question whether sticking to one kind of practice is worth the price they often pay in lack of excitement.

The problem of burnout is particularly critical for people working in systems or in community agencies. With the emphasis in this kind of work on giving to others, there is often not enough focus on giving to oneself. Unfortunately, some who enter the helping professions have high hopes that are never realized. If they meet with constant frustration, see almost no positive change in their clients, and encounter obstacles to meeting their goals of helping others, their hopes may eventually be replaced by the despair and powerlessness that characterize many of their clients.

Some Causes of Burnout

There is no single cause of burnout; rather, it is a condition that results from a combination of factors. Burnout is best understood by considering the individual, interpersonal, and organizational factors that contribute to it. Recognizing the causes of burnout can be the first step toward dealing with it. Burnout can be caused by:

- Doing the same type of work with little variation, especially if this work seems meaningless
- Giving a great deal personally and not getting back much in the way of appreciation or other positive responses
- Lacking a sense of accomplishment and meaning in your work

- Being under constant and strong pressure to produce, perform, and meet deadlines—many of which may be unrealistic
- Working with a difficult population, such as highly resistant clients, involuntary clients, or those who show very little progress or change
- Conflict and tension among staff; an absence of support from colleagues and an abundance of criticism
- Lack of trust between supervisors and mental-health workers, creating conflict rather than teamwork toward commonly valued goals
- Not having opportunities for personal expression or for taking initiative in trying new approaches; a situation in which experimentation, change, and innovations not only are not rewarded but are actively discouraged
- Having unrealistic demands on your time and energy
- Having jobs that are both personally and professionally taxing without much opportunity for supervision, continuing education, or other forms of in-service training
- Unresolved personal conflicts beyond the job situation, such as marital tensions, chronic health problems, or financial problems

Rather than looking at burnout as something that may afflict you, consider the role you may play in increasing your risk of burnout. Certain personality traits and characteristics can increase your risk factor. Some individual factors such as a compelling need for approval, feeling unappreciated, and striving for unrealistically high goals can increase your risk for burnout. Interpersonal and organizational factors are also causes of burnout.

Individual Factors

Helpers play a role in creating their own burnout. The chances for burnout rise if the person is younger, less self-confident, impulsive, impatient, and dependent on others for approval and affection and has goals and aspirations that are out of tune with reality (Maslach, 1982).

The need to be needed can work for or against you. There is a considerable expenditure of energy in thinking about and taking care of those who need you. If this need is great, you may find yourself a prisoner of the demands that in some way you have created for yourself based on your own needs. As you are starting out and building a practice, you may be flattered by those who are seeking your help. Indeed, it feels psychologically affirming to be sought after and needed. It is possible to become impressed with the economic rewards associated with helping people. The temptation is there to not turn away people, for both emotional and financial reasons. Some helpers have a difficult time taking a vacation, especially when they figure the lost income. Soon these helpers forget that they, too, have needs, which are probably not being met because of their overinvolvement with others and their overcommitments. There are limits to how much you can take on without paying a price in terms of your physical, mental, and emotional health.

Feeling unappreciated. A major theme heard by those who are suffering from burnout is that they do not feel recognized for who they are or what they do, that they receive little positive feedback, and that they do not feel that their dedication is appreciated. In such a setting they are eventually bound to lose their striving for excellence. This lack of recognition is compounded by the fact that you may have entered the helping professions because of your need for recognition and appreciation. You may be sincerely devoted to helping others, yet your efforts may seem meager at times. You will hear more often about what you are failing to do and about your deficiencies than about what you have done well. If appreciation is lacking on the job, it is difficult over a period of time to know whether what you are doing really makes a difference to anyone. This process tends to erode both your ideals and your enthusiasm, which leads to demoralization.

The real challenge is to learn ways of working for your own appreciation and self-worth. Unless you want to depend on clients or colleagues to give you positive feedback and confirmation, it is imperative that you give yourself the appreciation that you might be seeking from others.

How your ideals can become dulled.   An important factor in burnout is whether your ideals are working for you or against you. In our experience, those who set high goals for themselves seem to have a high need for recognition. They also tend to have high expectations of others. As long as they feel satisfied by their efforts, their energy level remains high. But when they get stuck in routine patterns and do not see the fruits of their efforts, they are likely to experience a sense of restlessness.

Most professional providers were initially attracted to their careers in large part because of their hope of making a significant difference in the lives of others. One sign of burnout is the dulling of these ideals and the loss of caring about others. Learning the fine balance between idealism and realism is essential if you hope to survive as a helping professional. The idealism embodied in the desire to "save the world" can sometimes be transformed into feelings of cynicism. The ideals that you hold when you begin your career can be a positive force, and this idealism can also be a direct path toward burnout. Your idealism can result in brainstorming ideas that are translated into new projects. Yet if you are not careful, you can get carried away with your enthusiasm and immerse yourself in your work and projects. If your total worth as a person hinges on your projects' bearing fruit, you may experience personal devastation when they cease being rewarding.

The toll of devoting yourself to your profession is more pronounced if you are set on changing the system quickly and efficiently. You may believe that it is possible to revolutionize the system, only to find time and again that systems are rigid and resistant to change. Thus, when you fail to succeed in your attempts to remake the system, you are likely to experience a deep frustration, which can easily result in a "what's-the-use?" attitude toward future goals.

If you are set on challenging people who have been in a system for a long time, you will probably run into many roadblocks. In challenging others you may alienate many staff members. Rather than setting yourself up for eventual failure, focus your energies on learning how to take constructive action within a system. This entails first knowing how systems work and understanding the reasons for the particular structure of a system. If you are unrealistically idealistic, you can fight a losing battle trying to change those who are committed to the status quo and who will fight you on your every proposal. We will be talking about the futility of focusing on "them out there" while ignoring your own behaviors.

The problem of tarnished idealism increases as you come into contact with cynical colleagues who are threatened by your enthusiasm. A seasoned staff member may tear down your ideals and try to convince you that you, too, will harden yourself to painful reality. Your co-workers may tell you of all the things that simply won't work. It is difficult to stay creative and excited in a job environment where those around you are continually chipping away at your efforts to make a difference. If you constantly hear that your proposals for change won't work and if you are without real support for your ideas, you are likely to face psychological erosion, and you might eventually join the ranks of your soured peers. Faced with this onslaught of negative input, many beginners start to doubt themselves and their competence. If you are beginning as a helper, you probably already have many self-doubts, and if these doubts are reinforced, it is easier to feel disillusioned.

A young man we know recently graduated with a bachelor's degree in psychology and worked briefly in a residential home for adolescents. Paul was greatly disillusioned when he encountered deeply entrenched cynicism in this facility. He quickly learned that both the residents and the staff were committed to the status quo. The apathy he saw in the staff discouraged him and led him to wonder if he wanted to pursue this field.

If you work in an environment where you receive negative bombardment, you would do well to actively seek some source of support either in your job setting or away from it. It would be a mistake to wait for the agency to create this support for you, so ask colleagues to join you in making the time for regular meetings.

We encourage you to look at the factors in you that are most likely to cause burnout. A common denominator in many cases of burnout is the question of *responsibility*. Helpers may feel responsible for what their clients do or don't do; they may assume too much responsibility for the direction of therapy; or they may have extremely high expectations of themselves. How does this description apply to you? In what ways could your assumption of an inordinate degree of responsibility contribute to your burnout?

Interpersonal and Organizational Factors

Maslach (1982) writes about involvement with people as a main source of burnout. She contends that the hallmark of the syndrome is a shift in the way professionals view the people they are helping. They change from feeling positive and caring to feeling negative and uncaring. Continuous contact with clients who are unappreciative, upset, and depressed often leads helpers to view all recipients in helping relationships in negative terms. Practitioners may care less, begin to make derogatory comments about their clients, ignore them, and want to move away from them. Dehumanized responses are a core ingredient of burnout.

One counselor in an agency notices that she is on the path toward burnout when she becomes too involved with her clients' struggles. She commented:

"Sometimes I'm unable to escape personal issues that arise when my clients' problems trigger issues similar to my own. This affects me in a positive way in that it holds me accountable within my own life and keeps me moving toward the best person I can become. Sometimes it affects me negatively when I become overly self-critical."

There is a vicious circle operating here. If you get an abundance of negative reactions from others, you will tend to become self-critical and wonder if you are making any difference to those you are supposedly helping. Being critical of and unkind to yourself usually leads to being critical of and unkind to others.

The impact that other people have on burnout should not be overlooked. If you are part of an institutional setting, the quality of your contacts with co-workers and supervisors is extremely important. Co-workers can be helpful in providing support for you, but if there is no climate of trust and openness in the work setting, you become more vulnerable to burnout. If these relationships are strained and the atmosphere is hostile and unsupportive, the chances of burnout are increased.

When we consulted at a state mental hospital, we found many workers who were suffering from burnout. They claimed to have difficult clients, a difficult administration, and difficult colleagues. If you find yourself in a similar situation with this combination of factors, you are in trouble. What we attempted to teach these workers at the state facility was to seek out others with whom to talk.

THE EXPERIENCE OF BURNOUT

Burnout is not a simple phenomenon. Helpers are affected in many ways by the strains of constant interaction with people in need of help. As an example, consider the case of a counselor named Daniel, who is suffering from many of the symptoms of burnout.

Physically, Daniel is fatigued most of the time. He has accepted an increased caseload and works long hours. He exercises very little because of a lack of time, does not have time to eat regularly or properly, and is so wrapped up in his work that he does not sleep well. He finds it a real chore to get up in the morning. He suffers from headaches that just will not go away as well as a range of other health problems that stem from his stressful lifestyle.

Intellectually, Daniel has lost his curiosity and desire to question or learn. Although when he was in graduate school he enjoyed sharing and discussing ideas about human behavior and counseling, now he cannot be bothered by argumentation, discussion, and revision of his ideas. With all the pressures at work, he finds no time to read or take courses to keep abreast of developments in the field. Instead, he hopes to find quick remedies to deal with the crisis situations that he faces in his daily work.

Emotionally, Daniel has spent so much time focusing on the emotional needs of others that he has failed to recognize his own needs. At one time he was able to provide nurturance for others, yet by chronically neglecting his need for expression he has become indifferent in his professional life and withdrawn from those he loves in his personal life. He is isolated and unable to feel either pain or joy. He feels very alone at work, and he tends to blame himself for not doing well. Because he is not feeling a sense of personal accomplishment, his view of his own worth is also declining. He experiences an increasing sense of wanting to get away from demands and pressures.

Interpersonally, Daniel has lost interest in being with others. He feels "peopled out" and is gleeful when clients cancel. He sometimes "forgets" his appointments with clients and fails to show up for staff meetings. When he began his career, he had high hopes of making an impact on the lives of others. Now his ideals are tarnished, and his motivation is low. His job performance is deteriorating, and much of the time he is indifferent. His family is also suffering from his burnout, for he shrinks away from involvement with his wife and children. He just wants everybody to leave him alone and make no more demands on him. He feels emotionally dry and has little energy to listen to what they might want from him. Even minor requests are heard as demands that only burden him more.

Daniel has paid a steep price for ignoring the stressful circumstances that resulted in his indifference. Not only has he become an impaired professional but he is suffering in his personal life as well. By withdrawing from his friends, family, and co-workers, he has cut off all sources of possible nourishment.

THE IMPAIRED PROFESSIONAL

Burnout often contributes to the making of an impaired practitioner. Guy (1987) defines impairment as the "diminution or deterioration of therapeutic skills and abilities due to factors which have sufficiently impacted the personality of the therapist to result in potential incompetence" (p. 199). In their study of distressed psychologists, Thoreson, Miller, and Krauskopf (1989) found that approximately 10% of their sample had experienced frequent levels of distress in the following categories: depression (11%), recurrent physical illness (10%), problems with alcohol use (9%), and feelings of loneliness (8%). Their study seemed to indicate that at least a minority of psychologists experience distress levels to the point that it impairs their ability to function effectively as professionals.

Impaired practitioners clearly contribute to the suffering of their clients rather than alleviating it. For example, sexually exploitive behavior by counselors is often a manifestation of impairment (Emerson & Markos, 1996). Counselors who become sexually involved with clients show personality patterns similar to those of impaired counselors. These shared characteristics include:

- Fragile self-esteem
- Difficulty establishing intimacy in one's personal life
- Professional isolation
- A need to rescue clients
- A need for reassurance about one's attractiveness
- Substance abuse

Because a common characteristic of impairment is denial, professional colleagues may need to confront the irresponsible behavior of an impaired counselor. Herlihy (1996) suggests confronting the impaired counselor with sensitivity, respect, and preparedness.

Although the professional impairment associated with chronic burnout has received much publicity from professional groups, it appears that many individual helpers have avoided or denied its existence. In her discussion of professional impairment, Stadler (1990) writes that we know very little about its impact on clients and that there are few professionally sponsored avenues to help distressed counselors. Graduate training programs in the helping professions should prepare students for the disappointments they will encounter in the course of their training as well as in the jobs they eventually secure. Students can learn not only about the rewards and frustrations of helping others but also about the hazards of this profession. If they are not given adequate preparation, they may be especially vulnerable to early disenchantment and high rates of burnout, for they are saddled with unrealistic expectations.

According to Stadler (1990), impaired practitioners have lost the ability to resolve stressful events. She points to the ethical concerns that are raised when impaired helpers continue their professional work. Those therapists whose inner conflicts are consistently activated by client material may respond by trying to stabilize themselves rather than to facilitate the growth of their clients. Clearly, impaired practitioners contribute to the suffering of their clients rather than alleviating this suffering. It is ethically imperative that they recognize and deal with their impairment. We think that licensing boards could require personal therapy in cases where counselor impairment becomes obvious. Of course, we hope that practitioners themselves will realize that they need therapy for themselves and welcome the opportunity to deal with problems that are keeping them stuck in dysfunctional patterns.

This chapter has addressed the effects of stress that can lead to burnout and impairment. The condition of burnout should not be viewed as an incurable disease. Rather, it may be helpful to view it in much the same way as you would a virus that infects you because of a weakening of your immune system. As is true in the case of a virus, burnout may afflict you during different times in your life. You need not be helpless, for just as you are able to cure a disease resulting from a virus, you are also able to cope with the outcome of burnout. In the next chapter we address the issue of managing stress, preventing burnout, and retaining your vitality as a person and as a professional.

By Way of Review

- One of the hazards of the helping professions is that helpers are typically not very good at asking for help for themselves.
- It is wise to sensitize yourself to both the external and internal factors that contribute to your experience of stress.
- One of the major environmental sources of job stress is the friction that arises out of working in an organization.
- Studies of therapists' perceptions of client behaviors find the following to be the most stressful: suicidal statements, anger toward the helper, aggression and hostility, severe depression, apathy and lack of motivation, and premature termination.

- There is a heavy price to pay for being a professional caregiver. No one is immune from the cost of caring for others.
- Being a professional helper often reopens your own psychological wounds. If you are not willing to work on your unfinished business, you might reconsider whether you want to accompany clients on their journey of dealing with their past wounds.
- Most helpers enter their profession with a high degree of idealism. Later, these ideals are sometimes tempered with realism. The danger is that idealism can be transformed into cynicism, which is a step away from burnout.
- There is no single cause of burnout; rather, there are individual, interpersonal, and organizational factors that lead to it. Understanding these factors can help you learn how to prevent or cope with burnout.
- Burnout is often the result of the many demands placed on you by an agency. It is important to learn specific ways of surviving with dignity in an agency setting.
- The impaired professional is an issue that the helping professions seriously need to address. Those helpers who are addicted to drugs, for example, will certainly be limited in providing quality services to their clients. Impairment is frequently the result of long-standing patterns of being burned out and not dealing with the condition. Coping with stress effectively is a way to lessen the chances of becoming an impaired helper.

WHAT WILL YOU DO NOW?

1. Make a list of some of the factors that are most stressful in your life. Next, write down a few ideas of what you can do now to minimize at least some of these sources of stress. Develop a plan of action, and try it out for at least a week. Consider making a contract with someone so that you will be accountable for acting to reduce stress in your life.

2. Identify a few of the warning signs that you are not taking care of yourself or that you are close to burnout. For example, you might not be getting adequate sleep, you might be ignoring exercise, or you might be experiencing a variety of physical symptoms. Are you willing to assume responsibility for eliminating something that you are doing that is contributing to your level of fatigue?

3. Arrange an interview with a practicing professional, and ask this person these questions: "What are some of the major stresses you face in your work?" "What are some ways you deal with these stresses?" "What are your thoughts on preventing burnout?"

4. Reflect on the patterns of stress you experience in your life. Think about your responses to the sources-of-stress checklist and the other information presented in this chapter. How do you think stress affects all areas of your life? What are you likely to do to cope with these sources of stress? In your journal, keep track of some stressful activities for a few weeks. Think about practical ways to minimize your stress in a few situations, especially by changing your reactions to them. Try out these new ideas, and write down your observations.

5. For the full bibliographic entry for each of the sources listed below, consult the References and Reading List at the back of the book.

For a discussion of the signs and symptoms of impaired helpers see Emerson and Markos (1996). For ideas for dealing with an impaired colleague see Herlihy (1996).

For readings on burnout, see Freudenberger, with Richelson (1980), Maslach (1982), and Pines, Aronson, with Kafry (1981). For a discussion of how stress affects your health, see Rice (1992); G. Corey and M. Corey (1997); and Corey, Corey, and Corey (1997). See Kottler (1993) and Guy (1987) for discussions of how stress affects the personal and professional lives of helpers. Kottler's (1997) edited book, *Finding Your Way as a Counselor*, contains a number of excellent articles on topics pertaining to the special demands of those in the helping professions.

Chapter 13

The Challenge of Retaining Your Vitality

FOCUS QUESTIONS

1. What are some specific ways in which you cope with the stresses you experience? How effective is your stress management?
2. Helpers sometimes engage in a self-defeating internal dialogue. For instance, they may expect that they will be perfect and may burden themselves with fears of making mistakes. What are some examples of your own internal dialogue that may not serve you well? How good are you at challenging self-defeating attitudes and beliefs?
3. It has been said that either you control stress or stress controls you. How would you apply this maxim to yourself at this time in your life?
4. How well do you utilize your time? What are some ways to better organize your time to achieve your priorities?
5. What major demands do you expect to face in the organization where you will work? How can you keep your individuality and integrity and at the same time keep your job?
6. What are some specific ways to lessen the chances of burnout? How can you remain alive both as a person and as a helper?

AIM OF THE CHAPTER

In the last chapter we examined how stress affects you in both your personal and your professional life and how chronically stressful patterns put you on a path toward burnout. This chapter deals with the challenge you face as a helper in retaining your vitality. We will focus on specific strategies for coping with stress effectively but, even more, on developing attitudes, thought patterns, and specific action plans geared to changing your lifestyle so you will be oriented toward health. Staying alive as a person and as a professional is not something that happens automatically; it is the result of a commitment to acquiring habits of thinking and action that promote soundness of mind and body.

It is unrealistic to think that you can eliminate stress from either your personal life or your professional life, but you do not have to be the victim of stress. You can recognize how you are being affected by stress and make decisions about how to think, feel, and behave in stressful situations. You can become aware of your destructive reactions to stress and learn constructive ways of coping with it. In short, you can learn to manage and control stress rather than being controlled by it.

It is important to sensitize yourself to both the external and internal factors that contribute to negative physical and psychological reactions. We will present a variety of strategies for coping with stress and burnout, and we encourage you to develop your own set of strategies for managing stressful experiences. We are merely introducing you to the subject of stress management and urge you to select at least one book from the suggested readings listed at the end of this chapter to use as your guide.

AN INTEGRATED MODEL FOR COPING WITH STRESS

The general framework of this section follows the model for coping with stress presented by Matheny, Aycock, Pugh, Curlette, and Cannella (1986). These authors designed a major study that attempted to synthesize the research on methods of coping. They define coping as "any effort, healthy or unhealthy, conscious or unconscious, to prevent, eliminate, or weaken stressors, or to tolerate their effects in the least hurtful manner" (p. 509). Their model includes both *preventive* and *combative* strategies. Although we use their framework as a basis for this discussion, we also draw from other authors and from our own experiences.

Preventive Strategies

There are three general strategies for preventing stress: (1) avoiding or reducing stressors, (2) altering stress-inducing behavior patterns, and (3) developing coping resources.

Avoiding or reducing stressors.   One fundamental way to prevent stress is to avoid stressors. You can escape stressors by physically removing yourself from the stressful situation. Although stress accompanies the pursuit of some of your key goals, many stresses are unnecessary for your success, and these you can seek to avoid. This strategy might entail changing jobs, getting out of a destructive relationship, or taking some other direct action. For example, a mental-health worker told us that he had come to feel trapped in his 40-hour-a-week job as a counselor in a community agency. He was feeling the stresses of a heavy caseload and was fragmented by his many tasks. Rather than merely complaining about his job, he arranged to cut back to half time so he could spend more time at home with a new baby and could pursue other professional interests. Even though he had to do some convincing of administrators at his agency to cut back his hours and still retain his position, and even though his family had to adjust to less income, he was not willing to continue to feel overwhelmed and do nothing about it.

You may not be able to take such extreme measures as this person did. If you find yourself in a similar situation and cannot afford to reduce your work hours or do not want to leave your job, you can still look for ways to reduce factors that cause you needless stress. You might devise ways of developing some projects at work that are especially meaningful to you. Or you might find ways to work creatively with others as a part of your position. For example, we know of some helpers who have teamed up and combined their programs on the wards of the hospitals where they work. Others have taken steps to co-lead groups. A social worker who led groups for outpatients teamed up with a music therapist, and the two found ways to combine their talents for the good of the clients and also keep themselves interested as professionals.

If you don't think of alternatives to reduce stressors at work, you may eventually stop functioning effectively and lose your job. You can look for better ways to control your work schedule, for example. Although you may not be able to avoid taking on difficult clients, you can avoid scheduling the more difficult ones back to back.

Modifying stress-inducing behaviors. A second preventive strategy is to work toward changing specific behaviors that produce stress. This strategy includes decreasing "Type A" behaviors such as excessive competitiveness, continual rushing, and hostility. Approaches to altering stress-inducing behavior patterns include a variety of methods known as cognitive restructuring. As we have said, much of your stress is determined by your beliefs about events. Sometimes you actually create your stress by clinging to outworn beliefs. If you can change self-destructive thinking into constructive thinking, you will go a long way toward eliminating needless stress. Working on a cognitive level involves efforts to reframe situations or events in such a way as to reduce their stress value. Reframing can be directed at changing the meaning of an event. Assume, for instance, that one of your clients stops coming for help. If you interpret her termination as a sign of your professional ineptitude, this event will certainly be a source of stress. Rather than making yourself totally responsible for your clients' outcomes, consider their role in making their therapy a success or a failure. If you hold to the conviction that you must be successful with every client, your belief will lead to much frustration. By challenging this belief and substituting more realistic beliefs, you can alter stressful events. Remember that the goal of coping is to help you appreciate that you do not have to be the victim of stress. As you increasingly realize that the ways in which you think, feel, and behave do contribute to your stress level, you are in a position to reduce this stress. We cover the topic of cognitive restructuring in more detail later in this chapter.

Developing resources for coping. A third approach to prevention consists of developing coping resources. One of these resources is a sense of physical health, which to a large extent depends on sound nutritional habits, regular physical exercise, getting enough rest, and the like. Psychological assets are other resources for coping, such as a sense of control, a belief in oneself, and confidence. Other resources include cognitive assets, such as functional beliefs and academic competencies, and social support, including a network of friends. You can do a lot to prevent stress by learning specific skills in the areas of assertiveness, time management, and relaxation. Resistance to stress is increased by an openness to change, a willingness to make commitments, and an appreciation that you can control your life. If you allow stress to overwhelm you and if you convince yourself that there is little you can do to change things, stress will control you.

Combative Strategies

The integrative model of coping (Matheny et al., 1986) outlines five combative strategies: (1) monitoring stressors and symptoms, (2) marshaling one's resources, (3) lowering stressful arousal, (4) using problem-solving methods, and (5) learning to tolerate those stressors that cannot be eliminated.

Self-monitoring.   Before you can change your behavior in stressful situations, you must first be aware of those situations and how you react to them. Although simply monitoring your stress may be of limited value, it is a prerequisite to using other methods of stress management. Self-monitoring will probably reveal that you increase your level of stress by (1) telling others stories about your stresses and (2) telling yourself over and over how stressful life is. One of the best ways to monitor stressful situations is by keeping a written record of your reactions to specific difficult situations each day. It is helpful to record the events that tend to produce stress for you and your behavior in these situations. Recording your thoughts, feelings, and actions in a variety of situations will give you clues to what stressors you most need to pay attention to. Once you detect patterns, you can begin to make some changes. Most books on stress management will provide you with specific hints on practical steps in this self-monitoring process.

Marshaling your resources.   After identifying a stressor, you need to draw on your resources and plan effective strategies for combat. You might make the mistake of underestimating your resources for dealing actively with stressful situations. For example, you might focus more on your deficits than on your personal strengths. It is important to remember that the aim of a stress-management program is not to eliminate stress but to cope with it in effective ways. Life without the challenge of stressful situations could be boring. The aim is to learn how to call on the many resources available to you so that you can combat unnecessary stress and maintain your zest for living.

Lowering stress arousal.   A number of means are available to reduce arousal that interferes with coping. For example, relaxation methods can be most useful in reducing tension. Other forms of tension reduction include play, vigorous physical exercise, and hobbies. Leisure is a good way to cope with stress. By allowing yourself to enjoy this time away from work, you will probably be in a better position to deal with stressors at work. You might find an activity such as gardening, meditating, practicing yoga, playing tennis, jogging, biking, knitting, or sitting in a park and watching ducks to be your way of relaxing.

In addition to these ways in which you can unwind and let go, you can also practice systematic relaxation training for about 20 minutes a couple of times a day. Of course, you need to grant yourself the latitude to relax, and you must be convinced that practicing relaxation exercises is not a waste of valuable time. Relaxation training will not work unless you are willing to learn skills, practice them regularly, and apply them to everyday life situations that bring on stress. The following books have some excellent guidelines for relaxation training: Butler (1981), Charlesworth and Nathan (1984), and Meichenbaum (1985).

Using problem-solving methods.   One way to cope with stressful situations is to use problem-solving methods, which include assessing the problem, finding out relevant information, challenging limiting assumptions, and identifying alternative behaviors. Common to most writers' problem-solving methods are the following steps as discussed by Meichenbaum (1985):

- Identify the stressor as a problem to be solved.
- Set concrete and realistic goals, and identify specific steps necessary to reach these goals.
- Consider a wide range of possible courses of action.
- Consider how others might respond if they were asked to deal with a similar stress problem.
- Evaluate the pros and cons of each of the proposed solutions, and then rank these solutions from least practical to most practical.
- Rehearse and practice new behaviors by means of imagery and behavioral rehearsal.
- Experiment with the solution that appears to be most feasible.
- Expect some setbacks and failures, but reward yourself for honest efforts.
- Reconsider the original problem in the light of your attempt at problem solving.

As a way of making the problem-solving approach more concrete and personal, picture yourself working with clients who have been sent to you by the court. You find the resistance of these involuntary clients to be stressful, because you are constantly trying to convince them that counseling might be of benefit to them. One way to solve this problem would be to find another job. If you are not willing or able to take this step, consider how you might apply problem-solving strategies. First, you can identify realistic goals. Although you would prefer a caseload of clients who were motivated to change and were seeking your help, the chances are that you cannot magically transform your clients. One goal might be to approach these clients differently, inviting them to use you as a resource but not taking full responsibility for whether they decide to take advantage of their resources for change. Next, you could challenge them when they tell you that they are being "forced to see you." You might see them for one session to tell them what they can expect from the counseling sessions and what you expect from them. As a condition of continuing the sessions, you could insist that they develop a clear contract delineating what they are willing to do as their part of the relationship. You could make a proposal to your supervisor for alternatives to seeing such clients on an individual basis. You could make appropriate referrals. After generating many possible approaches and imagining how you and others might respond in these circumstances, you could try out some new strategies with clients to test these alternatives.

Adjusting to stress by using cognitive approaches.   When certain stressors prove difficult to eliminate, successful coping involves adjusting to them in the ways that are least harmful. Cognitive restructuring is one of the most promising combative strategies. A good deal of stress results from our beliefs and stressful mental sets, including negative self-talk and "catastrophic" thinking. Cognitive restructuring aims at demolishing negative self-programming and learning constructive self-talk. The aim is to change the meaning that stressful situations hold for you. You can accomplish this by being less self-critical when you do not have perfect performances and by convincing yourself that you are not alone in facing stress.

Combining Preventive and Combative Strategies

The integrated model of coping with stress combines preventive and combative strategies. Probably the best way to cope with stress is to develop a multi-pronged approach rather than limiting yourself to a single strategy. In getting involved in a stress-management program, it is important to tailor the techniques to your individual personality and unique situation. Good training programs do not promote a simple formula or a "cookbook" approach for coping with stress. An effective program should be future-oriented, preparing you to apply strategies to various stressful life situations as they arise. You also need to be prepared for inevitable setbacks, and it is essential to stick with your program if you hope to see results. Thus, your program should help you identify sources of possible failure and prepare for them.

One of the programs for preventing and reducing stress is stress-inoculation training (SIT), as developed and refined by Meichenbaum (1977, 1985). SIT is not a single strategy for coping but combines aspects of didactic teaching, Socratic discussion, cognitive restructuring, problem solving, relaxation training, behavioral rehearsal, imagery, self-monitoring, self-instruction, self-reinforcement, and efforts at changing the environment. It is designed to help people not only resolve immediate problems but also apply what they learn to dealing effectively with future stressful situations. In short, SIT is designed to build "psychological antibodies" that will increase one's resistance to stressors. It generally consists of 12 to 15 sessions, plus "booster" and follow-up sessions.

Ideally, taking a course on stress management utilizing the strategies outlined by Meichenbaum would be a good way to learn and apply specific coping skills. If you are interested in learning more about the details of SIT, we recommend that you read Meichenbaum's excellent short book, which is included in the References and Reading List at the end of the book. Taking a workshop on stress management would be another approach. If these options are not practical at this time, you could at least carefully select some self-help books, of which there are an increasing number. As with many other endeavors, merely reading about stress management is not enough to combat some of the stresses you face. It is essential that you regularly practice the stress-management techniques that you read about.

COGNITIVE APPROACHES TO STRESS MANAGEMENT

Our beliefs largely determine how we interpret events. Thought of in this way, events are not the cause of our stress; rather, the meaning we give to these events is what is crucial. Albert Ellis, the founder of rational emotive behavior therapy

(REBT) and a precursor of cognitive therapy, is fond of citing the following quotation by the Stoic philosopher Epictetus: "Men are disturbed not by things, but by the views that they take of them." In this section we draw heavily from the writings of Ellis and other cognitive therapists, especially Aaron Beck, Gary Emery, and Donald Meichenbaum. All of these therapists have developed approaches to help people become aware of their cognitions, the dialogue that goes on inside of them, and how their thinking affects how they feel and act. The cognitive approaches offer specific strategies to clients for challenging and changing self-defeating cognitions and for developing sound thinking that leads to less stressful living.

In some circumstances, you may engage in self-defeating thinking and ineffective self-talk. If you can recognize the nature of your irrational beliefs and understand how they lead to problems, you can begin to convert self-defeating cognitions into self-enhancing ones. In much of the rest of this chapter we discuss cognitive approaches that shed light on how you create much of your own stress by the beliefs you hold and the statements you make to yourself. Because you have this capacity to create stress, you also have the means to lessen its impact. We describe some cognitive strategies that can be employed to retain your vitality on both the personal and professional levels. Our examples will be geared primarily to situations that you are likely to encounter in your work as a helping professional.

The A-B-C Theory

Ellis has developed what he calls his A-B-C theory of irrational thinking (Ellis, 1995). This theory explains the relationship among events, beliefs, and feelings. According to Ellis, your interpretations of events are frequently more important than what occurs in reality. He calls A an Activating event, B one's Belief system, and C the emotional Consequence. Consider the situation of applying for a new job in an agency and going through an interview. Let's imagine the worst scene. The director of the agency who interviewed you kindly tells you that she does not think you would fit well in the agency. She is not really impressed with your training and experience. You do not get this job, which you badly wanted. The activating event (A) in this case is the situation of being rejected. The (C) is the emotional consequences you experience. If you feel depressed, hurt, let down, and even devastated, the chances are that you hold what Ellis would term "irrational beliefs" about not having been accepted. For example, your beliefs (B) about this rejection might be some combination of the following thoughts: "It is absolutely horrible that I didn't get this job, and it surely proves that I'm incompetent." "I should have gotten this job, and this rejection is unbearable." "I must succeed at every important endeavor, or I'm really worthless." "I failed in this interview; it's a sure sign that I will fail in any other interview I might have." "This rejection means I'm a total failure."

Rational emotive and other cognitive-behavioral therapies are grounded on the premise that emotional and behavioral disturbances are originally learned by the inculcation of irrational beliefs from significant others during our childhood, as well as by our creative inventing of irrational dogmas and superstitions. However, we actively reinstill false beliefs by the processes of autosuggestion and self-repetition (Ellis, 1995). It is largely our own repetition of these early-indoctrinated irrational thoughts, rather than a parent's repetition, that keeps dysfunctional attitudes alive within us. Therefore, we mainly have ourselves to hold accountable when we feel and act miserably over our performance as helpers.

Ellis (1988) contends that we have the power to control our emotional destiny. He suggests that when we are upset, it is well to look to our hidden dogmatic "musts" and absolutistic "shoulds." For Ellis, practically all human misery and serious emotional turmoil is unnecessary. We create, both consciously and unconsciously, the ways we think and, hence, the ways we feel in a variety of situations. Because we have the capacity for self-awareness, we can observe and evaluate our goals and purposes and, thus, can change them. We can usually change our feelings, no matter what happens to us. We are able to decide to feel differently about a situation and, therefore, stubbornly refuse to make ourselves severely anxious or depressed about anything (Ellis, 1988, 1995; Ellis & Bernard, 1986; Ellis & Dryden, 1987; Ellis & Harper, 1975; Ellis & Yeager, 1989).

Those of us who are human-services providers often incorporate a wide range of dysfunctional beliefs that impair our capacity to function as effectively as we might with those who seek our assistance. For example, at times we may distort the processing of information, which can easily lead to faulty assumptions and misconceptions. Some of these common distortions are described by Beck and Weishaar (1995): forming conclusions based on an isolated event (selective abstraction); holding extreme beliefs on the basis of a single incident and applying them inappropriately to dissimilar events or settings (overgeneralization); overestimating the significance of negative events (magnification and exaggeration); and relating external events to ourselves, even when there is no basis for making this connection (personalization).

To complete the A-B-C model of Ellis, we look briefly at D-E-F. D is the process of actively and forcefully Disputing irrational beliefs that lead to negative emotional reactions, many of which are stressful. E consists of Effective and rational new beliefs. If you are successful in this process of disputing and in substituting constructive thinking for destructive thinking, then you have a new F, which is a new Feeling. Thus, instead of feeling depressed about a loss, you can put it in a new perspective and feel appropriately disappointed. Instead of feeling devastated by the lack of universal approval, you can feel appropriately hurt if a significant person rejects you. By changing your beliefs, you also change your feelings, which is a useful way of learning to reduce stress.

Identifying Self-Defeating Internal Dialogue

As a helper, you can complicate your life through the process of telling yourself that you must be all-knowing, superhuman, totally congruent, and perfect. If you feel depressed, agitated, or otherwise miserable about the job you are doing, it is essential that you examine your basic assumptions and beliefs to determine how they are influencing what you are doing and how you are feeling. As you become attuned to identifying your faulty thinking, you are in a position to change such patterns (Beck, 1976, 1987; Corey, 1996b; Ellis & Dryden, 1987; Kottler & Blau, 1989; Meichenbaum, 1986). Here are a few statements that we often hear helping professionals utter: "I am fully responsible for my clients' outcomes." "I must be successful with every client." "If a client discontinues, it's always my fault." "I should be able to help my clients more." "I must always be available for anyone who needs me." "If a client is in pain, I should take it away." "I should know everything." "If I make a mistake, that means I'm a failure." "Referring a client means that I'm inadequate." "If a couple divorces, I was not helpful enough." "I depend on my clients to love and appreciate me to feel worthwhile."

Statements such as these could go on and on, but as you can see, most of them refer to feelings of inadequacy, a nagging belief that one should be more, and a chronic sense of self-doubt. By assuming the giant share of responsibility for your clients, you are relieving them of the responsibility to direct their own lives, in addition to creating stress for yourself.

At this juncture you might go back over the above irrational beliefs and underline those statements that you hear yourself making. Do you tend to make any other related statements, especially with regard to your role in assuming responsibility for being the "perfect" helper? What are some examples of other things you say to yourself that often get you into trouble? What are some other beliefs you hold that tend to create stress for you?

Changing Distorted and Self-Defeating Thinking

Emery (1981), a cognitive therapist, has proposed the three A's as a method of challenging and changing self-defeating thinking: *awareness*, *answering*, and *action*.

Awareness is an essential prerequisite for any type of behavioral change. For example, you can pay attention to any mood changes. Being alert to your body can offer other clues. Noticing those times when your confidence appears to fade can be helpful. Another sign is difficulty concentrating or making decisions. It is important to monitor your thoughts so that you can become aware of how your thinking influences your behavior and your feelings.

Answering your negative thinking and learning how to dispute irrational beliefs is the next step in changing self-defeating thinking into rational thinking. Here are some common examples of faulty thinking:

1. *"Catastrophizing."* One type of irrational thinking involves giving the worst possible meaning to an event. You might say, for example: "I just knew something terrible would happen. Because I took a vacation, one of my clients overdosed on drugs. If I had stayed home, this wouldn't have happened."
2. *Self-blame* involves a total self-condemnation rather than criticism of a specific behavior. Thus, you might say, "Because my client overdosed on drugs, I'm a worthless therapist, and I deserve to suffer."

3. *Overgeneralizing* involves a negative absolutistic evaluation. If you failed with a given client, for instance, you might make the mistake of overgeneralizing by saying to yourself, "I always fail at anything that's important." Or you could say: "See what happened when I decided to take my vacation. I wasn't available when someone needed me, and I let that person down."

4. *All-or-nothing thinking.* Another form of faulty thinking is seeing life in either/or categories rather than taking into account the full continuum of possibilities. Thus, you might say to yourself: "Either I'm a success, or I'm a failure. Either I'm the perfect therapist, or I'm worthless."

5. *Language errors and negative thoughts.* Your choice of words and negative thinking often produce stress. By becoming aware of the quality of your language, you can get some idea of how your self-talk influences you. Here are some examples of negative thinking:

- "I *must* act competently in all situations, and I *must* win people's approval."
- "I *can't stand* making mistakes. They prove I'm a total failure."
- "I *must* be brilliant, and I *must* perform well at all times. If I'm ever less than brilliant, this is *horrible.*"
- "I *should* always put the interests of other people before my own. My mission is to help others, and I *shouldn't* be selfish."
- "I *ought* to be available when anybody needs me. If I'm not, this shows that I'm not a caring person and that I've probably chosen the wrong profession."

Learning how to answer and to dispute irrational beliefs entails identifying your core negative thoughts. As you review the above list, think about the statements you might be inclined to make. How often do you arouse stress in yourself with such thoughts? After you have identified a few core irrational beliefs, begin to answer them. Answering faulty beliefs is best done by vigorous disputation. One method for disputing irrational beliefs is illustrated in these examples wherein we provide a dysfunctional belief, a disputation, and a constructive belief.

SELF-STATEMENT: I should always be available for anyone who needs me. If I'm not, this shows that I'm not a caring person.

DISPUTATION: Why must I always be available? Where is it written that if I am not always there when a client wants me I am not a caring person?

CONSTRUCTIVE BELIEF: Although I want to be responsible, there are limits. Sometimes clients may have exaggerated needs. There are times when I may not be emotionally available for all clients.

SELF-STATEMENT: I should be able to do everything well, which means being perfect. Either I'm the perfect helper, or I am worthless.

DISPUTATION: Where did I pick up this belief? Does it make any sense that I should do everything well the first time? Can I do some things poorly and still be outstanding in other areas?

CONSTRUCTIVE BELIEF: Although I like doing well, I can accept imperfection in myself. I can tolerate mistakes. I do not have to be perfect to be capable. Since perfection is an unrealistic ideal, I will be "perfectly satisfied" with being a fallible human.

SELF-STATEMENT: I should always put the interests of other people before my own.

DISPUTATION: Who told me this? Is it really wrong to be concerned about myself? Can't I have self-interests and still be interested in others?

CONSTRUCTIVE BELIEF: I can't show more interest in others than I have for myself. If I don't take care of myself, the chances are slim that I'll be able to be concerned about the interests of others.

As you have seen, awareness is the first step in self-change, followed by learning how to answer and dispute self-defeating thinking. However, merely identifying faulty beliefs and learning to make functional statements do not alone ensure change. For change to occur, it is essential that you take *action*. You need to test reality and act on your new thoughts and beliefs. For example, assume that you have convinced yourself that your failure to get a job does not mean that you are a failure as a person. You can act on this belief by taking the risk of applying for a job that you might want. If you are afraid of getting people's disapproval, you can put yourself in situations where approval will not always be forthcoming. If you have convinced yourself that making a mistake as a helper is not horrible, you can allow yourself to make a mistake and not feel devastated. Rather than avoiding doing new things that you have wanted to do, you might seek out some of these new ventures and take the chance of being less than perfect. It is important for you to realize that at times you will have to force yourself to act in new ways that are not comfortable for you if you hope to challenge some self-limiting assumptions. For instance, if you have been avoiding giving talks to community groups because you are afraid that you will look like a fool, it might be important to challenge yourself by giving some of these speeches in spite of your fears. The point is that your new beliefs need to be put into action, and this is the hard part in making these changes.

A key point of this chapter has been that if you hope to prevent stress from controlling you, you need to take an active stance in recognizing how your stresses do lead to personal depletion and how, as you saw in the last chapter, they eventually lead to burnout. If you give of yourself continually and ignore all the signs of stress and the toll it is taking, you will eventually find that your well runs dry.

After reading this chapter, we hope you will make some decisions about specific ways you can better manage stress in your life. You can begin by monitoring how you are affected by stress, and you can follow up by applying some of the specific preventive and combative strategies for stress management that we have discussed. Perhaps one of the major challenges you will face is to retain your vitality and a sense of personal power in the organization where you work. The multiple demands from the agency and your clients can make it difficult to retain a spirit of believing that you are making a difference. The next section examines some ways to maintain your enthusiasm within an organization.

RETAINING YOUR POWER
AND VITALITY IN AN ORGANIZATION

Although we cannot prescribe a universal method of getting along in the agency where you work, we can present some strategies we have found helpful and ask you to determine how appropriate these strategies are for you. In addition, we hope you can think of other ways of preserving your individuality while working as part of a system.

Your first opportunity to assert your individuality is in the job interview. People being interviewed for a position often confine themselves to answering the questions asked of them. However, job interviews can be mutual exchanges in which you explore the requirements and expectations of a position and assess its suitability for yourself. It is important to recognize that accepting a position with an agency entails agreeing to work within a certain philosophical framework. By asking relevant questions, you begin to assume a stance of power, for you are exploring how much you want a particular job and what price you're willing to pay for it.

Our experience has been that most established organizations resist major attempts at change, yet small and subtle changes can be quite significant. If you devote most of your energy to trying to change the people who defend the status quo, your positive programs may become a lesser priority. You will need to decide for yourself how much energy you're willing to expend on dealing with the resistive forces you encounter. If you attempt radical, systemwide changes, you may feel overwhelmed or paralyzed. If you focus instead on making changes within the scope of your position, you'll stand a better chance of extending your influence. For instance, a social worker whose goal is to correct fundamental inequities in the social-welfare system may soon feel discouraged and helpless. By directing his attention to ways of dealing more humanely with the people he comes in contact with, he may experience a sense of power and accomplishment as he makes less grandiose but still significant changes. To take another example, a school counselor may give up in exasperation if she directs most of her efforts to changing her colleagues' view of their role. If she concentrates instead on defining her own role so that she can do the kind of counseling she believes in, she may succeed in making a smaller but still meaningful change.

Another way to assume the power to make changes is to learn the reasons for the policies of the organization for which you work. Perhaps there are good reasons why certain rules have been established, even if they seem to restrict your freedom in your job. However, if a policy is not in the best interest of your clients, you can begin to challenge the assumptions on which it is based. You can suggest alternative policies, and you can find out whether others on the staff share your view. Forming alliances with colleagues can put you in a better position to suggest changes than operating in isolation.

People often remain powerless because they do not establish their priorities and work on them systematically. In the following section, we consider time management as one strategy for organizing and best using your time to meet your priorities. We've found it helpful to first determine what we *most* want to accomplish in a given position. We recognize that we don't have total autonomy while we're associated with a particular organization, and so at times we're willing to negotiate and compromise. By ordering our priorities, we can decide which compromises we can make without sacrificing our integrity and which positions cannot be compromised in good faith. Knowing what we consider to be most important puts us in a much better position to ask for what we want. In addition, good communication with directors and supervisors is essential. We try to keep the people to whom we report informed about how we're using our time and why. Many times a proposal fails to be accepted not because it's unsound but because the person responsible for approving it has not been adequately informed of its rationale or design. Because supervisors or directors are the ones who will be on the receiving end of any complaints, they may thwart a plan because they haven't been convinced of its merit.

One essential element in learning how to work effectively in any organization is to realize that you are a vital part of that system, that "the institution" is not something that can be divorced from you. This awareness implies that your relationships with other staff members are a central part of the system. Ignoring this reality and attempting to function in isolation will probably diminish your effectiveness. More positively, colleagues can be nourishing and supportive, and your interactions with them can give you a fresh perspective on some of your activities. Furthermore, as we mentioned, genuine relationships with your co-workers can be a way of gaining power to make changes.

Unfortunately, although interactions with others in the institution can be energizing, they can also be debilitating. Instead of developing support groups within an agency, some people form cliques, harbor unspoken hostility, and generally refuse to confront the conflicts or frictions that keep the staff divided. There are often hidden agendas at staff meetings, and only superficial matters are discussed while real issues are kept secret. We want to underscore the importance of finding ways to establish working relationships that enrich your professional life instead of draining your energy. It is ironic that professional helpers, who are supposed to be experts in teaching others to establish nourishing relationships, often complain that they miss meaningful contacts with their colleagues. If you feel isolated, you can decide to take the initiative and arrange for helpful interactions with others on the staff. There are resources that can nourish you, if you reach out for them.

In thinking about the questions we pose below, clarify your position on ways in which you could increase your chances of assuming power in an organization, as well as remaining true to your principles:

- What questions would you raise in a job interview?
- What experiences have you had in encountering resistance to ideas that you wanted to put into practice?
- What would you do if the organization you worked for instituted some policies to which you were strongly opposed?
- What would you do if you believed that some fundamental changes needed to be made in your institution but your colleagues disagreed?
- What would you do if your supervisor continually blocked most of your activities, despite your efforts to keep him or her informed of the reasons for them?

- How would you attempt to make contact with other colleagues if members of your staff seemed to work largely in isolation from one another?
- If your staff seemed to be divided by jealousies, hostilities, or unspoken conflicts, what do you think you would do about the situation?
- What do you consider to be the ethics involved in staying with a job after you've done everything you can to bring about change, but to no avail? (Consider that you are being asked to do things that are against your basic philosophy.)

In working in an agency or an institution, your key challenge will be to maintain your own centeredness and a sense of your priorities. It is easy to become engulfed in the demands placed on you by the agency and, in the process, lose your own perspective on how your professional life fits into your total life plan. You can lose the sense of balance that is needed to maintain your own physical and psychological well-being unless you make the time for personal reflection and find ways to keep your centeredness. One way to put what you are doing in perspective is to learn the skills of time management. We suggest that you consider the value of a time-management program as a key strategy in coping with the stresses of working within any system. The next section discusses that approach.

TIME MANAGEMENT AS A STRATEGY FOR COPING WITH STRESS

We often hear students complaining that there are simply not enough hours in the day and night to do everything they want to do. Ask yourself the degree to which you are satisfied with how you are balancing your needs for work and for leisure. How well do you manage to meet your responsibilities at school, at work, and at home? Are you able to keep up with your studies and still maintain a social life? Is life only work, or do you make any time for play? Is life only play, and do you put off work lest it get in the way of your fun? Time is one thing we have in common, for we all have the same amount of it. Yet how you manage this time to your best advantage is a very individual matter. We offer you some suggestions for ways of keeping better track of what you are doing, what you want to be doing, and what you might do differently. If you'd like further suggestions on time-management strategies, we especially recommend Rice (1992) and Charlesworth and Nathan (1984).

Before you continue reading, spend a few minutes taking the following time-management inventory. It will help you assess the danger signals of poor allocation of time. Read each statement, decide whether it is more true or more false as it applies to you, and rate it accordingly with a T or an F.

_____ 1. I often feel confused and unsure of where I'm going.
_____ 2. At the end of most days I'm amazed at how little I've accomplished.
_____ 3. I have a hard time getting to important tasks and sticking with them.
_____ 4. I often find myself taking on tasks because I'm the only one who can do them.

___ 5. I often feel overwhelmed because I try to do too much in too little time.

___ 6. No matter how much I do, I feel that I'm always behind and never quite caught up.

___ 7. I find that I'm working longer and longer and sometimes wonder if I'm accomplishing much.

___ 8. I frequently miss deadlines.

___ 9. I simply have too many irons in the fire.

___ 10. It's very easy for me to put off until tomorrow what I know needs to be done today.

___ 11. I'm bothered by many unscheduled interruptions when I'm trying to do important work.

___ 12. I'm aware of hurrying much of the time and often feel hassled.

___ 13. I just don't have time to attend to important things, because I get lost in dealing with one crisis after another.

___ 14. I tend to be a perfectionist, and this leaves me never feeling satisfied with what I'm accomplishing.

___ 15. I feel guilty about leaving work behind me.

See whether there are any patterns in the way you are using your time. Are you able to identify particular ways in which you are wasting time? What most gets in the way of your effectively using what time you have? If at the end of a day you often find yourself wondering where your time went, you can probably benefit by doing a time study. Several times a day, stop to record what you have done in each half-hour period and how much time it took. At the end of each week simply look for patterns. Ask yourself questions such as "Where is most of my time going?" "Am I enjoying most of the things I do?" "Is there a way that I could cut out some of the things I'm doing, especially if they're not meaningful?" Merely identifying patterns will be an important first step in finding the areas in which you need to improve your managing of time.

After you have made this inventory of how you use your time, the next step is to find some positive way to stop wasting time. Here are a few suggestions for effective time management:

- Identify your long-range goals, specifying what personal changes you want to make, what kind of interpersonal relationships you'd like to develop and maintain, what activities you'd like to engage in, what projects you'd like to accomplish, and so forth.
- Break down your long-range goals into subgoals that can be accomplished in a shorter period. It might be helpful to prioritize your goals, from most important to least important.
- Realize that if you plan well today you are likely to be more relaxed tomorrow. Allocate your time according to your priorities. Build recreation time into your schedule.
- Learn to thin out your schedule somewhat. Realize that you probably won't be able to do all that you need or want to do in any given week. Therefore, focus on what you see as most essential, and prune those activities that are cluttering your life.

- Avoid procrastination. Keeping a schedule of what you have to do and when it must be done can give you some sense of pacing yourself. If you know that waiting until the very end causes you stress and makes you function poorly, you could at least experiment with getting certain assignments or tasks completed before the last minute.
- If you become aware of activities that distract you from doing the important things in your life, write down these time wasters and ways to avoid them. Then, before you engage in these activities again, pause to ask yourself if you are willing to use your time in such a manner.
- Learn to delegate. Rather than convincing yourself that you are the only one who can do certain tasks, learn to ask for help and to assign specific tasks to others. Even if some tasks do not get done as well as they might if you had done them yourself, ask yourself if this isn't a better arrangement.
- Reflect when others ask you to take on new projects. Before you say yes, make sure that you really want to accept such a project.
- Try to do a task only once. Rather than dealing with paperwork several times, make a quick decision the first time a document comes your way. If you can throw it away rather than filing it, do so.

Effective use of time is not something that simply happens to you. Instead, it is a skill that you acquire and refine. It is essential to write down your goals and then plan how to spend the time you have. You might organize your schedule by having a "to-do list" that ranks activities from high priority to low. At the end of each week and each month, review your activities in light of your long-range and short-range goals to determine whether you are putting your time to best use. If you practice a systematic approach to time management, you will probably find that you have more time to use in ways that are meaningful to you.

Here are a few suggestions for developing a systematic approach to managing your time:

- Schedule fixed responsibilities first—classes, work hours, and so forth—then work your study times and other activities around the fixed commitments.
- Figure out your peak-performance, high-energy times and schedule difficult and high-priority tasks then. Adjust your schedule around the times when you get the most done and when you'll have the fewest interruptions.
- Leave some unscheduled time for yourself and for unexpected tasks and opportunities.
- Try out your plan for a couple of weeks to see how well it works for you, but be open to revising it. Plans are designed to help you manage your life, not to control you. Realize that it takes time to break old habits and to establish new and more functional ones.
- Create a long-term to-do list that includes all major projects and other critical dates for the term. Put all the due dates on a semester calendar or schedule.
- Schedule time to do some of the things you enjoy doing. Including yourself in your schedule is one important step in preventing burnout, a topic that we take up next.

OTHER STEPS IN THE PREVENTION OF BURNOUT

Because professional burnout is an internal phenomenon that becomes obvious to others only in its advanced stages, you should take special care to recognize your own limits. How you approach your tasks and what you get from doing them are more important than how much you're doing. Ultimately, whether you experience burnout depends on how well you monitor the effects that the stresses of your work have on you and on the quality of your helping.

As you saw in the last chapter, many sources contribute to the process of burnout, so it stands to reason that many paths can be taken to combat it. You can do much personally to lessen the chances of burning out or to restore yourself. Individual strategies alone, however, are not enough. You need to make effective use of others as a source of support, which requires that you learn certain interpersonal skills. There is also the organizational level to consider. Institutions certainly do contribute to burnout, and they can develop strategies for its prevention. This section considers some of the individual, interpersonal, and organizational strategies for coping with the ongoing problem of professional burnout.

You Have Control over Yourself

We have suggested that to a large extent you create your own stress by the interpretation you give to events. Although you cannot always control these events, you can control how you react to them and the stance you take toward your life. If you are responsible for contributing to your physical and emotional exhaustion, you can also take action to change this condition. An important step is to realize that you are not an omnipotent being and that you cannot be the eternal giver to the universe. If you attempt this impossible dream, you ought to be prepared for the price you'll pay. Become attuned to the danger signals that you are being depleted, and take seriously your own need for nurturing and for recognition. What follows are some thoughts on what you can do to lessen the chances that you will get stuck in the rut of disillusionment. We do not present these ideas dogmatically but more in the spirit of encouraging you to develop your own strategy for keeping yourself alive personally and professionally.

- Examine your behavior to determine if it is working for you. You can ask yourself: "Is what I am doing what I really want to be doing? If not, why am I continuing in this direction?" "What are some things I want to be doing professionally that I am not doing? Who or what is stopping me?" "Am I accepting projects that I really want to reject? If so, why is it so difficult for me to say no?" Once you have answered some of these questions for yourself in an honest way, decide what action to take. For example, if you often say yes when you really want to firmly say no, you can begin to change this behavior.
- Look at your expectations to determine whether they are realistic. Although you may have initially become a helper because you wanted to create a better world, it is essential to temper your ideals with reality if you

are to avoid continual frustration. You may expect that you can be all things to all people, and you may think that it is your mission in life always to be available for anyone who needs you. These self-expectations will eventually wear you down. Even though it is hard to accept, there are clients whom you will not be able to help. Regardless of how much you have to offer others, there is a limit to what you can give.

- Recognize that you can be an active agent in your life. If you allow yourself to get into a rut of hopelessness and helplessness, you will feel that your destiny is out of your control.
- Find other sources of meaning besides your work. These activities and interests can help you at least temporarily escape from job stresses and keep a balance in your life.
- Granted that there are some unpleasant aspects about your job that may be difficult to change, you can approach your work differently. You can rearrange your schedule to reduce your stress. If you have some exceptionally difficult clients, for example, you can avoid seeing them one after the other. You can also look for new ways to bring your talents and interests to your work—for example, by exchanging jobs with a colleague for a time. If you stop blaming the institution for your problems and start assuming more control of your own destiny, this shift alone can make a key difference.
- It is easy to become overwhelmed by thinking about all the things that you feel powerless to change. Instead, focus on the aspects of your work that you have the power to change. Creativity grinds to a halt when most of your time is spent thinking of all that you cannot do rather than thinking about what you are able to do, within the limits that are imposed on you.
- Learn your own limits, and strive to avoid overextending yourself in an agency. Others might not make this easy, so it will take considerable self-discipline to maintain your limits. This means that you will have to struggle with clients who demand things from you that you are not willing to give. The same is true for those who employ you. If you have ignored setting limits, it may be extremely difficult to change this pattern, but it is not impossible.
- Look to colleagues and friends. Don't try to internalize all of your concerns and deal with them alone. Colleagues who face the same realities as you on the job can provide you with new information, insights, and perspectives. In the helping professions, the companionship of colleagues can be your greatest asset.
- Create a support group. If you wait for the system to organize a formal support group for you and your co-workers, you may have a long and frustrating wait. You can take the initiative to organize your colleagues to listen to one another and provide help. Do not get caught in the trap of using these meetings as mere gripe sessions. Instead, come up with alternative ways of approaching problems, and think of new ways to find hope.

Rather than wait until you are hit with a chronic case of burnout, recognize the early signs, and take remedial action quickly. Don't deceive yourself into thinking that only your colleagues will burn out while you will retain your unbounded enthusiasm forever. According to Maslach (1982), it's never too early to be thinking of ways to prevent burnout. She stresses that detecting the first signs of burnout is critical, for the condition can be dealt with more effectively in the initial stages. During the formative stages the symptoms are not so severe, the individual is still committed and caring, and there is more receptivity to change. In the course of many interviews as part of her research on burnout, Maslach heard a constant refrain of "Why didn't anyone tell me that this was what I was in for?" Over and over she found that helpers were ignorant and ill-prepared to cope with the emotional stresses of being a helping professional. They simply had not been made aware of the potential difficulties involved in working with people.

Several people in the healing professions told us of their personal strategies to prevent burnout:

- "To prevent burnout, I try to exercise daily, take personal time out with friends, go to personal therapy, and talk with co-workers and supervisors."
- "I plan my schedule carefully and make sure not to overextend myself. I take time off for vacations."
- "I take time out for myself to have fun. I do things like reading junk novels, shopping, spending time with my family, and going on vacations, and I always pat myself on the back for all my accomplishments."
- "I learn to say no and set limitations for myself. I try to allow as much time for play as I do for work, and I always try to leave my job at work."
- "I try to manage my time well. I reward myself with little presents. I take time off to go for a bike ride, go out for dinner, or take a bubble bath."
- "I don't bring work home with me. I try to leave my paperwork at school. I also take days off to relax when I need them."
- "I prevent burnout by doing a variety of things such as teaching, taking personal time out, writing, spending time with colleagues doing workshops, and spending lazy time off by being nonproductive."
- "I do my best to focus on those work activities where I can see results. Since I can do only so much with the time I have, I look for ways to get involved in projects that seem personally meaningful."
- "One strategy for coping with the resistance of administrators and colleagues is to deal with it much as I deal with the resistance of my clients. It helps me keep my perspective if I don't take the resistance I encounter personally."

A couple, both social workers, remind themselves continually not to become overwhelmed by the myriad of demands, not to lose sight of why they are in the agency, and not to get lost by being a cog in the production line. They have managed to temper their idealism by accepting that they cannot do everything they wanted to do. They are continuing to learn to cut down rather than taking on more and more. To prevent getting caught in a comfortable rut, they are creative in finding ways to vary their activities. They work with children and adults, co-lead groups, supervise interns, teach, and give in-service presentations. They attempt to develop a tolerant perspective when the agency acts in a petty way, which they do partly by keeping a sense of humor. They both assess their priorities and maintain limits. To be sure, this is not a simple matter but, instead, involves a commitment to self-assessment and an openness to change.

Ways of Staying Alive Personally and Professionally

What can you do not only to prevent yourself from becoming burned out but also to promote your wellness from a holistic perspective? Perhaps the most basic way to retain your vitality as a person and as a professional is to realize that you are not a bottomless pit and cannot give and give without replenishing your reserve. People often ignore signs that they are becoming depleted. They may view themselves as having unlimited capacities to give, and at the same time they may not pay attention to taking care of their needs for nurturing, recognition, and support. However, simply recognizing that you cannot be a universal giver without getting something in return is not enough to keep you alive as a person and a professional. What is needed is an action plan and the commitment to carry out this plan. Learning to cope with personal and professional sources of stress generally involves making some fundamental changes in your lifestyle. At this point, take some time to ask yourself what basic changes, if any, you are willing to make.

Your personal strategy.   The following is a list of suggestions for dealing with burnout. Of course, you need to find your own way of remaining vital as a professional; our purpose in presenting this list is to stimulate you to think of your own methods of preventing or treating burnout. After you think about each suggestion, rate each one by using the following code: A = this approach would be very meaningful to me; B = this approach would have some value for me; C = this approach would have little value for me.

_____ 1. Think of ways to bring variety into my work.
_____ 2. Become involved in peer-group meetings where a support system is available.
_____ 3. Find other interests besides my work.
_____ 4. Attend to my health, and take care of my body by exercising and eating well.
_____ 5. Determine whether what I am doing is meaningful or draining.
_____ 6. Do some of the things now that I plan to do when I retire.
_____ 7. Take time for myself to do some of the things that I enjoy doing.
_____ 8. Avoid assuming an inordinate amount of responsibility.
_____ 9. Attend a personal-growth group or some type of personal therapy experience to work on my level of vitality.
_____ 10. Travel or seek new experiences.
_____ 11. Read stimulating books, and do some personal writing.
_____ 12. Exchange jobs for a time with a colleague.
_____ 13. Find nourishment with family and friends.
_____ 14. Work at modifying repetitively stressful situations.
_____ 15. Find a person who will confront and challenge me and who will encourage me to look at what I'm doing.

_____ 16. Take short focusing and relaxing breaks during the day.

_____ 17. Learn to ask for what I want, even though I may not always get it.

_____ 18. Learn how to work for my own affirmation of my worth rather than looking for external validation.

_____ 19. Make time for my spiritual development.

_____ 20. Rearrange my schedule to reduce stress.

_____ 21. Learn my limits, and learn to set my limits with others.

_____ 22. Pursue some hobbies or do things I truly enjoy.

_____ 23. Get enough rest and sleep.

_____ 24. Take the initiative to begin new projects that have meaning to me.

_____ 25. Become active in a professional organization.

It may help to keep in mind that burnout is not always acute; rather, it is a cumulative process. You can handle only so much stress, and eventually you must pay the price in terms of your physical and psychological health. Recognizing the signs that you are on a path toward impairment demands a high level of honesty. You need to be alert to the subtle indications and then be willing to take action to remedy a situation that will inevitably result in burnout. It would be good to reflect on ways in which you can take care of yourself, as well as being concerned with being a helper to others.

Our personal experiences with preventing burnout.   We would like to share with you our own struggles with burnout and the measures we take to keep ourselves fresh. First of all, even though we are aware of the dangers of burnout, we are not immune to it. At different times throughout our professional lives we have lost a sense of enthusiasm, become cynical, felt depressed, and wanted to withdraw and get away from it all. We have come to realize that the answer does not lie merely in cutting out activities that we don't enjoy. Much of what we do professionally we like very much, and we have to remind ourselves that we cannot accept all the attractive projects that we may be interested in. The psychological and financial rewards, however high and tempting, do not always compensate for the emotional and physical depletion that results from an overscheduled professional life. At one time, for example, we scheduled as many as six weeklong residential groups a year, all of which were held at our home. Although these groups were professionally rewarding, it took a great deal of energy to lead them, and it necessitated rearranging our personal life. Now we limit ourselves to two of these weeklong groups, both of which we do in the summer when we have fewer demands from our regular jobs. In another instance we became aware that too many of our "vacations" were coupled with professional commitments such as giving a workshop or attending a convention. Although we see this mixture as a good balance, we nevertheless realized that we missed real vacations that were separate from any professional commitments.

Another way in which we attempt to prevent burnout is to pay attention to the early signals that we are overextending ourselves, and we involve ourselves in diverse projects. We engage in a variety of professional tasks, such as teaching, consulting, doing groups and workshops, and writing books. Besides offering our services to others, we recognize our need for input from others in the field, and we attend workshops for our own personal and professional development. Being aware of the demands that our profession puts on us, we are highly conscious of living a healthy lifestyle. Therefore, we pay attention to our nutritional habits, and no matter how busy we are, we make the time that we need for adequate rest and regular exercise. As part of our lifestyle, we made the decision to live in a remote mountain community. But this remoteness and our busy schedules kept us, at times, from seeing our friends and colleagues. We had to realize that we could easily separate ourselves too much from relationships that were much needed and a source of joy and support for us. Thus, we made extra efforts to schedule blocks of time with our friends and to maintain and to nourish these valued relationships.

BY WAY OF REVIEW

- Because it is next to impossible to eliminate stress from your life, the crucial question is "Does stress control you, or do you control stress?"
- You do not have to be the victim of stress, for you have the capacity to recognize situations that lead to stress, and you can make decisions about how you will think, feel, and behave in response to these situations.
- Preventive strategies for coping with stress include avoiding or reducing stressors, altering stress-inducing behavior patterns, and acquiring coping skills.
- There are also combative strategies for coping with stress. Self-monitoring is the first step in developing an effective stress-management program.
- Some of the most useful ways of managing stress are the cognitive approaches. These include changing your distorted self-talk, learning time-management skills, and applying them to daily life in a systematic fashion.
- Learning to recognize and cope with the reality of professional burnout is essential for your survival as a helper. Intense involvement with people over a period of time can lead to physical and psychological exhaustion.
- Because burnout is not something that suddenly happens to you, recognizing the early signs is an important step toward prevention.
- If you work in an agency, it is a challenge to retain your integrity, sense of direction, enthusiasm, and vitality. It is important to learn specific ways of surviving with dignity in an organization.
- If you work in an environment where there is a great deal of negativity, it is good to seek sources of positive support, both on your job and at home.
- Just as there are many sources of burnout, there are multiple ways to prevent and combat it. Individual, interpersonal, and organizational strategies can be devised.

WHAT WILL YOU DO NOW?

1. Make a poster that contains the essence of a cognition that is producing stress in your life. For instance, if you tell yourself "I must be perfect in everything I try," create a poster that captures this idea. Now, make another poster that challenges this idea, such as "It's human to be imperfect, and since I'm human,

it's OK for me to be imperfect!" Try acting as if you really believed your counter-message poster for at least a week, and record how you are doing in different situations.

2. If you have trouble doing everything that you want with the time you have available, consider trying the time-management strategies that we described. Keep a written record of what you do in the coming week. At the end of the week, review your activities, and ask yourself if you are spending the time you have in the ways you want.

3. Find a person in the helping professions who is willing to be interviewed about burnout. Focus your discussion with this person on what he or she does to keep alive personally and professionally. Questions to consider are "What do you find to be the major source of burnout?" "What do you do to prevent burnout?"

4. Think about how you are when you are at work and when you are on vacation. Ask someone who knows you in both situations to describe you in these situations. Does this person see you as the same in both contexts, or different? Use this exercise as a way of thinking about how your work affects your personal life.

5. Consider Covey's (1990) statement in *The Seven Habits of Highly Effective People* that "the self-renewal process must include balanced renewal in all four dimensions of our nature: the physical, the spiritual, the mental, and the social/emotional" (p. 301). Identify some specific ways you can achieve greater balance in your life to continue your self-renewal process. In your journal write down some ideas about patterns that you may want to change to enhance the balance in your life. Then make an action plan that will assist you in coping with stress by using some of the preventive and combative strategies discussed in this chapter.

6. For the full bibliographic entry for each of the sources listed below, consult the References and Reading List at the back of the book.

See Kottler (1997) for various articles on topics such as feeling lost as a counselor, helpers confronting themselves, making a difference, recognition, transitions and transformations, and reaching out. In this book, individuals address the challenges they have faced in retaining their vitality in the helping professions.

See Charlesworth and Nathan (1984) for a practical guidebook for coping with stress. See Corey, Corey, and Corey (1997) for chapters dealing with issues such as taking care of your health, time management, stress management, and coping with crisis. Also see G. Corey and M. Corey (1997) for ideas on self-renewal and retaining your vitality. For cognitive techniques in learning ways of disputing dysfunctional beliefs that often lead to stress, see Ellis (1988), Meichenbaum (1985), and Emery (1981). For time management, see Lakein (1974).

Concluding Comments

You can get into a powerless stance if you become overly ambitious and try to fill the bill of an "ideal helper." Remember that the challenges we have presented throughout these chapters do not have to be addressed immediately or all at once. You will always want to accomplish more than there is time for, so identify clear priorities of what you most want to accomplish. Setting priorities is essential if you want to maintain a sense of stability. At this point, we encourage you to dream and allow yourself to envision the helper you want to become. You can begin now to reach your visions by becoming an active and questioning student and by putting yourself fully into your fieldwork activities. We hope you will become excited by your journey of self-exploration as you learn about the helping professions.

The process of becoming a helper is intrinsically related to the process of becoming a person. In this book we have emphasized the importance of looking at your life and of understanding your motivations. Although it is not essential for you to be problem-free, we have stressed the importance of being a model for your clients. Reflect on whether what you do in your own life is what you encourage for your clients. If you urge your clients to take the risks that growth entails, it is essential that you do this in your own life.

This is a good time to reflect on the personal meaning this book has held for you. Do you still think the helping professions are for you? What do you think you can bring to your work? How might your work affect your personal life? What are the greatest challenges you expect to face? Do you now have a different perspective on the concerns that were addressed in this book? At this point, what do you see as your major strengths and some of your limitations? What steps could you take to work on your limitations? How can you build on your strengths?

Now that you have completed the book, read the focus questions at the beginning of each chapter again. Can you answer all of these questions now? Have your answers to some of these questions changed as you have acquired new knowledge from the book and in your course? We highly recommend that you also look at the key points at the end of each chapter in the *By Way of Review* section as a way to consolidate your key learnings. Finally, from the *What Will You Do Now?* section at the end of each chapter, choose one activity that is meaningful to you and that you are willing to pursue. Challenge yourself to extend your learning experience by taking the initiative to complete these projects on your own. If you have been keeping a journal, continue to write about the experiences you are having in your training program as a way to extend the self-reflection process. Best of luck in your continuing journey!

Appendix

A GUIDE TO PROFESSIONAL ORGANIZATIONS

It is a good idea while a student to begin your identification with state, regional, and national professional associations. To assist you in learning about student memberships, here is an annotated listing of some of the major national professional organizations along with a summary of their student membership benefits.

American Counseling Association (ACA)

The ACA has 56 state branches and 4 regional branch assemblies. Students qualify for a special annual membership rate of $59.50 and half the rate for membership in any of the 16 member associations or divisions. Student memberships are available to both undergraduate and graduate students enrolled at least half-time or more at the college level.

ACA membership provides many benefits, including a subscription to the *Journal of Counseling and Development* and a monthly newspaper entitled *Counseling Today*, eligibility for professional liability insurance programs, legal defense services, and professional development through workshops and conventions. A copy of ACA's *Code of Ethics and Standards of Practice* (1995) is available. ACA puts out a resource catalog that provides information on the various aspects of the counseling profession, as well as giving detailed information about membership, journals, books, home-study programs, videotapes, audio-tapes, and liability insurance. For further information, contact:

American Counseling Association
5999 Stevenson Avenue
Alexandria, VA 22304-3300
(703) 823-9800 or (800) 347-6647

National Board for Certified Counselors (NBCC)

The NBCC offers a certification program for counselors. National Certified Counselors (NCC) meet the generic professional standards established by the board and agree to abide by the *NBCC Code of Ethics* (1989). NCCs work in a variety of educational and social service settings such as schools, private practice, mental-health agencies, correctional facilities, community agencies, rehabilitation agencies, and business and industry. To qualify for an NCC, candidates must meet both the educational and professional counseling experience minimum requirements established by the NBCC. For a copy of the *NBCC Code of Ethics* (1989) and further information about becoming a National Certified Counselor, contact:

National Board for Certified Counselors
3-D Terrace Way
Greensboro, NC 27403
(910) 547-0607
(800) 398-5389 (application request line)

National Organization for Human Service Education (NOHSE)

The National Organization for Human Service Education's (NOHSE) focus is on supporting and promoting improvements in direct service, public education, program development, planning and evaluation, administration, and public policy. Members are drawn from diverse disciplines—mental health, child care, social services, gerontology, recreation, corrections, and developmental disabilities. Membership is open to human-service educators, students, fieldwork supervisors, and direct-care professionals. Student membership is $15 per year, which includes a subscription to the newsletter (*Link*), the yearly journal *Human Services Education*, and a discounted price for the yearly conference (held in October). For further information about membership in the National Organization for Human Service Education, contact:

> Douglas A. Whyte, Membership Chair
> Membership, NOHSE
> Community College of Philadelphia
> 1700 Spring Garden Street
> Philadelphia, PA 19130-3991
> (215) 751-8522 or (215) 751-8000

American Association for Marriage and Family Therapy (AAMFT)

The AAMFT has a student membership category. You must obtain an official application and include the names of at least two Clinical Members from whom the association can request official endorsements. You also need a statement signed by the coordinator or director of a graduate program in marital and family therapy in a regionally accredited educational institution verifying your current enrollment. Student membership may be held until receipt of a qualifying graduate degree, or for a maximum of five years. Members receive the *Journal of Marital and Family Therapy*, which is published four times a year, and a subscription to six issues yearly of *Family Therapy News*. For a copy of the *AAMFT Code of Ethics* (1991), membership applications, and further information, write to:

> American Association for Marriage and Family Therapy
> 1133 Fifteenth Street, N.W., Suite 300
> Washington, DC 20005-2710
> (202) 452-0109

National Association of Social Workers (NASW)

NASW membership is open to all professional social workers. The NASW Press, which produces *Social Work* and the *NASW News* as membership benefits, is a major service in professional development. NASW has a number of pamphlets available including these regarding practice standards:

- *Standards and Guidelines for Social Work Case Management for the Functionally Impaired*
- *Standards for the Practice of Clinical Social Work*
- *Standards for Social Work in Health Care Settings*
- *Standards for Social Work Practice in Child Protection*
- *Standards for Social Work Services in Long-Term Care Facilities*
- *Standards for Social Work Services in Schools*

For a copy of any of the above pamphlets, or for a copy of *The National Association of Social Workers Code of Ethics* (1996), or for information on membership categories and benefits, write to:

> National Association of Social Workers
> 750 First Street, N.E., Suite 700
> Washington, DC 20002-4241
> (202) 408-8600 or (800) 638-8799
> FAX (202) 336-8312

American Psychological Association (APA)

The APA has a Student Affiliates category rather than student membership. Journals and subscriptions are extra. Each year in mid-August or late August the APA holds a national convention. For further information or for a copy of the *Ethical Principles of*

Psychologists and Code of Conduct (1995), write to:

American Psychological Association
1200 17th Street, N.W.
Washington, DC 20036
(202) 955-7600

In addition to the national organization, there are seven regional divisions, each of which has an annual convention. For addresses or information about student membership in any of them, contact the main office of the APA or see a copy of the association's monthly journal, *American Psychologist*.

A number of APA publications may be of interest to you. The following can be ordered from:

American Psychological Association
Order Department
P. O. Box 2710
Hyattsville, MD 20784-0710
(703) 247-7705

1. *Specialty Guidelines for Delivery of Services by Psychologists*
   - "Delivery of Services by Clinical Psychologists"
   - "Delivery of Services by Counseling Psychologists"
   - "Delivery of Services by School Psychologists"
   - "Delivery of Services by Industrial/Organizational Psychologists"
2. *Careers in Psychology* (pamphlet)
3. *How to Manage Your Career in Psychology*
4. *Is Psychology the Major for You? Planning for Your Undergraduate Years*
5. *Graduate Study in Psychology and Associated Fields.* Information on graduate programs in the United States and Canada, including staff/student statistics, financial aid deadlines, tuition, teaching opportunities, housing, degree requirements, and program goals.
6. *Preparing for Graduate Study: Not for Seniors Only!*
7. *Ethnic Minority Perspectives on Clinical Training and Services in Psychology*
8. *Toward Ethnic Diversification in Psychology Education and Training*
9. *Ethical Principles in the Conduct of Research with Human Participants*
10. *Standards for Educational and Psychological Testing.* Revised standards for evaluating the quality of tests, testing practices, and the effects of test use. There are also chapters on licensure, certification, and program evaluation. New in this edition are chapters on testing linguistic minorities and the rights of test takers.

References

and Reading List

American Association for Marriage and Family Therapy. (1991). *AAMFT code of ethics.* Washington, DC: Author.

American Counseling Association (1995). *Code of ethics and standards of practice.* Alexandria, VA: Author.

American Psychological Association. (1993). Guidelines for providers of psychological services to ethnic, linguistic, and culturally diverse populations. *American Psychologist, 48*(1), 45–48.

American Psychological Association. (1995). *Ethical principles of psychologists and code of conduct.* Washington, DC: Author.

Anderson, M. J., & Ellis, R. (1988). On the reservation. In N. A. Vacc, J. Wittmer, & S. B. DeVaney (Eds.), *Experiencing and counseling multicultural and diverse populations* (2nd ed.) (pp. 107–126). Muncie, IN: Accelerated Development.

Anderson, S. K., & Kitchener, K. S. (1996). Nonromantic, nonsexual posttherapy relationships between psychologists and former clients: An exploratory study of critical incidents. *Professional Psychology: Research and Practice, 27*(1), 59–66.

Arredondo, P., Toporek, R., Brown, S., Jones, J., Locke, D., Sanchez, J., & Stadler, H. (1996). Operationalization of multicultural counseling competencies. *Journal of Multicultural Counseling and Devlopment, 24*(1), 42–78.

Association for Counselor Education and Supervision. (1993, Summer). Ethical guidelines for counseling supervisors. *Spectrum, 53*(4), 3–8.

Association for Specialists in Goup Work. (1989). *Ethical guidelines for group counselors.* Alexandria, VA: Author.

Association for Specialists in Group Work. (1991, Fall). Professional standards for the training of group workers. *Together, 20*(1), 9–14. Alexandria, VA: Author.

Association for Specialists in Group Work. (1992). Professional standards for the training of group workers. *Journal for Specialists in Group Work, 17*(1), 12–19.

Atkinson, D. R., Morten, G., & Sue, D. W. (Eds.). (1993). *Counseling American minorities: A cross cultural perspective* (4th ed.). Dubuque, IA: Brown & Benchmark.

Atkinson, D. R., Thompson, C. E., & Grant, S. K. (1993). A three-dimensional model for counseling racial/ethnic minorities. *The Counseling Psychologist, 21*(2), 257–277.

Attneave, C. L. (1985). Practical counseling with American Indian and Alaska native clients. In P. Pedersen (Ed.), *Handbook of cross-cultural counseling and therapy* (pp. 135–140). Westport, CT: Greenwood Press.

Austin, K. M., Moline, M. M., & Williams, G. T. (1990). *Confronting malpractice: Legal and ethical dilemmas in psychotherapy.* Newbury Park, CA: Sage.

Avila, D. L., & Avila, A. L. (1988). Mexican-Americans. In N. A. Vacc, J. Wittmer, & S. B. DeVaney (Eds.), *Experiencing and counseling multicultural and diverse populations* (2nd ed.) (pp. 289–316). Muncie, IN: Accelerated Development.

Baird, B. N. (1996). *The internship, practicum, and field placement handbook: A guide for the helping professions.* Upper Saddle River, NJ: Prentice-Hall.

Bartell, P. A., & Rubin, L. J. (1990). Dangerous liaisons: Sexual intimacies in supervision. *Professional Psychology: Research and Practice, 21*(6), 442–450.

Beck, A. T. (1976). *Cognitive therapy and the emotional disorders.* New York: New American Library.

Beck, A. T. (1987). Cognitive therapy. In J. K. Zeig (Ed.), *The evolution of psychotherapy* (pp. 149–178). New York: Brunner/Mazel.

Beck, A. T., & Weishaar, M. E. (1995). Cognitive therapy. In R. J. Corsini & D. Wedding (Eds.), *Current psychotherapies* (5th ed.) (pp. 229–261). Itasca, IL: F. E. Peacock.

Becvar, D. S., & Becvar, R. J. (1996). *Family therapy: A systemic integration* (3rd ed.). Needham Heights, MA: Allyn & Bacon.

Bednar, R. L., Bednar, S. C., Lambert, M. J., & Waite, D. R. (1991). *Psychotherapy with high-risk clients: Legal and professional standards.* Pacific Grove, CA: Brooks/Cole.

Bennett, B. E., Bryant, B. K., VandenBos, G. R., & Greenwood, A. (1990). *Professional liability and risk management.* Washington, DC: American Psychological Association.

Bergin, A. E. (1991). Values and religious issues in psychotherapy and mental health. *American Psychology, 46*(4), 393–403.

Bersoff, D. N. (1995). *Ethical conflicts in psychology.* Washington, DC: American Psychological Association.

Bersoff, D. N. (1996). The virtue of principle ethics. *The Counseling Psychologist, 24*(1), 86–91.

Bitter, J. R. (1987). Communication and meaning. Satir in Adlerian context. In R. Sherman & D. Dinkmeyer (Eds.), *Systems of family therapy: An Adlerian integration* (pp. 109–142). New York: Brunner/Mazel.

Bitter, J. R. (1988). Family mapping and family constellation: Satir in Adlerian context. *Individual Psychology: The Journal of Adlerian Theory, Research, and Practice, 44*(1), 106–111.

Borders, L. D. (1991). A systematic approach to peer group supervision. *Journal of Counseling and Development, 69*(3), 248–252.

Borders, L. D., & Leddick, G. R. (1987). *Handbook of counseling supervision.* Alexandria, VA: American Association for Counseling and Development.

Brammer, L. M. (1985). Nonformal support in cross-cultural counseling and therapy. In P. Pedersen (Ed.), *Handbook of cross-cultural counseling and therapy* (pp. 87–92). Westport, CT: Greenwood Press.

Brammer, L. M. (1993). *The helping relationship: Process and skills* (5th ed.). Boston: Allyn & Bacon.

Brockett, D. R., & Gleckman, A. D. (1991). Countertransference with the older adult: The importance of mental health counselor awareness and strategies for effective management. *Journal of Mental Health Counseling, 13*(3), 343–355.

Burke, M. T., & Miranti, J. G. (Eds.). (1995). *Counseling: The spiritual dimension.* Alexandria, VA: American Counseling Association.

Butler, P. E. (1981). *Talking to yourself: Learning the language of self-support.* San Francisco: Harper & Row.

Calfee, B. E. (1997). Lawsuit prevention techniques. In *The Hatherleigh guide to ethics in therapy.* New York: Hatherleigh Press.

Canter, M. B., Bennett, B. E., Jones, S. E., & Nagy, T. F. (1994). *Ethics for psychologists: A commentary on the APA ethics code.* Washington, DC: American Psychological Association.

Carlson, J., Sperry, L., & Lewis, J. A. (1997). *Family therapy: Ensuring treatment efficacy.* Pacific Grove, CA: Brooks/Cole.

Casey, K., & Vanceburg, M. (1985). *The promise of a new day: A book of daily meditations.* New York: Harper/Hazelden.

Charlesworth, E. A., & Nathan, R. G. (1984). *Stress management: A comprehensive guide to wellness.* New York: Random House (Ballantine).

Chiaferi, R., & Griffin, M. (1997). *Developing fieldwork skills: A guide for human services, counseling, and social work students.* Pacific Grove, CA: Brooks/Cole.

Clay, R. A. (1996a). Psychologists' faith in religion begins to grow. *APA Monitor, 27*(8), 1 & 48.

Clay, R. A. (1996b). Religion and psychology share ideals and beliefs. *APA Monitor, 27*(8), 47.

Conyne, R. K., Wilson, F. R., Kline, W. B., Morran, D. K., & Ward, D. E. (1993). Training group workers: Implications of the new ASGW training standards for training and practice. *Journal for Specialists in Group Work, 18*(1), 11–23.

Corey, G. (1995). *Theory and practice of group counseling* (4th ed.) and *Manual.* Pacific Grove, CA: Brooks/Cole.

Corey, G. (1996a). *Case approach to counseling and psychotherapy* (4th ed.). Pacific Grove, CA: Brooks/Cole.

Corey, G. (1996b). *Theory and practice of counseling and psychotherapy* (4th ed.) and *Manual.* Pacific Grove, CA: Brooks/Cole.

Corey, G., Corey, C., & Corey, H. (1997). *Living and learning.* Belmont, CA: Wadsworth.

Corey, G., & Corey, M. (1997). *I never knew I had a choice* (6th ed.). Pacific Grove, CA: Brooks/Cole.

Corey, G., Corey, M., & Callanan, P. (1998). *Issues and ethics in the helping professions* (5th ed.). Pacific Grove, CA: Brooks/Cole.

Corey, G., Corey, M., Callanan, P., & Russell, J. M. (1992). *Group techniques* (2nd ed.). Pacific Grove, CA: Brooks/Cole.

Corey, G., & Herlihy, B. (1996a). Client rights and informed consent. In B. Herlihy & G. Corey (Eds.), *ACA ethical standards casebook* (5th ed.) (pp. 181–183). Alexandria, VA: American Counseling Association.

Corey, G., & Herlihy, B. (1996b). Competence. In B. Herlihy & G. Corey (Eds.), *ACA ethical standards casebook* (5th ed.) (pp. 217–220). Alexandria, VA: American Counseling Association.

Corey, G., & Herlihy, B. (1996c). Counselor training and supervision. In B. Herlihy & G. Corey (Eds.), *ACA ethical standards casebook* (5th ed.) (pp. 275–278). Alexandria, VA: American Counseling Association.

Corey, G., & Herlihy, B. (1997). Dual/multiple relationships: Toward a consensus of thinking. In *The Hatherleigh guide to ethics in therapy* (pp. 193–205). New York: Hatherleigh Press.

Corey, M., & Corey, G. (1993). Difficult group members—difficult group leaders. *New York State Association for Counseling and Development, 8*(2), 9–24.

Corey, M., & Corey, G. (1997). *Groups: Process and practice* (5th ed.). Pacific Grove, CA: Brooks/Cole.

Cormier, S., & Hackney, H. (1993). *The professional counselor: A process guide to helping* (2nd ed.). Boston: Allyn & Bacon.

Covey, S. R. (1990). *The seven habits of highly effective people: Restoring the character ethic.* New York: Simon & Schuster (Fireside Book).

Crawford, I., Humfleet, G., Ribordy, S. C., Ho, F. C., & Vickers, V. L. (1991). Stigmatization of AIDS patients by mental health professionals. *Professional Psychology: Research and Practice, 22*(5), 357–361.

Cummings, N. A. (1995). Impact of managed care on employment and training: A primer for survival. *Professional Psychology: Research and Practice, 26*(1), 10–15.

D'Andrea, M., & Daniels, J. (1991). Exploring the different levels of multicultural counseling training in counselor education. *Journal of Counseling & Development, 70*(1), 78–85.

Devore, W. (1985). Developing ethnic sensitivity for the counseling process: A social-work perspective. In P. Pedersen (Ed.), *Handbook of cross-cultural counseling and therapy* (pp. 93–98). Westport, CT: Greenwood Press.

Dinkmeyer, D. C., Dinkmeyer, D. C., Jr., & Sperry, L. (1987). *Adlerian counseling and psychotherapy* (2nd ed.). Columbus, OH: Charles E. Merrill.

Donigian, J., & Malnati, R. (1997). *Systemic group therapy: A triadic model.* Pacific Grove, CA: Brooks/Cole.

Doyle, R. E. (1992). *Essential skills and strategies in the helping process.* Pacific Grove, CA: Brooks/Cole.

Dworkin, S. H., & Gutierrez, F. J. (1992). *Counseling gay men and lesbians: Journey to the end of the rainbow.* Alexandria, VA: American Association for Counseling and Development.

Egan, G. (1994). *The skilled helper: A problem-management approach to helping* (5th ed.). Pacific Grove, CA: Brooks/Cole.

Elkins, D. N. (1994, August). *Toward a soulful psychology: Introduction and overview.* Paper presented at the meeting of the American Psychological Association, Los Angeles.

Ellis, A. (1985). *Overcoming resistance: Rational-emotive therapy with difficult clients.* New York: Springer.

Ellis, A. (1986). Rational-emotive therapy approaches to overcoming resistance. In A. Ellis & R. Grieger (Eds.), *Handbook of rational-emotive therapy* (Vol. 2, pp. 246–274). New York: Springer.

Ellis, A. (1988). *How to stubbornly refuse to make yourself miserable about anything—yes, anything!* Secaucus, NJ: Lyle Stuart.

Ellis, A. (1995). Rational emotive behavior therapy. In R. J. Corsini & D. Wedding (Eds.), *Current psychotherapies* (5th ed.) (pp. 162–196). Itasca, IL: F. E. Peacock.

Ellis, A., & Bernard, M. E. (1986). What is rational-emotive therapy (RET)? In A. Ellis & R. Grieger (Eds.), *Handbook of rational-emotive therapy* (Vol. 2, pp. 3–30). New York: Springer.

Ellis, A., & Dryden, W. (1987). *The practice of rational-emotive therapy.* Secaucus, NJ: Lyle Stuart.

Ellis, A., & Harper, R. A. (1975). *A new guide to rational living.* North Hollywood, CA: Wilshire Books.

Ellis, A., & Yeager, R. J. (1989). *Why some therapies don't work.* Buffalo, NY: Prometheus Books.

Emerson, S., & Markos, P. A. (1996). Signs and symptoms of the impaired counselor. *Journal of Humanistic Education and Development, 34,* 108–117.

Emery, G. (1981). *A new beginning: How you can change your life through cognitive therapy.* New York: Simon & Schuster (Touchstone).

Erikson, E. (1963). *Childhood and society* (2nd ed.). New York: Norton.

Erikson, E. (1982). *The life cycle completed.* New York: Norton.

Essandoh, P. K. (1996). Multicultural counseling as the "fourth force." *The Counseling Psychologist, 24*(1), 126–137.

Faiver, C. M., Eisengart, S., & Colonna, R. (1995). *The counselor intern's handbook.* Pacific Grove, CA: Brooks/Cole.

Faiver, C. M., & O'Brien, E. M. (1993). Assessment of religious beliefs form. *Counseling and Values, 37*(3), 176–178.

Farber, B. A. (1983). Psychotherapists' perceptions of stressful patient behavior. *Professional Psychology: Research and Practice, 14*(5), 697–705.

Fassinger, R. E. (1991a). Counseling lesbian women and gay men. *The Counseling Psychologist, 19*(2), 156.

Fassinger, R. E. (1991b). The hidden minority: Issues and challenges in working with lesbian women and gay men. *The Counseling Psychologist, 19*(2), 157–176.

Foos, J. A., Ottens, A. J., & Hill, L. K. (1991). Managed mental health: A primer for counselors. *Journal of Counseling and Development, 69*(4), 332–336.

Forester-Miller, H., & Davis, T. E. (1995). *A practitioner's guide to ethical decision making.* Alexandria, VA: American Counseling Association.

Fraser, J. S. (1996). All that glitters is not always gold: Medical offset effects and managed behavioral health care. *Professional Psychology: Research and Practice, 27*(4), 335–344.

Freudenberger, H. J., with Richelson, G. (1980). *Burn out: How to beat the high cost of success.* New York: Bantam Books.

Fujimura, L. E., Weis, D. M., & Cochran, J. R. (1985). Suicide: Dynamics and implications for counseling. *Journal of Counseling and Development, 63*(10), 612–615.

Gabbard, G. (April, 1995). What are boundaries in psychotherapy? *The Menninger Letter,* Vol. 3, No. 4, pp. 1–2.

Garnets, L., Hancock, K. A., Cochran, S. D., Goodchilds, J., & Peplau, L. A. (1991). Issues in psychotherapy with lesbians and gay men: A survey of psychologists. *American Psychologist, 46*(9), 964–972.

Getz, J. G., & Protinsky, H. O. (1994). Training marriage and family counselors: A family-of-origin approach. *Counselor Education and Supervision, 33*(3), 183–200.

Gilliland, B. E., & James, R. K. (1997). *Crisis intervention strategies* (3rd ed.). Pacific Grove, CA: Brooks/Cole.

Gill-Wigal, J., & Heaton, J. A. (1996). Managing sexual attraction in the therapeutic relationship. *Directions in Mental Health Counseling, 6*(8), 4–15.

Glosoff, H. L., Corey, G., & Herlihy, B. (1996). Dual relationships. In B. Herlihy & G. Corey (Eds.), *ACA ethical standards casebook* (5th ed.) (pp. 251–257). Alexandria, VA: American Counseling Association.

Goldenberg, H., & Goldenberg, I. (1994). *Counseling today's families* (2nd ed.). Pacific Grove, CA: Brooks/Cole.

Goldenberg, I., & Goldenberg, H. (1996a). *Family therapy: An overview* (4th ed.). Pacific Grove, CA: Brooks/Cole.

Goldenberg, I., & Goldenberg, H. (1996b). *My family story: Told and examined* (4th ed.). Pacific Grove, CA: Brooks/Cole.

Goodman, R. W., & Carpenter-White, A. (1996). The family autobiography assignment: Some ethical considerations. *Counselor Education and Supervision, 35*(3), 230–238.

Gottlieb, M. C. (1990). Accusations of sexual misconduct: Assisting in the complaint process. *Professional Psychology: Research and Practice, 21*(6), 455–461.

Graham, D. L. R., Rawlings, E. I., Halpern, H. S., & Hermes, J. (1984). Therapists' need for training in counseling lesbians and gay men. *Professional Psychology: Research and Practice, 15*(4), 482–496.

Gray, L. A., & House, R. M. (1991). Counseling the sexually active clients in the 1990s: A format for preparing mental health counselors. *Journal of Mental Health Counseling, 13*(2), 291–304.

Grimm, D. W. (1994). Therapist spiritual and religious values in psychotherapy. *Counseling and Values, 38*(3), 154–164.

Guy, J. D. (1987). *The personal life of the psychotherapist.* New York: Wiley.

Haas, L. J., & Cummings, N. A. (1991). Managed outpatient mental health plans: Clinical, ethical, and practical guidelines for participation. *Professional Psychology: Research and Practice, 22*(1), 45–51.

Hackney, H., & Cormier, L. S. (1988). *Counseling strategies and interventions* (3rd ed.). Englewood Cliffs, NJ: Prentice-Hall.

Hamachek, D. (1988). Evaluating self-concept and ego development within Erikson's psychosocial framework: A formulation. *Journal of Counseling and Development, 66,* 354–360.

Hamachek, D. (1990). Evaluating self-concept and ego status in Erikson's last three psychosocial stages. *Journal of Counseling and Development, 68*(6), 677–683.

Hanna, S. M., & Brown, J. H. (1995). *The practice of family therapy: Key elements across models.* Pacific Grove, CA: Brooks/Cole.

Hanson, C. E., Skager, R., & Mitchell, R. R. (1991). Counselors in at-risk prevention services: An innovative program. *Journal of Mental Health Counseling, 13*(2), 253–263.

Hatherleigh guide to ethics in therapy. (1997). New York: Hatherleigh Press.

Herlihy, B. (1996). When a colleague is impaired: The individual counselor's response. *Journal of Humanistic Education and Development, 34,* 118–127.

Herlihy, B., & Corey, G. (1992). *Dual relationships in counseling.* Alexandria, VA: American Counseling Association.

Herlihy, B., & Corey, G. (1996a). *ACA ethical standards casebook* (5th ed.). Alexandria, VA: American Counseling Association.

Herlihy, B., & Corey, G. (1996b). Confidentiality. In B. Herlihy & G. Corey (Eds.), *ACA ethical standards casebook* (5th ed.) (pp. 205–209). Alexandria, VA: American Counseling Association.

Herlihy, B., & Corey, G. (1996c). Working with multiple clients. In B. Herlihy & G. Corey (Eds.), *ACA ethical standards casebook* (5th ed.) (pp. 229–233). Alexandria, VA: American Counseling Association.

Herlihy, B., & Corey, G. (1997a). *Boundary issues in counseling: Multiple roles and responsibilities.* Alexandria, VA: American Counseling Association.

Herlihy, B., & Corey, G. (1997b). Codes of ethics as catalysts for improving practice. In *The Hatherleigh guide to ethics in therapy* (pp. 39–59). New York: Hatherleigh Press.

Hern, B. G., & Weis, D. M. (1991). A group counseling experience with the very old. *Journal for Specialists in Group Work, 16*(3), 143–151.

Herr, E. L. (1991). Challenges to mental health counselors in a dynamic society: Macro-strategies in the profession. *Journal of Mental Health Counseling, 13*(1), 6–10.

Hersch, L. (1995). Adapting to health care reform and managed care: Three strategies for survival and growth. *Professional Psychology: Research and Practice, 26*(1), 16–26.

Ho, D. Y. F. (1985). Cultural values and professional issues in clinical psychology: Implications from the Hong Kong experience. *American Psychologist, 40*(11), 1212–1218.

Hoffman, M. A. (1991a). Counseling the HIV-infected client: A psychosocial model for assessment and intervention. *The Counseling Psychologist, 19*(4), 467–542.

Hoffman, M. A. (1991b). Training mental health counselors for the AIDS crisis. *Journal of Mental Health Counseling, 13*(2), 264–269.

Homan, M. (1994). *Promoting community change: Making it happen in the real world.* Pacific Grove, CA: Brooks/Cole.

Hotelling, K. (1991). Sexual harassment: A problem shielded by silence. *Journal of Counseling and Development, 69,* 497–501.

Hutchins, D. E., & Cole Vaught, C. G. (1997). *Helping relationships and strategies* (3rd ed.). Pacific Grove, CA: Brooks/Cole.

Hwang, P. O. (1995). *Other-esteem: A creative response to a society obsessed with promoting the self.* San Diego, CA: Black Forrest Press.

Ibrahim, F. A. (1991). Contribution of cultural worldview to generic counseling and development. *Journal of Counseling and Development, 70*(1), 13–19.

Ibrahim, F. A. (1996). A multicultural perspective on principle and virtue ethics. *The Counseling Psychologist, 24*(1), 78–85.

Ivey, A. E. (1992). Caring and commitment: Are we up to the challenge of multicultural counseling and therapy? *Guidepost, 34*(9), 16.

Ivey, A. E. (1994). *Intentional interviewing and counseling: Facilitating client development in a multicultural society* (3rd ed.). Pacific Grove, CA: Brooks/Cole.

Jaffe, D. T. (1986). The inner strains of healing work: Therapy and self-renewal for health professionals. In C. D. Scott & J. Hawk (Eds.), *Heal thyself: The health of health care professionals.* New York: Brunner/Mazel.

Jensen, J. P., & Bergin, A. E. (1988). Mental health values of professional therapists: A national interdisciplinary survey. *Professional Psychology: Research and Practice, 19*(3), 290–297.

Jones, C. L., & Higuchi, A. (1996). Landmark New Jersey lawsuit challenges "no cause" termination. *Practitioner Focus, 9*(2), 1 & 13.

Jones, L. (1996). *HIV/AIDS: What to do about it.* Pacific Grove, CA: Brooks/Cole.

Kain, C. D. (1996). *Positive HIV affirmative counseling.* Alexandria, VA: American Counseling Association.

Karon, B. P. (1995). Provision of psychotherapy under managed health care: A growing crisis and national nightmare. *Professional Psychology: Research and Practice, 26*(1), 5–9.

Kelly, E. W. (1994). The role of religion and spirituality in counselor education: A national survey. *Counselor Education and Supervision, 33*(4), 227–237.

Kelly, E. W. (1995a). Counselor values: A national survey. *Journal of Counseling and Development, 73*(6), 648–653.

Kelly, E. W. (1995b). *Spirituality and religion in counseling and psychotherapy.* Alexandria, VA: American Counseling Association.

Kilburg, R. R. (1986). The distressed professional: The nature of the problem. In R. R. Kilburg, P. E. Nathan, & R. W. Thoreson (Eds.), *Professionals in distress: Issues, syndromes, and solutions in psychology* (pp. 13–26). Washington, DC: American Psychological Association.

Kitchener, K. S. (1996). There is more to ethics than principles. *The Counseling Psychologist, 24*(1), 92–97.

Kottler, J. A. (1991). *The compleat therapist.* San Francisco, CA: Jossey-Bass.

Kottler, J. A. (1992). *Compassionate therapy: Working with difficult clients.* San Francisco, CA: Jossey-Bass.

Kottler, J. A. (1993). *On being a therapist* (rev. ed.). San Francisco, CA: Jossey-Bass.

Kottler, J. A. (Ed.). (1997). *Finding your way as a counselor.* Alexandria, VA: American Counseling Association.

Kottler, J. A., & Blau, D. S. (1989). *The imperfect therapist: Learning from failure in therapeutic practice.* San Francisco, CA: Jossey-Bass.

Kottler, J. A., & Brown, R. W. (1996). *Introduction to therapeutic counseling* (3rd ed.). Pacific Grove, CA: Brooks/Cole.

Kramer, S. A. (1990). *Positive endings in psychotherapy: Bringing meaningful closure to therapeutic relationships.* San Francisco, CA: Jossey-Bass.

Kreiser, J. S., Domokos-Cheng Ham, M. A., Wiggers, T. T., & Feldstein, J. C. (1991). The professional "family": A model for mental health counselor development beyond graduate school. *Journal of Mental Health Counseling, 13*(2), 305–314.

Kübler-Ross, E. (1993). *AIDS: The ultimate challenge.* New York: Macmillan, Collier Books.

Lakein, A. (1974). *How to get control of your time and your life.* New York: New American Library (Signet).

Lauver, P., & Harvey, D. R. (1997). *The practical counselor: Elements of effective helping.* Pacific Grove, CA: Brooks/Cole.

Lawson, D. M., & Gaushell, H. (1988). Family autobiography: A useful method for enhancing counselors' personal development. *Counselor Education and Supervision, 28*(2), 162–167.

Lawson, D. M., & Gaushell, H. (1991). Intergenerational family characteristics of counselor trainees. *Counselor Education and Supervision, 30*(4), 309–321.

Lee, C. C. (1991). New approaches to diversity: Implications for multicultural counselor training and research. In C. C. Lee & B. L. Richardson (Eds.), *Multicultural issues in counseling: New approaches to diversity* (pp. 209–214). Alexandria, VA: American Association for Counseling and Development.

Lee, C. C., & Richardson, B. L. (1991a). *Multicultural issues in counseling: New approaches to diversity.* Alexandria, VA: American Association for Counseling and Development.

Lee, C. C., & Richardson, B. L. (1991b). Problems and pitfalls of multicultural counseling. In C. C. Lee & B. L. Richardson (Eds.), *Multicultural issues in counseling: New approaches to diversity* (pp. 3–9). Alexandria, VA: American Association for Counseling and Development.

Lewis, J. A., & Lewis, M. D. (1989). *Community counseling.* Pacific Grove, CA: Brooks/Cole.

Loar, L. (1995). Brief therapy with difficult clients. *Directions in Mental Health Counseling,* 5(12), 3–11.

Loesch, L. C. (1988). Preparation for helping professionals working with diverse populations. In N. A. Vacc, J. Wittmer, & S. B. DeVaney (Eds.), *Experiencing and counseling multicultural and diverse populations* (2nd ed.) (pp. 317–340). Muncie, IN: Accelerated Development.

Long, V. O. (1996). *Communication skills in helping relationships: A framework for facilitating personal growth.* Pacific Grove, CA: Brooks/Cole.

Lorion, R. P., & Parron, D. L. (1985). Countering the countertransference: A strategy for treating the untreatable. In P. Pedersen (Ed.), *Handbook of cross-cultural counseling and therapy* (pp. 79–86). Westport, CT: Greenwood Press.

Luciano, M. J., & Merris, C. (1992). *If only you would change.* Nashville, TN: Nelson.

Lum, D. (1996). *Social work practice and people of color: A process-stage approach* (3rd ed.). Pacific Grove, CA: Brooks/Cole.

Margolin, G. (1982). Ethical and legal considerations in marital and family therapy. *American Psychologist, 37*(3), 788–801.

Marino, T. W. (1996). The challenging task of making counseling services relevant to more populations. *Counseling Today,* pp. 1 & 6.

Martin, D. G., & Moore, A. D. (1995). *First steps in the art of intervention: A guidebook for trainees in the helping professions.* Pacific Grove, CA: Brooks/Cole.

Maslach, C. (1982). *Burnout: The cost of caring.* Englewood Cliffs, NJ: Prentice-Hall (Spectrum).

Matheny, K. B., Aycock, D. W., Pugh, J. L., Curlette, W. L., & Cannella, K. A. S. (1986). Stress coping: A qualitative and quantitative synthesis with implications for treatment. *The Counseling Psychologist, 14*(4), 499–549.

Mattson, D. L. (1994). Religious counseling: To be used, not feared. *Counseling and Values, 38*(3), 187–192.

May, R. (1983). *Discovery of being.* New York: Norton.

McCarthy, P., Sugden, S., Koker, M., Lamendola, F., Maurer, S., & Renninger, S. (1995). A practical guide to informed consent in clinical supervision. *Counselor Education and Supervision, 35*(2), 130–138.

McClam, T., & Woodside, M. (1994). *Problem solving in the helping professions.* Pacific Grove, CA: Brooks/Cole.

McGoldrick, M., & Gerson, R. (1989). Genograms and the family life cycle. In B. Carter & M. McGoldrick (Eds.), *The changing family life cycle: A framework for family therapy* (2nd ed.) (pp. 164–189). Boston: Allyn & Bacon.

Meara, N. M., Schmidt, L. D., & Day, J. D. (1996). A foundation for ethical decisions, policies, and character. *The Counseling Psychologist, 24*(1), 4–77.

Meichenbaum, D. (1977). *Cognitive behavior modification: An integrative approach.* New York: Plenum.

Meichenbaum, D. (1985). *Stress inoculation training.* New York: Pergamon Press.

Meichenbaum, D. (1986). Cognitive behavior modification. In F. H. Kanfer & A. P. Goldstein (Eds.), *Helping people change* (3rd ed.) (pp. 346–380). New York: Pergamon Press.

Meier, S. T., & Davis, S. R. (1997). *The elements of counseling* (3rd ed.). Pacific Grove, CA: Brooks/Cole.

Miller, G. A. (1992). Integrating religion and psychology in therapy: Issues and recommendations. *Counseling and Values, 36*(2), 112–122.

Miller, G. M., & Larrabee, M. J. (1995). Sexual intimacy in counselor education and supervision: A national survey. *Counselor Education and Supervision, 34*(4), 332–343.

Miller, I. J. (1996). Managed health care is harmful to outpatient mental health services: A call for accountability. *Professional Psychology: Research and Practice, 27*(4), 349–363.

Miranti, J., & Burke, M. T. (1995). Spirituality: An integral component of the counseling process. In M. T. Burke & J. G. Miranti (Eds.), *Counseling: The spiritual dimension*. Alexandria, VA: American Counseling Association.

Modrak, R. (1992). Mass shootings and airplane crashes: Counselors respond to the changing face of community crisis. *Guidepost: AACD Newsletter, 34*(8), 4.

Morrissey, M. (1996). Supreme Court extends confidentiality privilege. *Counseling Today,* pp. 1, 6, 10.

Mosak, H., & Shulman, B. (1988). *Life style inventory*. Muncie, IN: Accelerated Development.

Myers, J. E. (1990). Aging: An overview for mental health counselors. *Journal of Mental Health Counseling, 12*(3), 245–259.

Myers, J. E., Poidevant, J. M., & Dean, L. A. (1991). Groups for older persons and their caregivers: A review of the literature. *Journal for Specialists in Group Work, 16*(3), 197–205.

National Association of Social Workers (1996). *Code of ethics*. Washington, DC: Author.

National Board for Certified Counselors (1989). *Code of ethics*. Alexandria, VA: Author.

National Organization for Human Service Education (1995). *Ethical standards of the National Organization for Human Service Education*. Philadelphia: Author.

Nelson-Jones, R. (1993). *Lifeskills helping: Helping others through a systematic people-centered approach*. Pacific Grove, CA: Brooks/Cole.

Neukrug, E. S. (1994). *Theory, practice, and trends in human services: An overview of an emerging profession*. Pacific Grove, CA: Brooks/Cole.

Newman, R. (1996). Supreme Court affirms privilege. *APA Monitor, 27*(8), 44.

Newman, R., & Bricklin, P. M. (1991). Parameters of managed mental health care: Legal, ethical, and professional guidelines. *Professional Psychology: Research and Practice, 22*(1), 26–35.

Nichols, M. P., & Schwartz, R. C. (1995). *Family therapy: Concepts and methods* (3rd ed.). Boston: Allyn & Bacon.

Nolan, E. J. (1978). Leadership interventions for promoting personal mastery. *Journal for Specialists in Group Work, 3*(3), 132–138.

Nye, R. D. (1996). *Three psychologies: Perspectives from Freud, Skinner, and Rogers* (5th ed.). Pacific Grove, CA: Brooks/Cole.

Okun, B. F. (1997). *Effective helping: Interviewing and counseling techniques* (5th ed.). Pacific Grove, CA: Brooks/Cole.

Olarte, S. W. (1997). Sexual boundary violations. In *The Hatherleigh guide to ethics in therapy*. New York: Hatherleigh Press.

Patterson, C. H. (1985). *The therapeutic relationship: Foundations for an eclectic psychotherapy*. Pacific Grove, CA: Brooks/Cole.

Patterson, C. H. (1989). Values in counseling and psychotherapy. *Counseling and Values, 33*, 164–176.

Peck, M. S. (1978). *The road less traveled: A new psychology of love, traditional values and spiritual growth*. New York: Simon & Schuster (Touchstone).

Pedersen, P. (1990). The multicultural perspective as a fourth force in counseling. *Journal of Mental Health Counseling, 12*(1), 93–94.

Pedersen, P. (1991a). Concluding comments to the special issue. *Journal of Counseling and Development, 70*(1), 250.

Pedersen, P. (1991b). Multiculturalism as a generic approach to counseling. *Journal of Counseling and Development, 70*(1), 6–12.

Pedersen, P. (1994). *A handbook for developing multicultural awareness* (2nd ed.). Alexandria, VA: American Counseling Association.

Pines, A., & Aronson, E., with Kafry, D. (1981). *Burnout: From tedium to personal growth.* New York: Free Press.

Ponterotto, J. G., Casas, J. M., Suzuki, L. A., & Alexander, C. M. (1995). *Handbook of multicultural counseling.* Thousand Oaks, CA: Sage.

Pope, K. S., Keith-Spiegel, P., & Tabachnick, B. G. (1986). Sexual attraction to clients: The human therapist and the (sometimes) inhuman training system. *American Psychologist, 41*(2), 147–158.

Pope, K. S., Sonne, J. L., & Holroyd, J. (1993). *Sexual feelings in psychotherapy: Explorations for therapists and therapists-in-training.* Washington, DC: American Psychological Association.

Pope, K. S., & Vasquez, M. J. T. (1991). *Ethics in psychotherapy and counseling: A practical guide for psychologists.* San Francisco, CA: Jossey-Bass.

Powers, R. L., & Griffith, J. (1986). *The individual psychology client workbook.* Chicago: The Americas Institute of Adlerian Studies.

Powers, R. L., & Griffith, J. (1987). *Understanding life-style: The psycho-clarity process.* Chicago: The Americas Institute of Adlerian Studies.

Prieto, L. R. (1996). Group supervision: Still widely practiced but poorly understood. *Counselor Education and Supervision, 35*(4), 295–307.

Purkey, W. W., & Schmidt, J. J. (1996). *Invitational counseling: A self-concept approach to professional practice.* Pacific Grove, CA: Brooks/Cole.

Quackenbos, S., Privette, G., & Klentz, B. (1986). Psychotherapy and religion: Rapprochement or antithesis? *Journal of Counseling and Development, 65*(2), 82–85.

Remley, T. (1996). The relationship between law and ethics. In B. Herlihy & G. Corey (Eds.), *ACA ethical standards casebook* (5th ed.) (pp. 285–292). Alexandria, VA: American Counseling Association.

Rice, P. L. (1992). *Stress and health* (2nd ed.). Pacific Grove, CA: Brooks/Cole.

Ridley, C. R. (1995). *Overcoming unintentional racism in counseling and therapy: A practitioner's guide to intentional intervention.* Thousand Oaks, CA: Sage.

Riger, S. (1991). Gender dilemmas in sexual harassment policies and procedures. *American Psychologist, 46*(5), 499–505.

Rodolfa, E. R., Kitzrow, M., Vohra, S., & Wilson, B. (1990). Training interns to respond to sexual dilemmas. *Professional Psychology: Research and Practice, 21*(4), 313–315.

Rutter, P. (1989). *Sex in the forbidden zone.* Los Angeles: Jeremy Tarcher.

Saeki, C., & Borow, H. (1985). Counseling and psychotherapy: East and West. In P. Pedersen (Ed.), *Handbook of cross-cultural counseling and therapy* (pp. 223–229). Westport, CT: Greenwood Press.

Sage, G. P. (1991). Counseling American Indian adults. In C. C. Lee & B. L. Richardson (Eds.), *Multicultural issues in counseling: New approaches to diversity* (pp. 23–36). Alexandria, VA: American Association for Counseling and Development.

Salisbury, W. A., & Kinnier, R. T. (1996). Posttermination friendship between counselors and clients. *Journal of Counseling and Development, 74*(5), 495–500.

Satir, V. (1983). *Conjoint family therapy* (3rd ed.). Palo Alto, CA: Science and Behavior Books.

Satir, V. (1989). *The new peoplemaking.* Palo Alto, CA: Science and Behavior Books.

Satir, V., & Baldwin, M. (1983). *Satir: Step by step.* Palo Alto, CA: Science and Behavior Books.

Satir, V., Bitter, J. R., & Krestensen, K. K. (1988). Family reconstruction: The family within— a group experience. *Journal for Specialists in Group Work, 13*(4), 200–208.

Schultz, D., & Schultz, S. E. (1994). *Theories of personality* (5th ed.). Pacific Grove, CA: Brooks/Cole.

Seppa, N. (1996, August). Supreme Court protects patient-therapist privilege. *APA Monitor, 27*(8), 39.

Sheehy, G. (1976). *Passages: Predictable crises of adult life.* New York: Dutton.

Sheehy, G. (1992). *The silent passage.* New York: Random House.

Sheehy, G. (1995). *New passages: Mapping your life across time.* New York: Random House.

Shulman, B., & Mosak, H. (1988). *Manual for life style assessment.* Muncie, IN: Accelerated Development.

Slaikeu, K. A. (1990). *Crisis intervention: A handbook for practice and research.* Boston: Allyn & Bacon.

Sleek, S. (1994, December). Ethical dilemmas plague rural practice. *APA Monitor, 25*(12), 26–27.

Sleek, S. (1995, July). Group therapy: Tapping the power of teamwork. *APA Monitor, 26*(7), 1, 38–39.

Smith, D., & Fitzpatrick, M. (1995). Patient-therapist boundary issues: An integrative review of theory and research. *Professional Psychology: Research and Practice, 26*(5), 499–506.

Smith, D. C., & Maher, M. F. (1991). Group interventions with caregivers of the dying: The "Phoenix" alternative. *Journal for Specialists in Group Work, 16*(3), 191–196.

Sonne, J. L., & Pope, K. S. (1991). Treating victims of therapist-patient sexual involvement. *Psychotherapy, 28,* 174–187.

Stadler, H. A. (1990). Counselor impairment. In B. Herlihy & L. B. Golden (Eds.), *AACD ethical standards casebook* (4th ed.) (pp. 177–187). Alexandria, VA: American Association for Counseling and Development.

Stake, J. E., & Oliver, J. (1991). Sexual contact and touching between therapist and client: A survey of psychologists' attitudes and behavior. *Professional Psychology: Research and Practice, 22*(4), 297–307.

Stewart, D. W. (1995). Termination. In D. G. Martin & A. D. Moore (Eds.), *First steps in the art of intervention: A guidebook for trainees in the helping professions* (pp. 157–170). Pacific Grove, CA: Brooks/Cole.

Stoltenberg, C. D., & Delworth, U. (1987). *Supervising counselors and therapists: A developmental approach.* San Francisco, CA: Jossey-Bass.

Stone, M. L., & Waters, E. (1991). Accentuate the positive: A peer group counseling program for older adults. *Journal for Specialists in Group Work, 16*(3), 159–166.

Sue, D., & Sue, D. W. (1991). Counseling strategies for Chinese Americans. In C. C. Lee & B. L. Richardson (Eds.), *Multicultural issues in counseling: New approaches to diversity* (pp. 79-90). Alexandria, VA: American Association for Counseling and Development.

Sue, D. W. (1990). Culture specific strategies in counseling: A conceptual framework. *Professional Psychology: Research and Practice, 21*(6), 424–433.

Sue, D. W. (1992). The challenge of multiculturalism: The road less traveled. *American Counselor, 1*(1), 6–14.

Sue, D. W. (1996). Ethical issues in multicultural counseling. In B. Herlihy & G. Corey (Eds.), *ACA ethical standards casebook* (5th ed.) (pp. 193–200). Alexandria, VA: American Counseling Association.

Sue, D. W., Arredondo, P., & McDavis, R. J. (1992). Multicultural counseling competencies and standards: A call to the profession. *Journal of Counseling and Development, 70*(4), 477–486.

Sue, D. W., Bernier, Y., Durran, A., Feinberg, L., Pedersen, P. B., Smith, E. J., & Vasquez-Nuttal, E. (1982). Position paper: Cross-cultural counseling competencies. *The Counseling Psychologist, 10*(2), 45–52.

Sue, D. W., Ivey, A., & Pedersen, P. (1996). *A theory of multicultural counseling and therapy.* Pacific Grove, CA: Brooks/Cole.

Sue, D. W., & Sue, D. (1985). Asian-American and Pacific Islanders. In P. Pedersen (Ed.), *Handbook of cross-cultural counseling and therapy* (pp. 141–146). Westport, CT: Greenwood Press.

Sue, D. W., & Sue, D. (1990). *Counseling the culturally different: Theory and practice* (2nd ed.). New York: Wiley.

Sumerel, M. B., & Borders, L. D. (1996). Addressing personal issues in supervision: Impact of counselors' experience level on various aspects of the supervisory relationship. *Counselor Education and Supervision, 35*(4), 268–286.

Szasz, T. (1986). The case against suicide prevention. *American Psychologist, 41*(7), 806–812.

Tabachnick, B. G., Keith-Spiegel, P., & Pope, K. S. (1991). Ethics of teaching: Beliefs and behaviors of psychologists as educators. *American Psychologist, 46*(5), 506–515.

Thoreson, R. W., Miller, M., & Krauskopf, C. J. (1989). The distressed psychologist: Prevalence and treatment consideration. *Professional Psychologist: Research and Practice, 20*(3), 153–158.

Tice, C., & Perkins, K. (1996). *Mental health issues and aging: Building on the strengths of older persons.* Pacific Grove, CA: Brooks/Cole.

Tjeltveit, A. C. (1986). The ethics of value conversion in psychotherapy: Appropriate and inappropriate therapist influence on client values. *Clinical Psychology Review, 6,* 515–537.

Vacc, N. A., & Clifford, K. F. (1988). Individuals with a physical disability. In N. A. Vacc, J. Wittmer, & S. B. DeVaney (Eds.), *Experiencing and counseling multicultural and diverse populations* (2nd ed.) (pp. 169–188). Muncie, IN: Accelerated Development.

Vasquez, M. J. T. (1996). Will virtue ethics improve ethical conduct in multicultural settings and interactions? *The Counseling Psychologist, 24*(1), 98–104.

Watts, R. E., Trusty, J., Canada, R., & Harvill, R. L. (1995). Perceived early childhood family influence and counselor effectiveness: An exploratory study. *Counselor Education and Supervision, 35,* 104–110.

Wehrly, B. (1995). *Pathways to multicultural counseling competence: A developmental journey.* Pacific Grove, CA: Brooks/Cole.

Weikel, W. J. (1990). A multimodal approach in dealing with older adults. *Journal of Mental Health Counseling, 12*(3), 314–320.

Whiston, S. C., & Emerson, S. (1989). Ethical implications for supervisors in counseling of trainees. *Counselor Education and Supervision, 28*(4), 318–325.

White, J. L., & Parham, T. A. (1990). *The psychology of blacks: An African-American perspective* (2nd ed.). Englewood Cliffs, NJ: Prentice-Hall.

Wilcoxon, S. A., Walker, M. R., & Hovestadt, A. J. (1989). Counselor effectiveness and family-of-origin experiences: A significant relationship? *Counseling and Values, 33*(3), 225–229.

Wittmer, J., & Remley, T. P., Jr. (1994, Summer). A counselor-client contract. *NBCC News-Notes, 11*(1), 12.

Wolfgang, A. (1985). The function and importance of nonverbal behavior in intercultural counseling. In P. Pedersen (Ed.), *Handbook of cross-cultural counseling and therapy* (pp. 99–105). Westport, CT: Greenwood Press.

Woodside, M., & McClam, T. (1994). *An introduction to human services* (2nd ed.). Pacific Grove, CA: Brooks/Cole.

Wrenn, C. G. (1962). The culturally encapsulated counselor. *Harvard Educational Review, 32,* 444–449.

Wrenn, C. G. (1985). Afterword: The culturally encapsulated counselor revisited. In P. Pedersen (Ed.), *Handbook of cross-cultural counseling and therapy* (pp. 323–329). Westport, CT: Greenwood Press.

Wubbolding, R. E. (1988). *Using reality therapy.* New York: Harper & Row (Perennial Library).

Wubbolding, R. E. (1996). Working with suicidal clients. In B. Herlihy & G. Corey (Eds.), *ACA ethical standards casebook* (5th ed.) (pp. 267–274). Alexandria, VA: American Counseling Association.

Yalom, I. D. (1983). *Inpatient group psychotherapy.* New York: Basic Books.

Yalom, I. D. (1995). *The theory and practice of group psychotherapy* (4th ed.). New York: Basic Books.

SUBJECT INDEX

Abandonment, as grounds for malpractice suits, 147, 149
A-B-C theory of irrational thinking, 330–331
Abortion, 156, 158, 160, 170–171, 291
Abuse:
  child, 35, 125, 149, 209, 212, 251, 289
  of the elderly, 35, 209
  of power in the supervisory relationship, 144–145
  psychological, of clients, 35
  sexual, of clients, 141, 147, 311
  spousal, 35
Acquired immune deficiency syndrome (AIDS):
  and confidentiality, 128–129
  duty to protect sexual partners, 128–129
  helper's role in client advocacy, 207
  helper's role in educating the public, 207, 210, 219–220
  helper's role in influencing policy-makers, 212
  and isolation, 216, 217
  and patients' anger, 217–218
  prevention through education as priority in, 219–220
  resistance within the helper, 60
  as special concern for helpers, 215–221
  special needs of clients with AIDS virus, 216–218
  stigma of, 216–217
  working with AIDS patients, effect on helpers, 218–219, 232
Action strategies:
  in cognitive therapy, 334
  importance of, 76–78

Active listening, 33, 68, 246, 248
Adlerian lifestyle assessment, 264
Adolescence, developmental stage of, 294–295
Adoption, 162, 171
Adulthood:
  early, 295–298
  late, 302–303
  middle, 298–301
Affairs in marriage, helper's stance on, 96, 127, 156, 163–164, 165, 301
African American/Black clients, 177, 182
Alcoholics Anonymous, 59
American Association for Marriage and Family Therapy (AAMFT), 118, 133, 142, 349
American Counseling Association (ACA), 118, 119, 122, 123, 126, 128, 129, 131–132, 133, 137, 142, 143, 144, 157, 173, 180, 348
American Indian clients, 177, 184, 187, 189, 198
American Psychological Association (APA), 118, 133, 141, 237, 349–350
American Red Cross, 233
Anger, 93, 239, 269, 270, 275, 276, 281, 290, 320
  in clients with AIDS virus, 217–218
Approval, need for, 71
Asian American clients, 177, 184, 186, 187, 189
Assertiveness:
  cultural assumptions about, 188
  and supervision, 42, 45
Assessment, 69

TO THE OWNER OF THIS BOOK:

We enjoyed writing *Becoming a Helper,* 3rd Edition, and it is our hope that you have enjoyed reading it. We'd like to know about your experiences with the book; only through your comments and the comments of others can we assess the impact of this book and make it a better book for readers in the future.

School: _____

Instructor's name: _____

1. What did you like *most* about the book? _____

_____

_____

_____

2. What did you like *least* about the book? _____

_____

_____

_____

3. How useful were the suggested activities and annotated reading lists at the end of the chapters?

_____

_____

4. In what course did you use this book? _____

_____

5. In the space below, or in a separate letter, please tell us what it was like for you to read this book and how you used it; please include your suggestions for revisions and any other comments you'd like to make about the book.

Optional:

Your name: _____ Date: _____

May Brooks/Cole quote you, either in promotion for *Becoming a Helper*, 3rd Edition, or in future publishing ventures?

Yes: _____ No: _____

Sincerely,

Marianne Schneider Corey
Gerald Corey

FOLD HERE

NO POSTAGE
NECESSARY
IF MAILED
IN THE
UNITED STATES

BUSINESS REPLY MAIL
FIRST CLASS   PERMIT NO. 358   PACIFIC GROVE, CA

POSTAGE WILL BE PAID BY ADDRESSEE

ATT: *Marianne Schneider Corey & Gerald Corey*

Brooks/Cole Publishing Company
511 Forest Lodge Road
Pacific Grove, California 93950-9968

FOLD HERE

Brooks/Cole is dedicated to publishing quality books for the helping professions. If you would like to learn more about our publications, please use the mailer to request our catalogue.

Name: _____

Street Address: _____

City, State, and Zip: _____

FOLD HERE

BUSINESS REPLY MAIL

FIRST CLASS   PERMIT NO. 358   PACIFIC GROVE, CA

POSTAGE WILL BE PAID BY ADDRESSEE

ATT: *Human Services Catalogue*

Brooks/Cole Publishing Company
511 Forest Lodge Road
Pacific Grove, California 93950-9968

FOLD HERE

IN-BOOK SURVEY

At Brooks/Cole, we are excited about creating new types of learning materials that are interactive, three-dimensional, and fun to use. To guide us in our publishing/development process, we hope that you'll take just a few moments to fill out the survey below. Your answers can help us make decisions that will allow us to produce a wide variety of videos, CD-ROMs, and Internet-based learning systems to complement standard textbooks. If you're interested in working with us as a student Beta-tester, be sure to fill in your name, telephone number, and address. We look forward to hearing from you!

In addition to books, which of the following learning tools do you currently use in your counseling/human services/social work courses?

_____ **Video** _____ in class _____ school library _____ own VCR

_____ **CD-ROM** _____ in class _____ in lab _____ own computer

_____ **Macintosh disks** _____ in class _____ in lab _____ own computer

_____ **Windows disks** _____ in class _____ in lab _____ own computer

_____ **Internet** _____ in class _____ in lab _____ own computer

How often do you access the Internet? _____

My own home computer is:

_____ Macintosh _____ DOS _____ Windows _____ Windows 95

The computer I use in class for counseling/human services/social work courses is:

_____ Macintosh _____ DOS _____ Windows _____ Windows 95

If you are NOT currently using multimedia materials in your counseling/human services/social work courses, but can see ways that video, CD-ROM, Internet, or other technologies could enhance your learning, please comment below:

_____

_____

_____

Other comments (optional): _____

_____

Name _____

Address _____

Telephone number (optional): _____

You can fax this form to us at (408) 375-6414; e:mail to: info@brookscole.com; or detach, fold, secure, and mail.

FOLD HERE

BUSINESS REPLY MAIL

FIRST CLASS   PERMIT NO. 358   PACIFIC GROVE, CA

POSTAGE WILL BE PAID BY ADDRESSEE

ATTN: ___MARKETING_____

Brooks/Cole Publishing Company
511 Forest Lodge Road
Pacific Grove, California 93950-9968

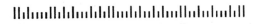

FOLD HERE